Lecture Notes in Biomathematics

Managing Editor: S. Levin

65

Immunology and Epidemiology

Proceedings of an International Conference held in Mogilany, Poland, February 18–25, 1985

Edited by G. W. Hoffmann and T. Hraba

WILLIAM MADISON RANDALL LIBRARY UNC AT WILMINGTON

Springer-Verlag
Berlin Heidelberg New York Tokyo

Editorial Board

M. Arbib H.J. Bremermann J.D. Cowan W. Hirsch S. Karlin
J.B. Keller M. Kimura S. Levin (Managing Editor) R.C. Lewontin R. May
J.D. Murray G.F. Oster A.S. Perelson T. Poggio L.A. Segel

Editors

Geoffrey W. Hoffmann
Departments of Physics and Microbiology, The University of British Columbia
Vancouver, B.C., V6T 1W5, Canada

Tomáš Hraba
Institute of Molecular Genetics, Czechoslovak Academy of Sciences
142 20 Prague, Czechoslavakia

Mathematics Subject Classification (1980): 92-02, 92-06, 92A07, 92A15

ISBN 3-540-16431-6 Springer-Verlag Berlin Heidelberg New York Tokyo
ISBN 0-387-16431-6 Springer-Verlag New York Heidelberg Berlin Tokyo

This work is subject to copyright. All rights are reserved, whether the whole or part of the material is concerned, specifically those of translation, reprinting, re-use of illustrations, broadcasting, reproduction by photocopying machine or similar means, and storage in data banks. Under § 54 of the German Copyright Law where copies are made for other than private use, a fee is payable to "Verwertungsgesellschaft Wort", Munich.

© by Springer-Verlag Berlin Heidelberg 1986
Printed in Germany

Printing and binding: Beltz Offsetdruck, Hemsbach/Bergstr.
2146/3140-543210

QR185
.5
.I46
1986

PREFACE

In February 1985 a small international meeting of scientists :ook place at the recreation resort of the Polish Academy of Sci- nces in Mogilany, near Cracow, Poland. The initiative for holding he workshop came from a working meeting on mathematical immunology nd related topics at the International Institute for Applied Sys- ems Analysis in Laxenburg, Austria, in November 1983. In addition o representatives of IIASA, delegates of the IIASA National Member rganizations (NMO) of Czechoslovakia, Italy, and the Soviet Union ook part in that working meeting. The participants came to the onclusion that IIASA could play an important role in facilitating he development of research in this field. The first step that they ecommended to IIASA was to organize a workshop on mathematical mmunology. The purpose of the workshop was to review the progress hat has been made in applying mathematics to problems in immunology nd to explore ways in which further progress might be achieved, specially by more efficient interactions between scientists working n mathematical and experimental immunology. Some National Member rganizations contributed to the success of the workshop by nominat- ng further participants working in this or related fields. For nstance, thanks to a suggestion of the British NMO, the meeting lso included analyses of the interactions between the immune state f a population and epidemiological phenomena.

There were 33 participants at Mogilany from 11 countries, amely Canada, Czechoslovakia, Federal Republic of Germany, Hungary, apan, Netherlands, Poland, Sweden, United Kingdom, USA, and USSR. his volume is a selection of the papers presented at the meeting.

Most of the papers in this collection consider problems at the ellular or higher levels of organization. Cellular immunology is a iscipline that might sometimes seem to lack a widely accepted heoretical basis, apart from the essential tenet of clonal selec- ion and the generally agreed existence of T cells and B cells. The ontroversial nature of many aspects of cellular immunology, ogether with the rapid progress currently being made, makes it one f the most exciting areas of science today. It is important to ote that all cellular immunologists, including those of both the xperimental and the mathematical varieties, are theoretical immu- ologists. The design of each new experiment is a theoretical task nd is based on a theoretical view of the immune system, which for ost immunologists is a rapidly evolving function of time.

283378

Some experimental cellular immunologists are still skeptical concerning the role to be played by mathematics in immunology. There seems however to be a trend towards widespread acceptance of a role for mathematics in this field. The phenomena encompassed by cellular immunology are already so numerous, and often so confusing, that there is also a growing willingness on the part of many experimentalists to welcome professional model builders to the discipline. In fact, there is no choice; it would be irresponsible of us to fail to utilize the tools of mathematics and the powerful modern computers that have become available, and which so far have not been utilized in this area to the extent that they might be. This is due largely to the very limited contacts between investigators in experimental and mathematical immunology. The Mogilany meeting was successful in this respect because scientists of both of these groups participated and explored possibilities for closer collaboration.

In this volume we have a collection of papers giving a representative picture of important problems of mathematical immunology. The introductory chapter gives a brief overview of the various levels at which the immune system can be studied and points out some of the main ways in which the application of mathematics has been important. We hope this will help the contributions made at Mogilany to be seen in a wider context.

The Mogilany meeting was jointly sponsored by the International Institute for Applied Systems Analysis, the Polish Academy of Sciences and the Institute of Control and Systems Engineering of the Academy of Mining and Metallurgy, Cracow, Poland.

G. W. Hoffmann
Los Alamos

T. Hraba
Prague

October 1985

CONTRIBUTORS

Roy M. Anderson	Department of Pure and Applied Biology, Imperial College, London University, England
A. L. Asachenkov	Department of Numerical Mathematics, USSR Academy of Sciences, Moscow, USSR
L. N. Belykh	Department of Numerical Mathematics, USSR Academy of Sciences, Moscow, USSR
Rob J. de Boer	Bioinformatics Group, University of Utrecht, Utrecht, The Netherlands
Michael Chow	Department of Microbiology, University of British Columbia, Vancouver, British Columbia, Canada
Anwyl Cooper-Willis	Department of Microbiology, University of British Columbia, Vancouver, British Columbia, Canada
J. Doležal	Institute of Information Theory and Automation Czechoslovak Academy of Sciences Prague, Czechoslovakia
Wulf Dröge	Institut für Immunologie und Genetik, Deutsches Krebsforschungszentrum, Heidelberg, West Germany
[illegible]. Farooqi	Department of Electrical and Computer Engineering, Oregon State University, Corvallis, Oregon, U.S.A
[illegible]. Haas	Borstel Research Institute, Borstel, West Germany
[illegible]. Heilig	Department of Electrical and Computer Engineering, Oregon State University, Corvallis, Oregon, U.S.A
Geoffrey W. Hoffmann	Departments of Physics and Microbiology, University of British Columbia, Vancouver, British Columbia, Canada
Pauline Hogeweg	Bioinformatics Group, Universiy of Utrecht, Utrecht, The Netherlands
[illegible]. Hraba	Institute of Molecular Genetics, Czechoslovak Academy of Sciences, Prague, Czechoslovakia
[illegible]an Ince	Department of Infectious Diseases, University Hospital, Leiden, The Netherlands

Miloš Jílek
Institute of Microbiology, Czechoslovak Academy of Sciences, Prague, Czechoslovakia

J. T. Jodkowski
Department of Physical Chemistry, Medical School of Wrocław, Wrocław, Poland

C. Łaba
Department of Clinical Immunology, Institute of Immunology and Experimental Therapy, Polish Academy of Sciences, Wrocław, Poland

A. Lange
Department of Clinical Immunology, Institute of Immunology and Experimental Therapy, Polish Academy of Sciences, Wrocław, Poland

G. I. Marchuk
Department of Numerical Mathematics, USSR Academy of Sciences, Moscow, USSR

Angela McLean
Department of Pure and Applied Biology, Imperial College, London University, London, England

Seth Michelson
Department of Radiation Medicine and Biology Research, Rhode Island Hospital, Providence, Rhode Island, U.S.A.

R. R. Mohler
Department of Electrical and Computer Engineering, Oregon State University, Corvallis, Oregon, U.S.A

Daniela Přikrylová
Institute of Microbiology, Czechoslovak Academy of Sciences, Prague, Czechoslovakia

J. W. Vaupel
International Institute for Applied Systems Analysis, Laxenburg, Austria

A. I. Yashin
International Institute for Applied Systems Analysis, Laxenburg, Austria

S. M. Zuev
Department of Numerical Mathematics, USSR Academy of Sciences, Moscow, USSR

TABLE OF CONTENTS

PART I

OVERVIEW

THE STRUCTURE OF MATHEMATICAL IMMUNOLOGY

G. W. Hoffmann
Departments of Physics and Microbiology[1]
University of British Columbia
Vancouver, B.C., Canada V6T 1W5
and
Theoretical Biology and Biophysics
Los Alamos National Laboratory
Los Alamos, NM 87545, U.S.A.

and

T. Hraba
Institute of Molecular Genetics
Czechoslovak Academy of Sciences
142 20 Prague, Czechoslovakia

Mathematical immunology is a young (some might even say immature) but nevertheless wide-ranging discipline. In order to put the papers of this book into a broader context, we here give a brief, necessarily sketchy, overview of some of the main areas of mathematical immunology, not all of which were represented at the Mogilany conference. A more comprehensive overview of the range of the subject may be gained from the collective contents of several monographs and collections of papers on mathematical immunology (1-6).

Within the immune system there are events at many different levels. Table I gives these levels with some examples of processes that take place at each of them. At least some events at each level have been subjected to mathematical analysis.

Perhaps the most fundamental interaction that has been treated mathematically is the interaction of antigen and antibody (5), an event at the molecular level in our hierarchy. The paper of Žaba _et al_. (page 224) belongs to this category. It is concerned with a computer program for the evaluation of a radio-immune assay for the determination of circulating immune complexes. A very difficult aspect of the modelling of the interactions between antigen and antibodies is the spectrum of affinities in a given normal serum. This has been studied in detail by the Italian group (7).

---
[1] Permanent address

TABLE I

THE VARIOUS LEVELS OF PROCESSES IN THE IMMUNE SYSTEM

Level	Processes
Molecular	Antigen-antibody interactions Complement binding
Cellular	Antigen-cell interactions Antibody mediated cell lysis or cytotoxicity Immunoglobulin binding to cellular Fc receptors Complement binding to cellular receptors Complement cascade Antigen-antibody-cell interactions (IgE)
Intercellular	Antigen presenting cell-lymphocyte interactions T cell-B cell interactions T cell-T cell interactions Cellular cytotoxicity Cell adherence
Organism	Cellular population dynamics of immunocytes Network regulatory phenomena Immunity to infections Tumor immunity Transplantation immunity and tolerance Allergic diseases Autoimmune diseases Acquired immune deficiency
Population	Immunological aspects of epidemiology

The cellular level concerns interactions between single cells and molecules. The molecules involved can be antibody, antigen, or specific or nonspecific factors produced by lymphocytes and macrophages. Detailed thermodynamic and kinetic models have been developed, and the contributions of the Los Alamos group have been particularly important. For example, the success of mathematical models in both qualitatively and quantitatively accounting for bell-shaped histamine release curves is one of the most elegant achievements of mathematical immunology to date (8).

Events at the single cell level were described at Mogilany by Ince (page 229), who is concerned with the electrophysiology of macrophages. Ince points out that the role of ion channels in the cells of the immune system is poorly understood, but he nevertheless is optimistic that such studies will eventually contribute to our understanding of host defence mechanisms.

The next level is intercellular; that is, it concerns the interactions of cells with cells. An example of such events is the interaction between killer cells and their targets; these interactions have been nicely modelled by Perelson and Macken (9). Further examples have been provided by Bell and Bongrand, who have been active in calculations of the forces involved in cell adhesion (10).

The results obtained from cell adhesion studies are vitally important for Mohler and coworkers, who are developing models of lymphocyte migration or "traffic" (see page 208). Experimentalists working on lymphocyte traffic collect dozens of experimental facts and numbers, each of which will become more meaningful when placed in the context of a comprehensive mathematical model.

Perhaps the most challenging problem of mathematical immunology, and the problem that is widely regarded as central to the field, is the task of describing the immune response itself in mathematical form. We would like to have a model that accounts for the various idiosyncracies of the system. Mathematical models that aim to do this are usually formulated as sets of differential equations that simulate the population dynamics of the various cells (helper T cells, suppressor T cells, B cells, etc.) and of molecules (antigens, antibodies, etc.). Many workers have tackled this problem. There has, however, been a lack of convergence in the approaches taken by various investigators. The difficulty lies in the fact that each investigator is both theorist (he reviews the literature and then makes a set of postulates about the system) and modeller (he then models what he has decided are the essential features of the system). There are almost as many sets of postulates as there are investigators, so it is no wonder that the mathematical models are as notable for their diversity as for anything else, and no "standard model" has emerged. This problem is thoroughly discussed by Jílek and Prikrylová (page 8) and by Hoffmann, Cooper-Willis, and Chow (page 15), who propose a systematic approach toward resolving the difficulty.

The overall state of immunity of an organism (the organismal level in our hierarchy) can be the sum of several types of immune reactions: the production of antibodies of various immunoglobulin classes, delayed hypersensitivity, and other types of cell-mediated immune reactions, and especially the cooperative and suppressive activity of T cells. Some of these components can be antagonistic in their biological effects. For example, lymphoid cells from a mouse manifesting transplantation immunity transfer this immune state to non-immune recipients. On the other hand, antibodies in sera of the same donors cause immunological enhancement, that is, prolongation of graft survival. Such effects are not well understood, and there is much experimental and modelling work to be done before such complexities are unravelled.

A good starting point for a theory of immune responses and immune responsiveness is a description of the immune system repertoire. The T cell repertoire is particularly important for the regulation of immune responses, and Dröge (page 32) describes a quasi-quantitative model of that repertoire.

Several authors describe immune response models consisting of sets of differential equations. Prikrylová presents a detailed model of T-dependent antibody responses (page 44). Hraba and Dolezal describe a system for the study of immunological tolerance (page 53). The development of their model has been characterized by a close interplay between the mathematical modelling and the planning of experiments.

Marchuk, Asachenkov, Belykh, and Zuev's paper (page 64) is concerned with the course of infectious diseases and the immune response. Their analysis, which is mathematically one of the more difficult ones, primarily treats immunity to viruses.

Models of tumor immunity and of tumor escape are described by Michelson (page 82) and by de Boer and Hogenweg (page 120). Tumor escape in the first model is due to antigenic modulation. The second model omits antigenic modulation, and tumor escape is ascribed to the initial size of the tumor and to its antigenicity.

Hoffmann, Cooper-willis, and Chow describe events that occur at the organismal level, that is, what happens when two immune systems react to each other. They describe a new symmetry relationship for such interactions, namely that the antibodies in an A anti-B serum are complementary to (have shapes that fit) the antibodies of a B anti-A serum (page 15).

The final level in our hierarchy of interactions concerns the relationship between epidemiology and the degree of immunity of individuals in a population. Anderson's contribution to this area (page 142) deals with immunology to parasites, while McLean (page 171) develops a model that she applies to the influence of immunity on the epidemiology of measles in developing countries. Finally, Yashin and Vaupel discuss the complexities for epidemiology resulting from inherent heterogeneity in populations (page 198).

References

1. G. I. Bell, A. S. Perelson, and G. H. Pimbley, eds. Theoretical Immunology. Marcel Dekker, 1978.

2. G. I. Marchuk, ed. Modelling and Optimization of Complex Systems, in Proceedings of the IFIP-TC7 Working Conference, Novosibirsk, USSR. Vol. 18 in Lecture Notes in Control and Information Sciences. Springer-Verlag, 1979.

3. C. Bruni, G. Doria, G. Koch, and R. Strom, eds. Systems Theory in Immunology. Vol. 32 in Lecture Notes in Biomathematics. Springer-Verlag, 1979.

4. G. I. Marchuk and L. N. Belykh, eds. Mathematical Modelling in Immunology and Medicine, in Proceedings of the IFIP TC7 Working Conference, Moscow, July 1982. North-Holland, 1983.

5. C. DeLisi. Antigen Antibody Interactions. Vol. 8 in Lecture Notes in Biomathematics. Springer-Verlag, 1976.

6. G. I. Marchuk. Mathematical Models in Immunology. Optimization Software, Publication Division, distributed by Springer-Verlag, 1984.

7. R. Strom, C. Bruni, A. Germani, G. Koch, and A. Oratore. Prob-lems in the Evaluation of Antibody Affinity Distribution During the Immune Response. Vol. 32 in Lecture Notes in Biomathematics. Springer-Verlag, 1979, pp. 104-113.

8. M. Dembo, B. Goldstein, A. K. Sobotka, and L. M. Lichtenstein. Degranulation of Human Basophils: Analysis of Histamine Release and Desensitization Due to a Bivalent Penicilloyl Hapten. J. Immunol. 123:1864-1872, 1979.

9. A. S. Perelson and C. A. Macken. Kinetics of Cell-Mediated Cytotoxicity: Stochastic and Deterministic Multistage Models. Math. Biosciences 70:161-194, 1984.

10. P. Bonard and G. I. Bell. Cell-Cell Adhesion: Parameters and Possible Mechanisms, in Cell Surface Dynamics: Concepts and Models (A. S. Perelson, C. DeLisi, and F. W. Wiegel, eds.). Marcel Dekker, 1984.

PART II

REGULATION

SOME NOTES ON MATHEMATICAL MODELLING OF THE IMMUNE RESPONSE

Miloš Jílek and Daniela Přikrylová
Institute of Microbiology, Czechoslovak Academy of Sciences,
142 20 Prague 4, Czechoslovakia

"Although the majority of theories in immunology have been non-mathematical, there are a variety of quantitative questions whose solutions require mathematical analysis and mathematically formulated models" (Bell and Perelson 1978). It is necessary to subjoin that not only quantitative but many qualitative questions, too, require appropriate mathematical solutions (e. g., by the use of kinetic logic - see Přikrylová and Kůrka 1984).

Mathematical models have been used in immunology since its beginning. However, the history of mathematical modelling of the course of the immune response and of its regulation is relatively short (not longer than 20 years). During this not very long time several hundreds of papers concerning the construction of mathematical models of the course of the immune response, mathematical analysis of these models and their computer simulation, comparison of properties of models and simulation results with experimental data have been published (see, e. g., reviews given by Bell and Perelson 1978, Mohler et al. 1980, DeLisi 1983).

Although mathematical modelling has not penetrated till now into the consciousness of the general immunological public it seems to be one of the most progressive and most perspective approaches of modern immunology.

The convocation of this workshop shows that there are some problems associated with this activity and that the confusion and vagueness of some concepts leads to misunderstanding between theoretical (or mathematical) and experimental immunologists. Some of these problems will be discused in the present contribution.

Possibilities and limitations of mathematical modelling and computer simulation of the immune response

There are three essential restrictions on the possibility of mathematical modelling and simulation of the immune response: contemporary immunological knowledge, available mathematical apparatus, and available computer systems.

Knowledge on the immune system is the basis on which any mathematical model of the immune system has to be built. Every model regards only a part of the real system. The quality of the model depends on the delimitation of this part (i. e., on the choice of system elements involved in the model) and on accepted assumptions concerning the immune response (i. e., on their choice within the framework of knowledge of the system).

The immune response is a very complex biological process, and, therefore, a considerable complexity of its mathematical model may be expected whatever kind of mathematical apparatus (e. g., systems of differential equations, stochastic processes, methods of mathematical logic, etc.) shall be used. However, the solving of complex models is very difficult and sometimes does not lead to satisfactory solution (e. g., when the model consists of a system of many differential or integral-differential equations, the problem of existence of the solution and its uniqueness is as a rule either unsolvable or solvable very strenuously, and "information on the qualitative properties of the model can only be surmised from numerical examples" (Merrill 1980); such information is, of course, highly incomplete, and the success of modelling than depends on the quality of choice of sets of parameter values and initial data. Therefore, the search for the simplest possible model is a general feature of the modelling of any biological process. On the other hand, however, the danger of oversimplification is not negligible (omitting of some important components of the modelled process).

Since a very complex process is modelled and simulated, also the choice of a suitable computation system must be carefully considered since insufficient hardware and/or software makes the use of the model very difficult.

Choice of assumptions (axioms) of the model with regard to the purpose of modelling

Mathematical models are constructed on the basis of accepted assumptions concerning the modelled reality. However, these assumptions are usually simplifying to a certain extent, and by the choice of assumptions we may define that part of the reality (or that part of knowledge of the reality) which is to be studied.

A model in which its elements represent molecules has, of course, properties different from those of a model in which its elements represent cells, in spite of the fact that both of them are models of processes which occur during the immune response.

As the model represents always only a part of the modelled reality it is important to distinguish between internal control (i. e., interrelations between components of the modelled system) and various external influences which can be stated explicitly (by the choice of appropriate parameter values).

Choice of adequate mathematical apparatus

The course of the immune response may be considered to be a realization of a stochastic process (e. g., differentiation and proliferation process of cells participating in the immune response may be modelled by any non-homogeneous multitype birth-and-death process, etc.). However, most mathematical models in immunology are deterministic (systems of differential or integral-differential equations are the most frequently used mathematical approximations to appropriate stochastic processes), as the use of stochastic processes as models of such a complex process as the immune response leads to considerable difficulties. But, when using deterministic approaches, we lose information concerning the variability of the process under study. This variability is usually not negligible and, sometimes, it may be of great interest; therefore the Monte Carlo simulation should be used at least in some cases.

Models of system behaviour and models of system structure

There are two basic properties of any system under study: Behaviour of the system, i. e., dependence of responses (outputs) on stimuli (inputs), and structure of the system, i. e., arrangement of elements of the system and their interrelations and interactions (let us mention that elements of the system may be - on another level of resolution - held and studied as particular systems).

Behaviour of the system may be sometimes modelled irrespective of its structure (e. g., the course of the immune response measured by the number of antibody forming cells or the amount of antibodies in sera may be well approximated by any polynom); the first model of the immune response (Hege and Cole 1966) is of this type (the model consists of the relationship between antibody and antibody forming cells, without profound immunological motivation of this relationship).

Most contemporary models (since the models of Bell 1970, and Jílek and Šterzl 1970) may be classified as models of the system, emanating from hypotheses concerning the structure of the system. The testing of the similarity between the structure of a modelled real system and the structure of its model is done by comparing the behaviour of the two systems. Search for critical points of the model in which disagreement between the behaviour of the two systems occurs leads to the planning of new experimental studies, formulation of higher-precision hypotheses concerning the immune response, and to development of the model.

Models of experiments and models-theories

Mathematical models in immunology may be classified also from another point of view than in preceding sections:

One group comprises mathematical models of experimental methods (e. g., DeLisi and Bell 1974 developed a model of hemolytic plaque formation). The substance of these models is a precise mathematical formulation of (more or less) known facts, and they are based on known (e. g., physico-chemical) laws. The purpose of these models is the elucidation of the functioning of modelled experimental methods and facilitation of design of experiments (e. g., in the choice of optimal exposure time, etc.).

Another group represents mathematical models of some partial event and processes (e. g., Bell 1978 developed a model of the molecula bridging between cells).

A third group involves mathematical models of the regulation of th immune response or of its substantial parts (models of humoral immune re sponse, models of cellular immune response, etc.). These models are base on hypotheses concerning the structure of the immune system, the functio of its individual components and their mutual relationships and interac tions during the immune response.

Comparison of simulation results with incomplete experimental data

While results of the simulation of the course of the immune respons have mostly continuous character, experimental data are usually collecte at discrete instants (very often at one or at a few instants only, e.g. on the 5th day after last immunization); the model may suggest any othe interpretation of experimental results than experimental data suggest a first sight, and it also facilitates the planning of new experiments con cerning the modelled reality.

This is not a specific feature of immunological experiments; let u hear a general account of this matter:

"The principal difficulty attached to the mathematical analysis o physiological and medical systems stems from the mismatch between th complexity of the processes in question and the limited data availabl from such systems, especially from in vivo studies. These limitation are essentially problems of measurement. 1) There are restrictions o the number of variables and parameters... Uncertainty will occur in suc measurement if the assumptions built into the model are not appropriate Also the frequency of measurement is restricted, for example, where bloc sampling is involved. 2) Many measurements are severely corrupted b noice, due to experimental error or unwanted physiological disturbances 3)... there are some variables... for which scales of measurement ar not clearly defined and only qualitative concepts are available." (Cobell et al. 1984) ooperation and responsibility of different experts in construction of he model

Assumptions of mathematical models of the immune response should be ased on contemporary immunological knowledge. It is evident that formu- ation of these assumptions may not be done by the mathematician alone; t would be probably best if the whole mathematical model was done by the mmunologist alone - however, few immunologists are sufficiently mathe- atically erudite.

Mathematical model of the immune response represents sometimes the ork of one author, but in many cases it results from the cooperation of team of authors - experts in different branches (biologist, mathema- ician, computer scientist, etc.). It is self-evident within the frames f the specialization of labour.

Sometimes, however, the competence and responsibility of individual oworkers is not clearly delimited, and the result of such cooperation s unfortunately stigmatized by evident misunderstanding: the mathemati- ian does not formulate biological assumptions correctly, the biologist oes not catechize the adequateness of mathematical assumptions and athematical formulations (e. g., of differential equations forming the odel), the part of the paper written by the mathematician does not cor- espond to the part written by the biologist (or vice versa), etc.

It follows that the immunologist participating in the construction f a mathematical model of the immune response should be able to at least ead a mathematically formulated model (of course, it is not necessary or him to know details of the appropriate mathematical theory).

nterpretation and extrapolation of the attained results of modelling nd simulation

By <u>interpretation</u> of a mathematical model and its simulation is eant their translation (inclusive of all consequences) into the natural anguage . Interpretation belongs undoubtedly to the most difficult ac- ivities when using mathematical models of biological processes. If the odel results from cooperation of mathematicians and biologists, the interpretation is one of the most important roles of biologists, whil mathematicians' role is to call biologists' attention to possible con- sequencies of the model and to look after the adequacy of the translatio into the natural language.

Extrapolation of results of modelling and simulation into the a yet experimentally uninvestigated region of reality may suggest desig of new experimental studies aimed at testing whether the model represent reality adequately even in the region into which the extrapolation i made. Extrapolation must not be held as substitution for unexecuted ex- periments (as was expected by some workers at the beginning of the er of mathematical models in immunology); this follows from the simplifyin assumptions underlying the basis of mathematical models.

. . .

The enumeration of problems given above is by no means complete and appropriate comments do not pretend to being absolutely correct. W only wanted to mention some problems discussed at our institute and o seminars on mathematics and biology we had organized in Prague - prob- lems which seem to be of some importance when trying to construct goo mathematical models of the immune response.

References

Bell, G. I.: Nature 228, 1970, 739-744.

Bell, G. I.: Science 200, 1978, 618-627.

Bell, G. I., Perelson, A. S., in: Theoretical Immunology. Marcel Dekker New York - Basel 1978, 3-41.

Cobelli, C., Carson, E. R., Finkelstein, L., Leaning, M. S.: Am. J. Physiol. 246, 1984, R259-R266.

DeLisi, C.: Ann. Rev. Biophys. Bioeng. 12, 1983, 117-138.

DeLisi, C. P., Bell, G. I.: Proc. Natl. Acad. Sci. 71, 1974, 16-20.

Hege, J. S., Cole, L. J.: J. Immunol. 97, 1966, 34-40.

Jílek, M., Šterzl, J., in: Developmental Aspects of Antibody Formation and Structure. Academia, Prague 1970, 963-981.

Lumb, J. R.: Immunology Today 4, 1983, 209-210.

Merrill, S. J., in: Modeling and Differential Equations in Biology. Marcel Dekker, New York - Basel 1980, 13-50.

Mohler, R. R., Bruni, C., Gandolfi, A.: Proc. IEEE 68, 1980, 964-990.

Přikrylová, D., Jílek, M., Doležal, J.: Kybernetika 20, 1984, 37-46.

Přikrylová, D., Kůrka, P., in: Simulation of Systems in Biology and Medicin ČSVTS, Prague 1984, 725/1-5.

ON PARADOXES AND PROGRESS IN THEORETICAL IMMUNOLOGY, AND EVIDENCE FOR A NEW SYMMETRY

Geoffrey W. Hoffmann, Anwyl Cooper-Willis and Michael Chow
Departments of Physics and Microbiology
University of British Columbia
Vancouver, British Columbia
Canada V6T 1W5

SUMMARY

A view is offered on how we might collectively and perhaps objectively judge which of a variety of theories of regulation are the best, and thus decide which theories should be adopted as standard models for more detailed work. A new theoretical symmetry relationship is then presented for pairs of anti-sera of the type A anti-B and B anti-A, together with experimental evidence validating the relationship. The evidence includes a new phenomenon relevant to transplantation immunology, that we call "reverse enhancement".

ON THE EVALUATION OF COMPETING THEORIES OF IMMUNOREGULATION

In an essay accompanying the invitation to attend this meeting, Asachenkov wrote that "The individual models of theoretical immunology develop relatively independently. This isolation is one of the main reasons why these models do not influence actively enough research on experimental and clinical immunology". We believe that Asachenkov has here made an important and valuable observation. Immunology is a very complex field, with a fluid theoretical basis. Each theorist is able to select a subset of the experimental data, make a set of postulates, and construct a mathematical model relevant to that subset, often calling it "a first step" towards a more comprehensive model. There is however so far very little evidence of a consensus developing from the various "first steps". Our occasional meetings seem to be too brief and too few and far between, to permit the very extensive discussions to occur, that might lead to some convergence in the model-building process. In view of this serious and seemingly persistent situation, we must ask what needs to be done.

An IIASA theoretical immunology project could certainly be a key step towards achieving the desired convergence, and this meeting could therefore be the beginning of a new phase in mathematical and theoretical immunology. In addition, we feel it might be worthwhile to think about whether an overall strategy can be devised, particularly with respect to systematically evaluating the merits and demerits of various models of immune regulation.

Can we jointly formulate a "theory of theories", that might help us to collectively and as objectively as possible reach a consensus as to which theories are best? If that were possible, we could then perhaps focus much of our collective efforts and talents on the analysis of the "standard models".

It might be possible to first reach agreement on a set of criteria, according to which theories of the immune response could be evaluated. Such a set is easily formulated, and might include the following:

1. Simplicity (Economy) in the Set of Postulates. This criterion is a statement of the Principle of Occam's Razor: "Other things being equal, a simple theory is preferable to a complex one". Simplicity is often notoriously difficult to define, and often exists mainly in the eye of the beholder, but attempts to assess the relative complexity of various models could certainly be made. Theorists are likely to differ with experimentalists in the assessment of what is, and what is not, simple.
2. Scope, Explanatory Power (Number and Diversity of Phenomena). The theory should obviously be as complete as possible. A group of theoretical immunologists might like to assemble a catalogue of phenomena, which it feels an adequate theory of immunoregulation should ideally be able to account for.
3. Predictive Power. Some experimentalists seem to subscribe to the view that this is the main or even the only criterion by which theories should be judged. "Sure", we once heard an experimental colleague say condescendingly, "theories are useful providing they lead to new experiments, to testable predictions". The implication was that the theories are otherwise useless. Our colleague seemed to have forgotten that Darwin's theory of evolution, perhaps the most influential of all theories in the natural sciences, was very strong in its explanatory power, and much weaker in its predictive power. Predictive power is nevertheless obviously very important.

4. <u>Paradoxes</u>. The phenomena, on which it is particularly important to concentrate our efforts, are the anomalies or paradoxes; phenomena which are not satisfactorily accommodated within the popular current theoretical framework(s). A scientific paradox formally exists when a theory is sufficiently complete, such that we can predict from the theory what should happen in a certain situation, but we experimentally observe a different result. The experimental result is then a paradox within that particular theoretical framework. The crucial roles that paradoxes can play in the development of science are exemplified by the Michelson-Morley experiment, which was a prelude to the theory of relativity, and the "Ultra-violet catastrophe" of black body radiation, which was a prelude to the development of quantum theory.

   At present there is no well-defined, consensus view on how the immune system is regulated, and various people with various theories consider various phenomena to be paradoxes. The phenomena that are explicitly described as paradoxes deserve particular attention, because they might be very important clues, pointing to aspects of the system that are being widely viewed in quite the wrong way. We are presently assembling a volume entitled "Paradoxes in Immunology" (1) which we hope will be useful in giving model builders a collection of particularly puzzling results. Twenty-seven immunologists (or groups of immunologists) describe phenomena, mostly immunoregulatory phenomena, that are difficult or impossible to understand within the current theoretical picture. Usually people discuss in print that which they understand. In this volume of paradoxes the authors take the opportunity to discuss phenomena they do not understand, which for constructing new models is much more challenging and potentially more useful. Such paradoxes might permit us to very efficiently select the better or best among alternative theories.

5. <u>Rigor</u>. The route from a set of postulates to demonstrating explanatory power, including the elucidation of paradoxes, and to making testable predictions, can be more or, alternatively, less rigorous. The more mathematical the route, the more rigorous it is, in general. The more rigorous it is, the better the theory, we would all concur. However, our feeling is that it is better to concentrate initially on scope and

subsequently on rigor, rather than being very concerned about rigor in the early stages of the development of a model.

Thank you for your patience in listening to these general remarks, which some of you might consider to be self-understood or even trivial. Whether trivial or not, we suggest that if an IIASA project in theoretical immunology is to be successful, the various models should be systematically subjected to comparative analyses along lines similar to those sketched above. We feel that extensive and systematic comparative evaluations of various models have not been made in the past, and that this is the main reason for the existence of the problem described by Asachenkov. A general framework, similar to the one we have outlined, might make it easier for us all to be perhaps a little less polite about each other's models, and thus accelerate our progress towards an adequate model of immunoregulation. An IIASA project in theoretical immunology could then contribute a great deal towards correcting the deficiency described by Asachenkov, and for that reason, among others, we strongly support the idea of such a project.

We now turn to some real science.

ON THE PRESENT STATUS OF IDIOTYPIC NETWORK THEORIES OF IMMUNOREGULATION.

The development of a theory of regulation of the immune system based on Niels Jerne's network hypothesis (2) is a great challenge for theoretical immunologists. Models of the network have been developed mainly by Richter (3), Ivanov, Janenko, Fontalin and Nesterenko (4), Herzenberg, Black and Herzenberg (5) and ourselves (6-8).

Jerne himself recognized from the outset the need for a mathematically precise formulation of what was a revolutionary vision, but a rather fuzzy theory, with regard to the details. As formulated by Jerne, the theory simply started from the view that the V regions of antibodies and the specific cellular receptors constitute a network of specifically recognizing and recognized components. Jerne then postulated that there were both specific stimulatory and suppressive interactions between V regions. But he conceded that "The weakness of this incipient network theory lies in its lack of precision... This leaves an ambiguity in the answer to the question whether the relations between two sets is suppressive or stimulatory, or partly one and partly the other, and thus permits us to postulate interactions that suit our explanatory needs", (2); and further, "To become meaningful, a more explicit formulation of the network and its functional features and parameters would be needed.... Questions as to the degree of stability of network modulations induced by antigen cannot be solved intuitively, as intuition is an unreliable substitute for mathematical demonstration" (9).

The explicit models with a mathematical component that have now been published include the asymmetric network models of Richter (1) and Ivanov _et al_. (3), and the symmetric model by ourselves (6,10). The asymmetric model of Herzenberg _et al_. has no mathematical underpinning. We have criticized the other models, mainly on the basis of the assumed asymmetry (6,10). Spouge recently contributed a new analytic treatment of the complexity-stability problem in the context of the symmetric theory (11), which had previously been analysed only using numerical techniques (7,10).

A NEW SYMMETRY RELATIONSHIP FOR IMMUNE SYSTEM NETWORKS

We here describe a simple new phenomenon, which can be understood without invoking any mathematics.

The symmetrical network theory is partly based on an experimentally well-established symmetry relationship, which we could call the "first symmetry" of immune system network theory. The first symmetry is the fact that if an idiotype P is recognized by a particular "anti-idiotype" Q, then P is simultaneously an anti-idiotype of the idiotype Q. This symmetry, which is illustrated in figure 1, has been demonstrated for both stimulation and killing (12,13). Consequences of first symmetry are that there is no fundamental regulatory distinction between paratopes and idiotopes as originally defined by Jerne, and the "internal image" is functionally identical with the "anti-idiotypic set".

First symmetry refers to interactions within a single immune system network. We will now derive a second symmetry, that concerns the interactions between two different immune system networks. It was discovered in the course of trying to understand an intriguing paradox that has attracted much attention, known as the "I-J paradox" (14-17). We will not attempt to review the I-J

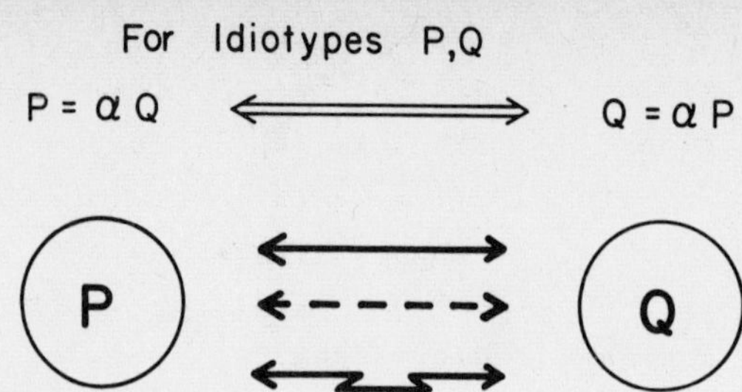

Fig.1. The first symmetry of immune system network theory. If idiotype P is anti-idiotypic to Q, this implies that idiotype Q is anti-idiotypic to P, and vice-versa. Stimulation (solid arrow), inhibition (broken line) and killing (jagged line) can all be bidirectional.

phenomenology in any detail. Suffice it to say that the paradox arose when molecular genetic studies showed that the genes for certain protein molecules, that seem to play a key role in immunoregulation, are not found in the part of the DNA where they had been expected on the basis of genetic studies. In line with the ideas of Schrader (18) and Tada (19), we considered the possibility that anti-I-J antibodies might have anti-anti-self specificity. That idea led us to a new symmetry relationship.

The theoretical result is derived by considering reciprocal immunizations with lymphoid cells of two strains of mice, A and B. This procedure amounts to confronting two immune system networks with each other. The set of cell-surface antigens expressed by A but not by B will be denoted by a, and the corresponding set of antigens expressed by B but not by A will be denoted by b. When lymphoid cells from A are injected into a B animal, the A cells that recognize b antigens in the host are stimulated and proliferate, while A cells of other specificities are not stimulated. There are then two sets of foreign entities that can be recognized by B, namely the a set of antigens, and the A anti-b receptors. Thus the immune response of B to A has two components, namely B anti-a (conventional anti-foreign) and B anti-(A anti-b), which is anti-anti-self. Similarly, the immune response of an animal A to B lymphoid cells consists of the two components A anti-b (or anti-foreign) and A anti-(B anti-a) (or anti-anti-self), as shown in figure 2.

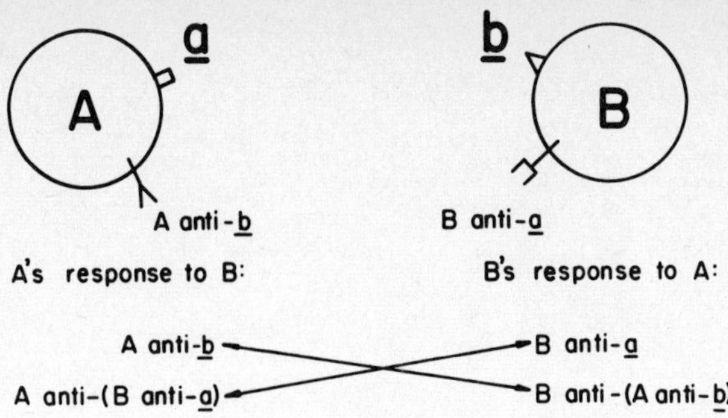

Fig. 2. The second symmetry of immune system networks. For two genetically dissimilar individuals A and B, the total immune response of A to B is complementary to the total immune response of B to A, when (and only when) anti-anti-self responses are included in the analysis.

It follows that the anti-foreign response in B is precisely complementary to the anti-anti-self response in A, and the anti-foreign response in A is complementary to the anti-anti-self response in B. Consequently the total response of A to B is complementary to the total response of B to A. In short, A anti-B is anti-(B anti-A).

We tested the validity of the above hypothetical "second symmetry" using the three H-2 congenic strains C57BL/10 ("B10"), B10.D2 and B10.BR. We raised three reciprocal pairs of anti-sera: B10 anti B10.BR and B10.BR anti-B10; B10.D2 anti B10.BR, and B10.BR anti B10.D2; and finally, B10 anti B10.D2 and B10.D2 anti B10. The anti-sera had cytotoxic titres against lymph node cells of the immunizing strain of at least 100. Typical inhibition results are shown in figure 3. We refer to the target cells as strain "B" and the lytic serum as A anti-B. For instance, in the first panel of fig. 3, A = B10.BR and B = B10. The important result was that we could inhibit the killing of the target cells by first mixing the lytic A anti-B serum with the reciprocal B anti-A serum. This was true even when the B anti-A serum was absorbed with A cells. Classically, of course, we would expect such an absorbed serum to have no specific activity at all. The negative controls for the inhibition are normal (non-immune) B serum, normal A serum, A anti-B and A anti-B absorbed B. We note that strong inhibition by B anti-A was observed in 5 of the 6 cases, with some inhibition in the sixth case. We also observed that a little inhibitory activity was

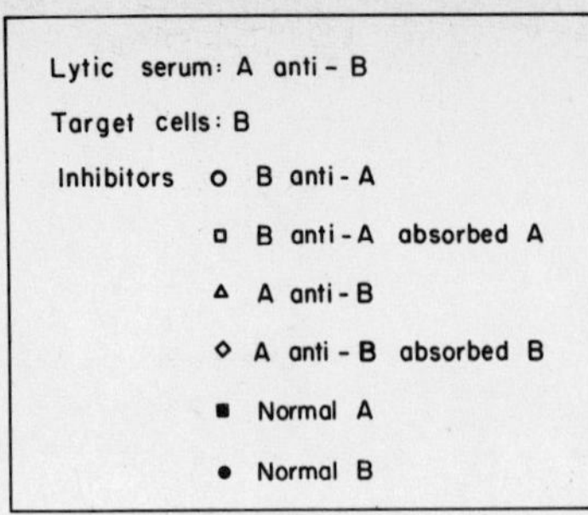

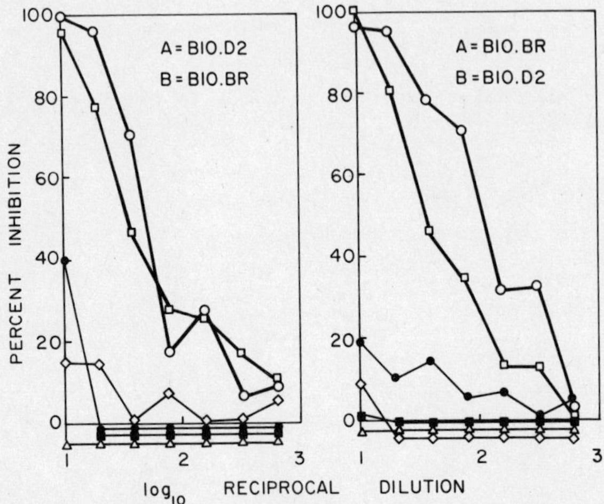

Fig. 3. Experimental tests of second symmetry using 6 B10 congenic hyperimmune antisera. The antisera were raised with 6 to 9 weekly injections of 10^7 spleen cells. In each of the panels, one of the sera, denoted by "A anti-B" was used as the lytic serum, to kill cells of strain "B". In each case the killing was inhibited by B anti-A serum, either absorbed against A cells (gluteraldehyde fixed) or not absorbed. The control sera were A anti-B, A anti-B absorbed B, sera from unimmunized A ("normal A") and sera from unimmunized B ("normal B"). Figure continued on next page.

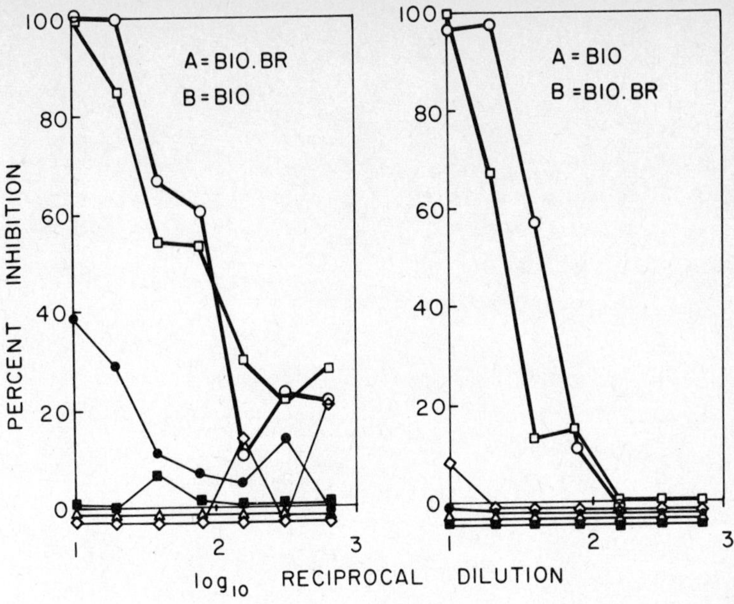

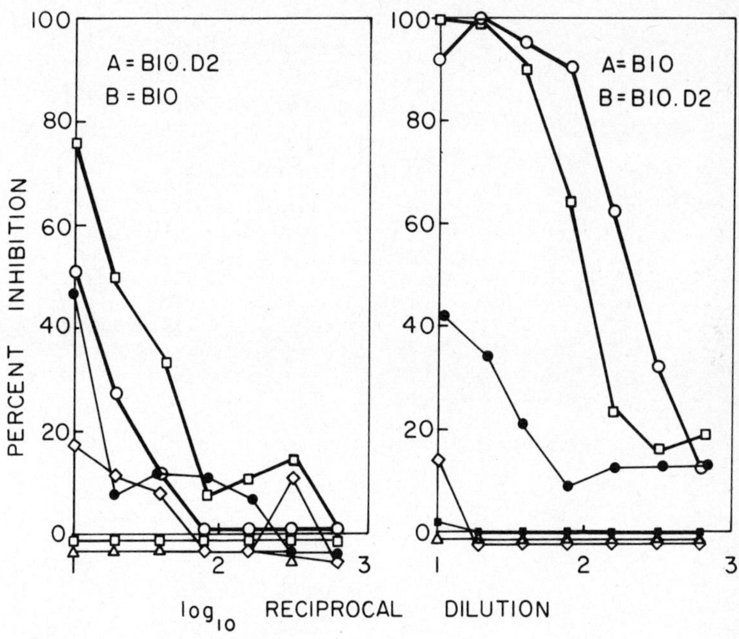

Fig. 3, continued.

present in several of the normal B sera. (This last aspect has not been investigated in any detail. It raises the interesting question of whether there is an anti-anti-self component in immune responses also to environmental antigens, and if so, why?)

The strains B10, B10.BR and B10.D2 are identical except for the H-2 complex. Similar results to those of figs. 3 and 4 were obtained in a study involving the three completely unrelated strains SJL, C57BL/6 and CBA.

Antibody is responsible for both the lytic and the inhibitory properties of the anti-sera, since absorption with goat anti-mouse immunoglobulin coupled to sepharose 4B removes both activities (Table 1).

Table 1

Lytic and Inhibitory Activities of Anti-sera before and after Absorption with Anti-Ig or Immunogen

Serum	Absorption	As lytic serum: % lysis of target cells	As inhibitor of lysis by reciprocal serum: % inhibition
Experiment 1			
CBA anti-B6	-	42.2	99.8
CBA anti-B6	Goat anti-mouse Ig	0.0	0.0
CBA anti-B6	B6 spleen cells	0.0	95.6
Experiment 2			
SJL anti-CBA	-	78.7	54.9
SJL anti-CBA	Goat anti-mouse Ig	0.0	0.0
SJL anti-CBA	CBA spleen cells	0.0	76.1

The two components of the antibody response are seen to be separated by absorption against lymphoid tissue of the immunizing strain, which removes the lytic but not the inhibitory activity of the antiserum. The simplest explanation for all these findings is, we believe, that the inhibition is indeed due to the presence in the B anti-A serum of B anti-A-anti-b (anti-anti-self) antibodies.

THE RELEVANCE OF SECOND SYMMETRY TO TRANSPLANTATION IMMUNOLOGY: REVERSE ENHANCEMENT.

If antibodies in a B anti-A serum inhibit A anti-B antibodies _in vitro_, it is obviously possible that they should inhibit an A anti-B response also _in vivo_. We showed that this is indeed the case by demonstrating that, for instance, CBA anti-SJL immune serum absorbed with SJL cells causes an enhancement of the survival of CBA skin grafts on SJL mice, as shown in figure 4(a). The results shown in figures 4(b) and 4(c) prove that the enhancing effect of the immune absorbed serum is specific. In the experiment of figure 4(b) the graft donor and recipients were interchanged, so that the donors were SJL mice, and the recipients were CBA. There was then no significant graft enhancement. In the experiment of figure 4(a) the survival of an irrelevant ("3rd party") graft is shown to be not enhanced by the serum.

Completely analogous results were obtained with an SJL anti-CBA serum absorbed with CBA Cells, as shown in figure 5.

The degree of specificity seen in these experiments was greater than that seen with the _in vitro_ assay, where a lot of cross-reactivity was very often seen with third party antisera (results not shown). The only speculation we can offer that might be a step towards accounting for this difference, is that the _in vivo_ effects could perhaps involve a different slice of the antibody affinity spectrum than the _in vitro_ assay, and the _in vivo_ effects can consequently be more specific. That is, however, clearly an incomplete rationale.

It has been known for a long time that hyperimmune serum can enhance the survival of various transplanted tissues in a wide variety of species (reviewed by Carpenter, d'Apice and Abbas (20), Voisin (21) and Morris (22). In the previous work however ("conventional enhancement", figure 11) antiserum directed against the graft gave enhanced graft survival, while here we used antiserum made in the graft donor strain against recipient lymphoid cells, and then absorbed with the same immunizing type of cells. Since the converse serum is used, we call this phenomenon "reverse enhancement" (fig. 6).

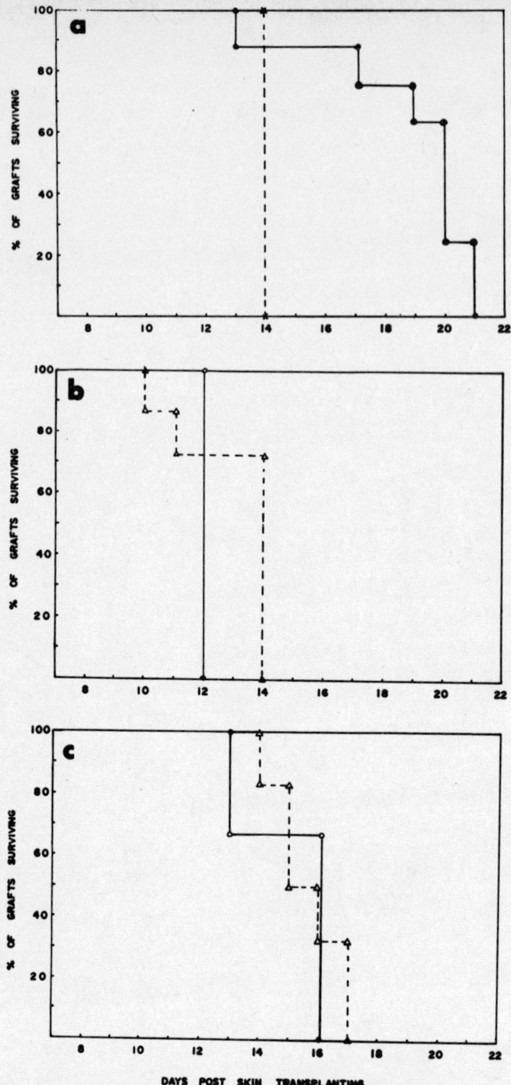

Fig. 4. (a) Enhancement of the survival of CBA grafts on SJL mice with CBA anti-SJL immune serum absorbed with SJL lymphoid cells. The control group of mice shown here (dashed line) received no serum, the experimental group received 5 µl immune absorbed serum on each of the days -4, -1 and 0 relative to grafting. The immune serum was raised with injections of 10^7 spleen and thymus cells at weekly intervals for 6 to 9 weeks. There were 5 to 8 mice in each group. (b) First specificity control. The CBA anti-SJL immune absorbed serum caused no enhancement of SJL grafts on CBA mice, that is, grafts in the opposite direction. Group with serum, solid line; group without serum, dashed line. (c) Second specificity control for the CBA anti-SJL immune absorbed serum. No enhancement is observed of an irrelevant graft, B10.D2, on an SJL mouse.

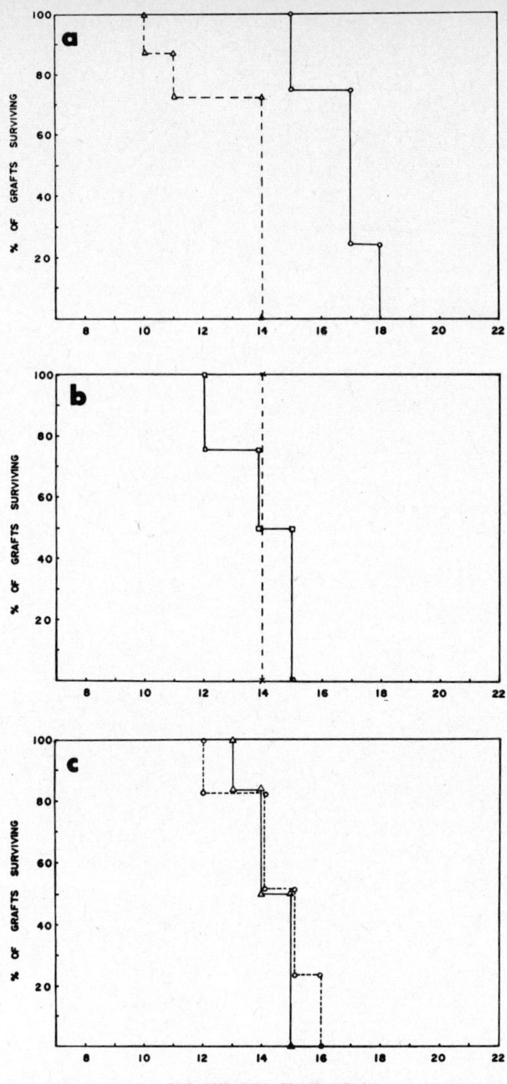

ig. 5. Enhancement of the survival of SJL grafts on CBA mice with JL anti-CBA immune serum absorbed against CBA lymphoid cells. The ontrol group shown here (dashed line) received no serum. The serum reparation and injection protocols were as given in caption to igure 4.

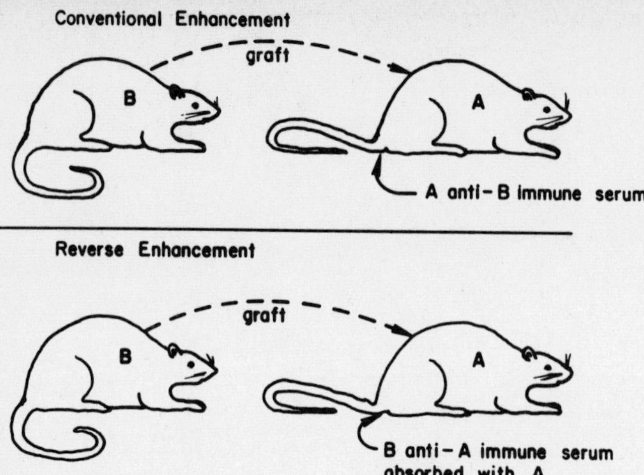

Fig. 6. The difference between conventional enhancement and reverse enhancement.

Reverse enhancement is potentially of importance for clinical immunology. There has recently been much interest in the use of xenogeneic organ transplants. Reverse enhancement might help to improve the success of such transplants. A xenogeneic organ donor could be made immune to tissue of the organ recipient, and then immune-absorbed serum from the donor could be injected into the organ recipient, near the time of the organ transplant. The same might be true in the case of at least some transplants from allogeneic donors. We have found that anti-anti-self antibody activity is produced equally efficiently when heavily irradiated (2000 rad) lymphoid spleen cells are used as immunogen. This suggests that radiation could be used to inactivate any pathogens resident in the graft recipient tissue sample, prior to that tissue sample being used to raise the required antiserum in the graft donor.

Our results using both *in vitro* and an *in vivo* assay system are consistent with the idea that the injection of allogeneic lymphoid cells routinely leads to the production of anti-anti-self antibodies in parallel with anti-foreign antibodies. The production of anti-anti-self antibodies is obviously of great advantage to the individual, since such antibodies cause a negative selection of anti-self clones and of clones that cross-react with both foreign and self antigens. The remaining anti-foreign antibodies cannot then cross-react with self. This constitutes a fail-safe mechanism, which ensures adequate specificity of immune responses to structures that are similar to self antigens. Thus we have a clear cut role for network regulation in helping the immune system to discriminate between self and nonself.

Ramseier and Lindenmann (23) and subsequently Binz and Wigzell (24) have previously shown that "anti-recognition structure" antibodies (that have anti-anti-self specificity in some of their experiments) can be produced with F1 and parental inbred animals, when the experiments are designed in such a way as to exclude the possibility of a conventional anti-foreign (i.e. anti-alloantigen) response. Our results show that appreciable amounts of anti-anti-self antibodies are routinely present in allo-antisera raised against completely unrelated strains, and their presence can be detected using quite simple assay systems.

We finally reiterate that the two new phenomena we have described, namely second symmetry and reverse enhancement, were discovered in the course of attempts to understand the I-J paradox. We feel that this illustrates the value of identifying the paradoxes in cellular immunology, and focussing attention on them, even if one does not necessarily resolve the paradoxes.

Acknowledgments

We thank Dr. Ed Levy of the Philosophy Department, University of British Columbia, for stimulating discussions on the philosophy of science aspects of this essay. Grant support from MRC Canada and NSERC Canada is gratefully acknowledged.

REFERENCES

1. "Paradoxes in Immunology", G. W. Hoffmann, J.G. Levy and G.T. Nepom, Editors, CRC Press, Boca Raton, Florida, 1986. (in press).
2. Jerne, N.K. "Towards a network theory of the immune system". Ann. Immunol., 125C (1974) 373-389.
3. Richter, P.H. "A network theory of the immune response". Eur. J. Immunol. 5, 350-354 (1975).
4. Ivanov, V.V., Janenko, V.M., Fontalin, L.N. and Nesterenko, V.G. "Modelling of idiotype-anti-idiotypic interactions of immune network with regard to distinctive subpopulations among lymphocytes" in "Mathematical Modelling in Immunology and Medicine". G.I. Marchuk and L.N. Belykh, Editors, North-Holland Publishing Co., Amsterdam 1983, pp. 141-149.

5. Herzenberg, L.A., Black, S.J. and Herzenberg, L.A. "Regulatory circuits and antibody responses". Eur. J. Immunol. 10, 1-11, 1980.
6. Hoffmann, G.W. "On Network Theory and H-2 Restriction", in Contemporary Topics in Immunology (N. Warner, Ed.) vol. 11, 1980, pp. 185-226.
7. Hoffmann, G.W. and Cooper-Willis, A. "Symmetry, complexity and stability in immune system network theory" in "Mathematical Modelling in Immunology and Medicine", G.I. Marchuk and L.N. Belykh, Editors, North-Holland Publishing Co., Amsterdam, 1983, pp. 31-42.
8. Gunther, N. and Hoffmann, G.W. "Qualitative dynamics of a network model of regulation of the immune system: A rationale for the IgM to IgG switch". J. Theoret. Biol. 44, 815-855 (1982).
9. Jerne, N.K. "Clonal selection in a lymphocyte network" in "Cellular Selection and Regulation in the Immune Response", G.M. Edelman, Ed., Raven Press, New York, 1974 pp. 39-48.
10. Hoffmann, G.W. "The Application of Stability Criteria in Evaluating Network Regulation Models", in "Regulation of Immune Response Dynamics", C. DeLisi and J.R.J. Hiernaux (Eds.), CRC Press, Boca Raton, Florida, 1982 pp. 137-162.
11. Spouge, J.L. "Increasing stability with complexity in a system composed of unstable subsystems". J. Math. Analysis and Applications, in press.
12. Urbain, J., Wailmart, C. and Cazenave, P.A. "Idiotypic regulation in immune networks" In Contemp. Topics in Molecular Immunology, vol. 8, eds. Inwan, F.P. and Mandy, W.J., pp. 113-148, Plenum Press, New York, 1981.
13. Cooper-Willis, A. and Hoffmann, G.W. "Symmetry of effector function in the immune system network". Mol. Immunol. 20 (8), 865-870, 1983.
14. Steinmetz, M., Minard, K., Horvath, S., McNicholas, J., Frelinger, J., Wake C., Mack, B. and Hood, L. "A molecular map of the immune response region from the major histocompatibility complex of the mouse". Nature (London) 300, 35-42, 1982.
15. Klein, J. and Nagy, Z.A. "Trouble in the J-land". Nature (London) 300, 12-13, 1982.
16. Munro, A. "The I-J paradox remains unsolved". Nature (London) 306, 537-538, 1983.

17. Sachs, D.L., Lynch, D.H. and Epstein, S.L. "The I-J dilemma: new developments". Immunology Today, 5, 94-95, 1984.

18. Schrader, J.W. "Nature of the T cell receptor. Both T cell receptor and antigen-specific T cell derived factors are coded for by V genes, but express anti-self idiotypes indirectly determined by major histocompatibility genes". Scand. J. Immunol. 10, 387-393, 1979.

19. Tada, T. "Are there unique I region-controlled determinants on T cells?" in "Paradoxes in Immunology", Hoffmann, G.W., Nepom, G.T. and Levy, J.G., eds., CRC Press, Boca Raton, Florida, 1986.

20. Carpenter, C.B., d'Apice, A.J.F., Abbas, A.K. "The Role of Antibodies in the Rejection and Enhancement of Organ Allografts". Advances in Immunol. 22, 1, 1976.

21. Voisin, G.A. "Role of antibody classes in the regulatory facilitation reaction". Immunol. Reviews, 49, 3, 1980.

22. Morris, P.J. "Suppression of rejection of organ allografts by alloantibody". Immunol. Rev., 49, 93, 1980.

23. Ramseier, H. and Lindenmann, J. "Aliotypic antibodies". Transpl. Rev. 10, 57-96, 1972.

24. Binz, H. and Wigzell, H. "Shared idiotypic determinants on B and T lymphocytes reactive against the same antigenic determinants. I. Demonstration of similar or identical idiotypes on IgG molecules and T cell receptors with specificity for the same alloantigens". J. Exp. Med. 142, 197-211.

Antigen recognition by T cells.-Towards a mathematical description of the T cell specificity repertoire.

Wulf Dröge
Institut für Immunologie und Genetik
Deutsches Krebsforschungszentrum
Im Neuenheimer Feld 280
D-6900 Heidelberg
West-Germany

The usefullness of mathematical equations as an adequate description for certain immunological phenomena is occasionally recognized even by experimentalists (see 1,2). A well known example is the mathematical treatment of antigen-antibody interactions and a more recent example is the paper by Matis et al. (3). Some theoretical implications of this and several related papers shall be discussed in this commentary. These considerations lead to a mathematical description of the T cell specificity repertoire.

For the purpose of this paper I shall distinguish the following groups of antigens: the self-antigens will be divided into self-major-histocompatibility antigens (self-MHA) and conventional self antigens (self-CA); and the foreign antigens will be divided similarly into foreign (allogeneic) MHA and foreign CA. The CA are defined as antigens which are not MHA and which are recognized by T cells only in combination with MHA.

I. Suppression of clonal proliferation by superoptimal concentrations of antigen.-Stimulation of T cell clones with intermediate affinity for self antigen as a predictable consequence.

The term "high dose tolerance" describes the well known phenomenon that high doses of antigen often induce a state of specific unresponsiveness. The antigen-dose-response curve in these cases has a clear-cut maximum. Two independent studies (3,4) now showed a similar dose-response curve for the proliferative response of antigen-specific

T cell clones against antigen pulsed antigen presenting cells (APC).

The experiments of Matis et al. (3) showed, moreover, that a given T cell clone can be stimulated by two different antigens, and that optimal stimulation is obtained with different concentrations of these two crossreactive antigens. For example, a concentration of 0.24 M pigeon cytochrome C was found to stimulate optimal proliferative responses in a given experimental situation whereas the concentration of 0.24 M tobacco hornworm moth cytochrome C was already inhibitory (3). The most obvious interpretation is that these antigens have different affinities to the antigen receptors of the clone. This pattern of responses of a single clone against two different antigens will certainly have its mirror image in the stimulatory effects of a given antigen on two different T cell clones. One can expect that a relatively high concentration of a given antigen will suppress a clone that bears receptors with high affinity to this antigen, but will stimulate cells with comparably lower (i.e. intermediate) affinity for this antigen. As the T cell system is always facing syngeneic APC with high concentrations of self antigen, one can expect that the stimulation of T cells with intermediate affinity to self antigens will be constantly occurring in vivo. This is indeed a very strong prediction, unless other mechanisms interfere with this process. The autologous MLR *in vitro* (5-8) and the intrathymic (10-13) and postthymic (14,15) proliferation of the T cell population or the development of self-H-2 specific CTL from nude mouse bone marrow cells (16) may be visible consequences of this phenomenon. A selective stimulation of T cells with intermediate affinities to self antigens has already been proposed to constitute the major force that generates the T cell repertoire (17-19). The generation of the T cell repertoire resembles according to this concept a heteroclitic immune response: most of the selected cells will have only intermediate affinity to the selecting antigen (i.e. self antigens) but high affinity to one or the other foreign antigen (i.e. a virus), against which they will eventually defend the organism.

II. Evidence that the T cell receptor recognizes antigen complexes consisting of one CA and one MHA molecule each.

Several laboratories have been able with the help of monoclonal antisera to identify structurally related clonotypic molecules on

T cells, which were subsequently shown to be the antigen receptors (20-24). These structures are disulfide-bridged heterodimers consisting of two chains with molecular weights of about 40 kd. Importantly, these receptors molecules were shown to be responsible for binding simultaneously conventional antigen (CA) and major histocompatibility antigen (MHA) (23).

In support of the conclusion that a single receptor binds simultaneously both, CA and MHA molecules, Matis et al. (3) have found that T cell proliferation is a function of the product of the concentrations of CA and MHA molecules. Accordingly, DNA synthesis has been found to be inhibited by an excess of either CA or MHA molecules. The mass action law predicts that the product of the concentrations of CA and MHA is proportional to the concentration of (hypothetical) complexes of CA and MHA. Therefore, this observation suggests (even though it does not prove) that the T cell receptor recognizes antigen complexes consisting of one CA and one MHA molecule each.

III. Experimental evidence suggesting that T cell receptors recognize unaltered MHA determinants on the CA/MHA complex.

The phenomenon that foreign CA determinants such as virus particles are recognized by T cells preferentially or exclusively in combination with self-MHA has been described many years ago and has been termed "self-restriction" (25). Self-restriction applies also to T cell tolerance of self-CA (26). It was also pointed out (25) that the phenomenon of self-MHA restriction may be based either upon the recognition of newly formed "neoantigenic determinants" which are formed by the interaction of CA and MHA ("altered self model"), or upon the recognition of unmodified determinants on both types of antigens ("dual recognition"). The experiments discussed in the previous section were not designed to distinguish between these two recognition modes.

However, recognition in a pure "altered self" mode appears to be very unlikely in the view of several sets of observations (25,27-35). All these observations showed in essence that animals which have been depleted of alloreactive cells with specificity for a given allogeneic haplotype recognize CA better in the context of self-MHA than in the context of MHA of the allogeneic haplotype. These observations indicated that the self-restrictedness (i.e. the preference for self-MHA) exists not only at the level of the activated effector T cells but already at the level of the precursor T cell repertoire before deliberate immunization. Recent evidence indicated that this applies also to normal animals (36). If the T cell population recognizes a foreign CA determinant (which it has not experienced before) preferentially in the context of self-MHA determinants, we must conclude that this self-MHA/CA complex must have something in common with the MHA determinants in the selecting environment before the encounter with this foreign CA determinant. In so far, there must be a component of "dual recognition" (see (37)). The T cell receptor must recognize usually unaltered self-MHA in complex with CA determinants. The combined conclusion from this and the preceding section is, therefore, that two distinct binding regions on a single T cell receptor usually recognize unaltered determinants on the CA and MHA molecules, respectively.This does not exclude that the same combination(s) of binding regions may occasionally accomodate foreign MHA or chemically modified MHA molecules also in an "altered self mode" as suggested by the crossreactivity patterns of cloned T cell lines (38-40).

IV. Theoretical conclusions from the available experimental information.

The combined information of the previous sections leads to several theoretical conclusions, which are illustrated graphically in Fig.1. I shall first come back to the main point of section I that the T cell system is constantly confronted with large numbers of autologous (syngeneic) APC, which are expected to stimulate T cells with intermediate affinity to self antigens into proliferation. The graphs a and b in Fig.1 illustrate the situation that cells with intermediate affinity to self antigens will optimally be driven into proliferation and therefore constitute a high relative frequency in the repertoire, whereas T cells with very low or very high affinity to self-antigens will be poorly stimulated and therefore be represented with a relatively low frequency in the T cell repertoire (see section I). The intensity of the shading illustrates the relative frequency of the T cells with the corresponding affinity. This probability profile will apply to the affinity to self-MHA (Fig.1a) and also to the affinity to self-CA

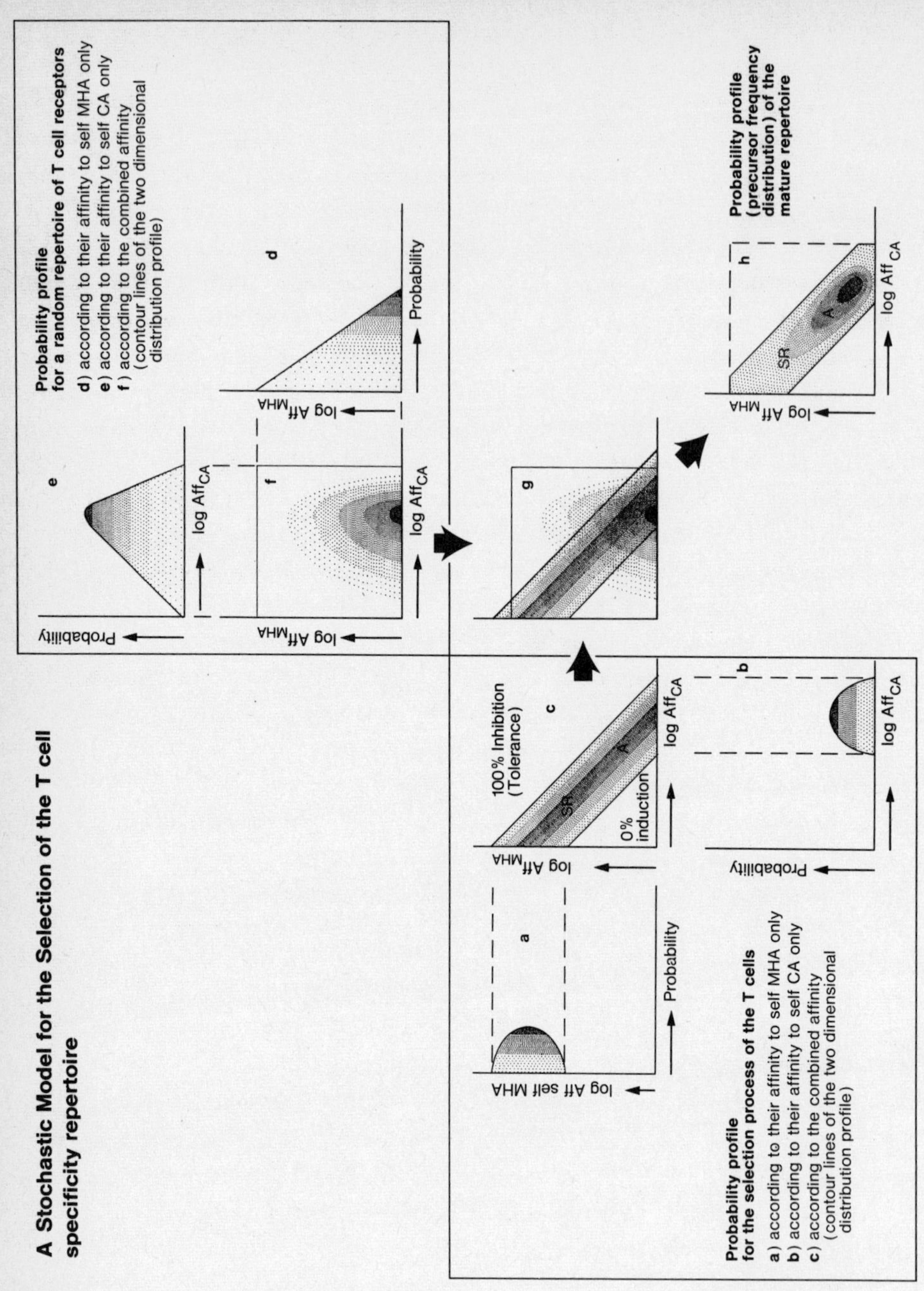

Legend to Fig. 1: A Stochastic Model for the Selection of the T cell specificity repertoire. For details see text.

(Fig.1b).

The main points of sections II and III were i) that T cells recognize complexes of CA and MHA and ii) that two distinct binding regions on a single T cell receptor recognize unaltered determinants on the CA and MHA molecules, respectively. In order to appreciate these points, it may be useful to compare the T cell receptor with the B cell receptor. The B cell receptor is known to bind antigen also with two binding regions, namely with the V regions of the immunoglobulin heavy and light chains, respectively. The major difference between T cell and B cell receptors may simply be that one of the two binding regions of the T cell receptor has been selected to recognize MHA determinants. Two points which are established for interactions between antigen and immunoglobulin molecules are expected to apply also to receptor-ligand interactions on the T cell: i) the consequence of a receptor-ligand interaction will depend exclusively on the affinity of the total interaction irrespective of how much the individual V-region contributes to the total binding energy, and ii) the total affinity is approximately the product of the affinities at the individual binding regions. (The binding energies at the two binding regions contribute approximately additively to the total binding energy.) The total affinity of the T cell receptor for the MHA/CA complex will be, therefore, approximately the product of the affinities of its two binding regions for the MHA and CA determinants, respectively:

$$A_{total} = A_{MHA} \cdot A_{CA}.$$

It is reasonable to assume that the selection for intermediate affinity to self antigen (see section I) is also based on this total affinity of the receptor:

$$P_{selection} = f\ (A_{total}) = f\ (A_{self\text{-}MHA} \cdot A_{self\text{-}CA}).$$

This equation simply states that all cells with a given constant product of affinities to self MHA and self CA, respectively, will have the same probability to be stimulated and selected by syngeneic APC, irrespective of the individual affinities of their binding regions for self MHA or for self CA. In Fig.1c, I have therefore plotted all T cells with all possible combinations of binding regions according to their affinities to self-MHA determinants (ordinate) and affinities to self-CA determinants (abscissa) on a logarithmic two-dimensional probability plot. It is easy to see that all points with a given constant total affinity to self antigens (i.e. with a given constant product of the individual affinities to self-MHA and self-CA determinants) are located on a straight diagonal line as shown in Fig.1c. Cells with intermediate affinities are, therefore, located on a diagonal band as illustrated by the shaded area in Fig.1c. Cells in the lower left corner of this two-dimensional probability plot have only a weak total affinity to complex self antigens and are therefore not adequately stimulated by autologous APC; and cells in the upper right corner have a high total affinity and are therefore also not stimulated or even rendered unresponsive (see Section I). The entire mature T cell repertoire may, therefore, be located on such a diagonal band.

The shaded area in Fig.1c illustrates only the probability distribution for the selection process and does not take into account the two dimensional frequency distribution of receptors in the original specificity repertoire. The relative frequency ($P_{original}$) of a certain type of cells in the original repertoire multiplied with the probability ($P_{selection}$) that this type of cells will be stimulated and selected into the mature repertoire is expected to give the relative frequency in the mature T cell specificity repertoire:

$$P_{mature} = P_{original} \cdot P_{selection}.$$

For the purpose of this paper it may be useful to assume that the original repertoire before the selection process is practically random. How would a random repertoire of receptors be distributed in the two-dimensional log-plot according to the affinities to self-MHA (ordinate) and to self-CA (abscissa)? The probability distribution with respect to the affinity for MHA determinants should be relatively simple and is schematically illustrated in Fig.1d: most receptors of a random repertoire are expected to have only low affinity to a given self-MHA (i.e. the probability for low affinity receptors is high), whereas receptors with high affinity to self-MHA determinants should be relatively infrequent (low probability of receptors with high affinity to self-MHA). Moreover, there should be a final upper limit for the affinity to self-MHA, because even the best fitting receptor would have only a final maximum affinity. The probability distribution profile for the affinity to self-CA is slightly more complicated (Fig.1e). In contrast to self-MHA, there are many self-CA determinants. The selection process (see Section I) is expected to operate according to the affinity to the best fitting self-antigen. For example, a receptor with high affinity to the best fitting self-antigen should be rendered tolerant. One can, therefore, expect that most of the receptors in a random repertoire will have intermediate or even relatively high affinity to the best fitting self-CA and only relatively few receptors will have low affinity to the best fitting self-CA (Fig.1e). On the other hand, few receptors will have very high affinity to self-CA and there is again an upper threshold for the affinity to self-CA, since even the best fitting receptor has only a maximum affinity. One can therefore predict a bell-shaped distribution profile as schematically shown in Fig.1e. The distribution profiles in Fig.1d and Fig.1e are essentially mirror images of the affinity distribution profiles of a random pool of antigens in relation to different populations of antibodies. If a random pool of antigens is facing only one or a few antibodies, one can expect that most interactions have low affinity and that only few antigens bind with high affinity to these antibodies. However, if there are many antibodies (as it is the case in the immune system) every antigen is likely to find an antibody with intermediate or high affinity to this antigen, and only few antigens will bind with very low or extremely high affinity to the best fitting antibody. The latter distribution would correspond to Fig.1e. Fig.1f describes the resulting two-dimensional distribution profile of a random repertoire of receptors in frequency contour lines according to their affinities to self-MHA, on the one hand, and self-CA, on the other hand. If this repertoire is subjected to a selection process with the probability distribution according to Fig.1c, one obtains the probability distribution shown in Fig.1h. This is expected to describe essentially the precursor frequency distribution of T cells in the mature repertoire.

The graphs f,c and h in Fig.2 correspond to Fig.1f,c and h and show some special examples to illustrate the shaping of the repertoire: the cells in the circled areas 1,2, and 3 are chosen to have the same relative frequency in the original repertoire, i.e. they are located on the same probability contour line in Fig.2f. The cells in areas 1 and 3 have practically 0% chance to be selected into the mature repertoire, whereas cells in area 2 will be optimally selected and appear in the mature repertoire with a finite probability (Figs. 2c and h). The cells in the circles 2 and 4, on the other hand, have the same probability to be selected into the repertoire. However, there are more cells in the original repertoire in area 4 than in area 2 (Fig.2f), and the mature repertoire will therefore also contain more cells in area 4 than in area 2 (Fig.2h).

One of the remarkable features of the expected mature repertoire (Fig.1h) is that typically self-restricted (SR) and alloreactive (A) T cells are located on two ends of one continuous spectrum of T cells with an unknown degree of overlap. T cell receptors with high affinity to typically foreign CA (i.e. with low affinity for self-CA) are located in the left end of this diagonal band (Fig.1h), and these

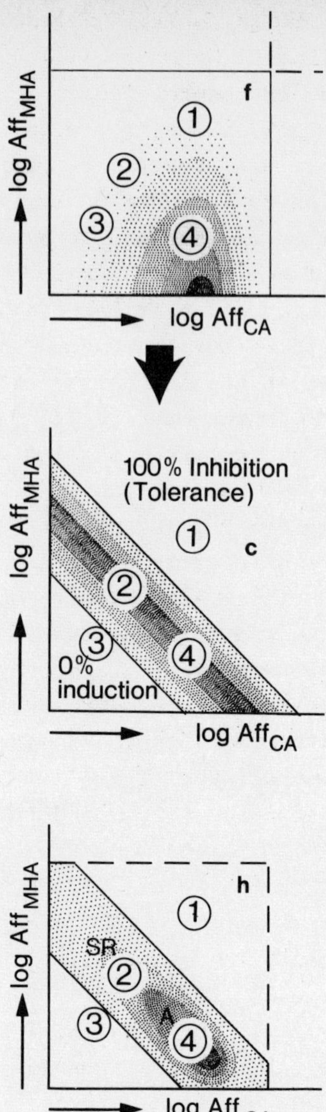

Legend to Fig.2: Examples to illustrate the shaping of the T cell repertoire by the selection process illustrated in Fig.1. For details see text.

T cells are expected (according to Fig.1h) to have a relatively high affinity to a given foreign CA in one binding region and a relatively high affintiy to self-MHA in the other binding site: these are typically self-restricted cells. On the other hand, the original random repertoire is expected to contain also binding sites with relatively high affinity to foreign (allogeneic) MHA determinants. Because of the well-known crossreactivity between allelic variants of MHA, one can expect that these binding sites have low or intermediate affinity to self-MHA. The mature repertoire is expected to contain receptors with low or intermediate affinities to self-MHA in the intermediate range and lower end of the diagonal band (Fig.1h); and these receptors are expected (according to Fig.1h) to have a second binding region with intermediate or high affinity to self-CA determinants including non-polymorphic CA determinants which are also present on allogeneic cells. These receptors are, therefore, expected to have one binding region with relatively high affinity to one or another allogeneic MHA determinant and a second binding region with relatively high affinity to non-polymorphic CA determinants which are also expressed on allogeneic cells. This leads to the conclusion that alloreactive T cells use indeed both binding regions to recognize the allogeneic cells.

The degree of self-restrictedness of an immune response against a given antigen will be determined by the ratio of "self-restricted" versus "allo-restricted" cells that are activated by this antigen. The probability profile in Fig.1h makes the prediction that the degree of self-restrictedness will be different for different antigens; and it will be the lower the more the antigen under test crossreacts with self-CA.

VI. Final conclusions

There is a good chance that the T cell repertoire will eventually be described (and precursor frequencies be calculated) by a simple probability function of the affinity to self-antigens and of the concentration of these antigens on the surface of autologous antigen presenting cells. This probability function will depend firstly on the shape of the original germ line repertoire of T cell receptors and secondly, on the selection which is provided by stimulatory and inhibitory processes which operate constantly in the T cell system.

REFERENCES

1.) Lumb, J.R. (1983) Immunology Today 4, 209.

2.) Giorno, R.C. (1983) Immunol. Today 4, 336.

3.) Matis, L.A., Glimcher, L.H., Paul, W.E., and Schwartz, R.H. (1983) Proc. Natl. Acad. Sci. 80, 6019.

4.) Lamb, J.R., Skidmore, B.J., Green, N., Chiller, J.M., and Feldmann, M. (1983) J. Exp. Med. 157, 1434.

5.) Howe, M.L., Goldstein, A.L., and Battisto, J.R. (1970) Proc. Natl. Acad. Sci. 67, 613.

6.) von Boehmer, H. and Byrd, W.J. (1971) Proc. of Aust. Soc. of Med. Res. 2, 462.

7.) Kuntz, M.M., Innes, J.B., and Weksler, M.E. (1976) J. Exp. Med. 143, 1042.

8.) Battisto, J.R. and Ponzio, N.M. (1981) Progr. Allergy 28, 160.

9.) Metcalf, D. Recent results in cancer research 5, (Springer, Berlin).

10.) Metcalf, D. and Wiadrowski, M. (1966) Cancer Res. 26, 483.

11.) Milchalke, W.D., Hess, M.W., Riedwyl, H., Stoner, R.D., and Cottier, H. (1969) Blood 33, 541.

12.) Bryant, B.J. (1971) J. Immunol. 107, 1791.

13.) Shortman, K. and Jackson, H. (1974) Cell. Immunol. 12, 230.

14.) Galli, P. and Dröge, W. (1980) Eur. J. Immunol. 10, 87.

15.) Rocha, B., Freitas, A.A., and Coutinho, A.A. (1983) J. Immunol. 131, 2158.

16.) Reimann, J. and Miller, R.G. (1983) J.Exp.Med. 158, 1672.

17.) Dröge, W. (1979) Immunobiology 156, 2.

18.) Dröge, W. (1981) Cell. Immunol. 57, 251.

19.) Dröge, W. (1981) Cell. Immunol. 64, 381.

20.) Allison, J.P., Mcintyre, B.W., and Bloch, D. (1982) J.Immunol. 129, 2293.

21.) Meuer, S.C., Fitzgerald, K.A., Hussey, R.E., Hodgdon, J.C., Schlossman, S.F., and Reinherz, E.L. (1983) J. Exp. Med. 157, 705.

22.) Haskins, K., Kubo, R. White, J., Pigeon, M., Kappler, J., and Marrack, P. (1983) J. Exp. Med. 157, 1149.

23.) Marrack, P., Hannum, C., Harris, M., Haskins, K., Kubo, R., Pigeon, M., Shimonkevitz, R., White, J., and Kappler, J. (1983) Immunol. Rev. 76, 131.

24.) Acuto, O., Meuer, S.C., Hodgdon, J.C., Schlossman, S.F., and Reinherz, E.L. (1983) J. Exp. Med. 158, 1368.

25.) Zinkernagel, R.M. (1978) Immunol. Rev. 42, 224.

26.) Groves, E.S. and Singer, A. (1983) J. Exp. Med. 158, 1483.

27.) Von Boehmer, H., Hudson, L., and Sprent, J. (1975) J. Exp. Med. 142, 989.

28.) Von Boehmer, H., and Sprent, J. (1976) Transplant. Rev. 29, 3.

29.) Zinkernagel, R.M., Callahan, G.N., Althage, A., Cooper, S., Klein, P.A., and Klein, J. (1978) J. Exp. Med. 147, 882.

30.) Bevan, M.J. (1977) Nature (London) 269, 417.

31.) Bevan, M.J. and Fink, P.J. (1978) Immunol. Rev. 42, 3.

32.) Katz, D.H. (1977) Cold Spring Harbor Symp. Quant. Biol. 41, 611.

33.) Sprent, J. (1978) Immunol. Rev. 42, 108.

34.) Waldmann, H. (1978) Immunol. Rev. 42, 202.

35.) Kruisbeek, A.M., Sharrow, S.O., and Singer, A. (1983) J. Immunol. 130, 1027.

36.) Good, M.F. and Nossal, G.J. (1983) Proc. Natl. Acad. Sci. 80,1693.

37.) Cohn, M. and Epstein, R. (1978) Cell. Immunol. 39, 125.

38.) Finberg, R., Burakoff, S.J., Cantor, H., and Benacerraf, B. (1978) Proc. Natl. Acad. Sci. 75, 5145.

39.) Levy, R.B., Gilheany, P.E., and Shearer, G.M. (1980) J. Exp. Med. 152, 405.

40.) Ben-Nun, A., Lando, Z., Dorf, M.E., and Burakoff, S.J. (1983) J. Exp. Med. 157, 2147.

MATHEMATICAL MODELLING OF THE IMMUNE RESPONSE: A MODEL OF THE PROLIFERATION CONTROL

Daniela Přikrylová
Institute of Microbiology, Czechoslovak Academy of Sciences
142 20 Prague 4, Czechoslovakia

The successful immune response to given antigen is manifested by elim- ination of antigen; generation of antibody forming cells and production o antibody (if humoral response) or cytotoxic cells (if cellular immunity) and generation of memory cells. Memory cells remain in the organism afte primary response, and they prove that the secondary response is more effi- cient. Such a process is the result of an intricate interaction within th multicomponent immune system. Although at the present time all major compo nents (cell populations) which take part in the immune response are prob ably known, the question how these components interact during the cours of the immune response has not been solved satisfactorily yet. In ou model we have tried to formulate the relations between cell population taking part in the immune response, which seemed to be substantial for it proper function.

The models which have been constructed in our department are base upon the assumption of two differentiation stages of cells (Sercarz an Coons 1962, Šterzl 1962). After first antigenic stimulus the immunocom petent cell is changed into an immunologically activated cell. This ac tivated cell is changed into a plasma cell forming antibody against give antigen if challenged with antigen again, or proliferates and after prolif eration it changes into a memory cell which is different from the immuno competent cell.

These models (Jílek and Šterzl 1970, 1971, 1973, Jílek and Klei 1979, Klein et al. 1980, 1982, Přikrylová et al. 1984) were constructe for antigens which are rapidly metabolized (e. g., sheep red blood cells where the binding of antigen with antibody during the primary respons is negligible, and the description of behaviour of the antigen by expo nential function suits well. These models involved the assumption tha the proliferation of immunologically activated cells stops after certai number of generations (Jílek and Šterzl 1970, 1971, 1973, Jílek and Klein 1979) or that the generation time extends (Klein et al. 1980, 1982).

In our present model the control of proliferation activity during the course of immune response is involved (the previous models are extended to include the population of T helper cells - growth factor producers). In this model the interaction between T cell and B cell subsets is mediated by a growth factor, and the presence of the growth factor (which is produced in the presence of a satisfactory antigen concentration) is necessary for proliferation of participating cells.

To extend the model to include other kinds of antigen than are rapidly eliminated (as assumed formerly) it was necessary to include the assumption of participation of antibody in the elimination of the antigen during the course of the immune response. The logical correctness of arrangement of such a complex model was tested by the method of kinetic logic (Přikrylová and Kůrka 1984) showing possible transition and final states of the system.

Mathematical model

The model is based on the following assumptions:

1) Cells:

Macrophages (Mf) - remain constant, produce IL 1 after antigenic stimulation.

T helpers - enter the system as H_x precursors, after antigenic stimulus they change into H_a sensitive to the second signal (IL 1, GF). GF (growth factor) effects a change of H_a into the proliferating H_y, while IL 1 effects a direct change of H_a into H_z; H_y after repeated antigenic signal become H_z producing GF.

B cells enter the system as precursors X, after antigenic stimulation they become A sensitive to the second signal (GF), thus changing into proliferating Y, which after repeated antigenic signal change into Ab producing Z cells. Without meeting the antigen again, and in absence of sufficient amount of GF, Y cells become memory cells M.

2) Signals:

Antigen (Ag)

a) external information labeling the cell which take part in immune response;

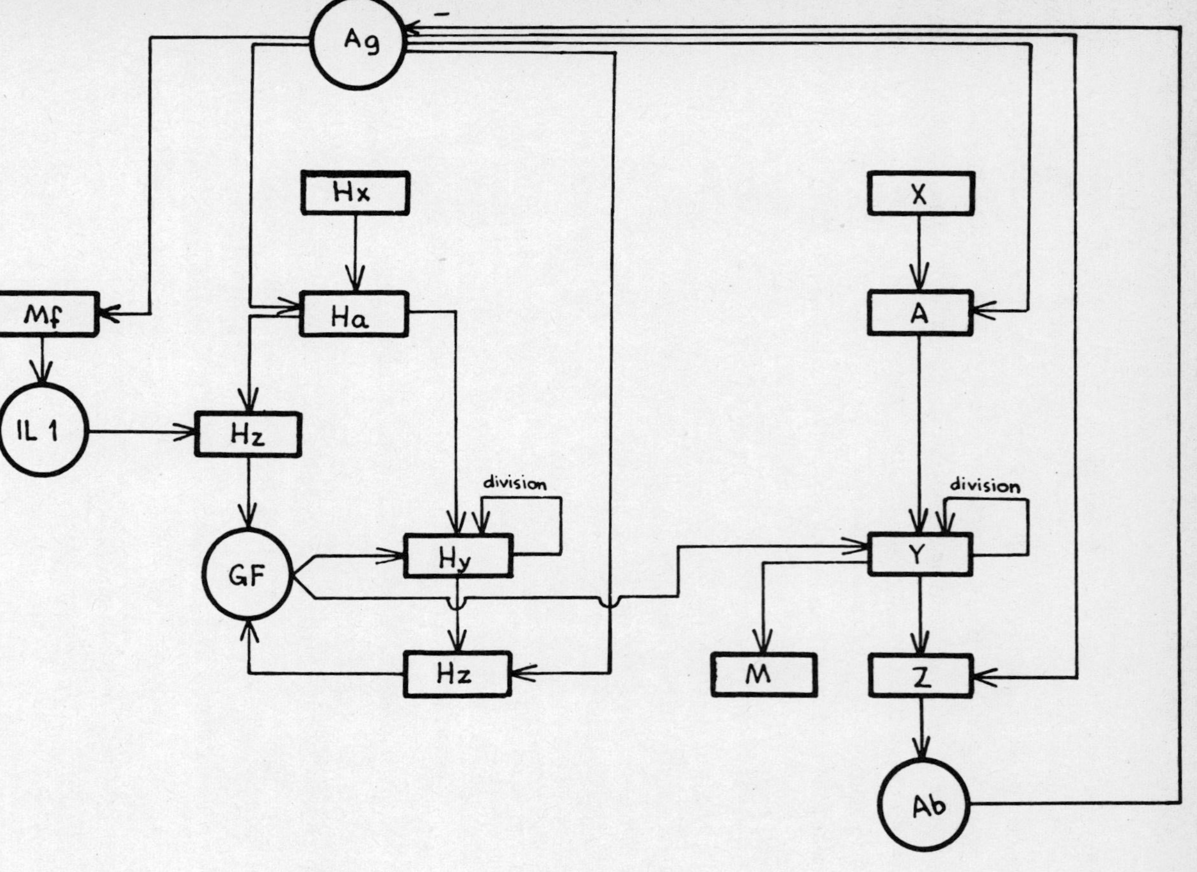

Fig. 1. Block diagram of the interactions during immune response.

ii) signal to the final differentiation (after proliferation and decrease of GF concentration).

IL 1 - initiates the lymphocyte response via stimulation of H_x to become H_z and to produce GF.

GF - signal for H_y and Y to proliferate.

Antibody (Ab) - participate in elimination of the antigen.

The control of the immune response depends on the absolute amounts of elements engaged in it (i. e., cells, antigen, cell products) as well as on their interrelations.

To model decision steps we have used particular switching functions.

Differential equations

$$H_x' = l_x - H_x(f_x + l_x/H_{x0})$$
$$H_a' = H_x f_x - H_a f_a$$
$$H_y' = H_a f_a f_g + H_y[(l_y f_p - m_y) - f_y(1 - f_p)]$$
$$H_z' = H_a f_a(1 - f_g) + H_y f_y(1 - f_p) - m_z H_z$$
$$X' = l_x - X(f_x + l_x/X_0)$$
$$Y' = X f_x + Y[(l_y f_p - m_y) - (1 - f_p)]$$
$$Z' = (Y + M) f_y(1 - f_p) - m_z Z$$
$$M' = Y(1 - f_y)(1 - f_p) + M[(l_y f_p - m_m) - f_y(1 - f_p)]$$
$$(IL1)' = l_i f_s - (m_i H_a + m_{if})IL1$$
$$(GF)' = l_f H_z - [m_f(H_a + H_y + Y + M) + m_{if}]GF$$
$$(Ag)' = (l_a - k m_{ab} Ab)Ag$$
$$(Ab)' = l_b Z - (m_b + m_{ab} Ag)Ab$$

Switching functions

Functions which approximate the changing probabilities of the realization of differentiation or proliferation signals were used in the standard form: $P\{Q\} = Q^2/(1 + Q^2)$. $P\{Q(t)\}dt$ is the probability that appropriate event occurs during the interval (t, t + dt).

$f_x = P\{Ag/[q_x(H_x + H_a + H_y + X + Y + M)]\}$ refers to the transition from H_x to H_y or from X to Y, respectively

$f_y = P\{Ag/[q_y(H_x + H_a + H_y + X + Y + M)]\}$ refers to the transition from H_y to H_z or Y to Z, respectively

$f_a = P\{GF/(q_a IL1)\}$ refers to the transition from H_a to H_y under conditi that transition from H_a to H_y or H_z will be realized

$f_g = P\{[IL1 + GF)/[q_i H_a + q_g(H_a + H_y + Y + M)]\}$ refers to the transitio from H_a to H_y or H_z

$f_p = P\{GF/[q_p \max(c, Ag)(H_a + H_y + Y + M)]\}$ refers to the proliferating fraction of appropriate cells

$f_s = P\{Ag/[q_s(H_x + H_a + X + Y + M)]\}$ refers to the production of IL1 by macrophages

Parameters

l_x... rate of precursors supply, l_y, l_a (>0)... proliferation rates, l_i l_f, l_b... rates of production, m_y, m_z, m_m... death rates, m_i, m_f, m_{ab}, k... binding rates, m_{if}, m_b, l_a (<0)... decay rates, q_x, q_y, q_a, q_g, q_i q_p, q_s, c... parameters of switching functions where q_x represents effi ciency of Ag presentation, q_y, q_s represent efficiency of Ag signal, q_a q_g, q_i represent sensitivity to signals, q_p represents relation between GF and Ag.

Estimation of parameter values

l_x, l_y, l_b, m_y, m_z, m_m, m_b were chosen on the basis of experimental fir ings from the literature; l_i, l_f, m_i, m_f, m_{if} were extrapolated from ou experiments; l_a, m_{ab}, k were tested within the broad spectra of values, and q_x, q_y, q_s, q_a, q_g, q_i, q_p were set during simulation runs.

Examples

The course of the primary response as well as that of the secondary response was simulated by the numerical integration of the system of differential equations. An example of computer simulation result is giver in Fig. 2. In this example following parameter values were used:

$l_x = m_y = q_x = q_y = 0.001$, $l_y = 0.05$, $l_b = 0.002$, $m_z = 0.02$, $m_m = 2\text{x}10^{-}$ $m_b = 0.005$, $l_i = 0.09$, $l_f = q_a = q_g = q_i = 0.1$, $m_i = m_f = 0.07$, $m_{if} =$ $= 0.007$, $l_a = -0.002$, $m_{ab} = 0.9$, $k = 2$, $q_s = 1\text{x}10^{-4}$, $q_p = c = 0.01$.

Initial values: $Ag = H_x = X = 1$, $H_a = H_y = H_z = Y = Z = M = IL1 = GF =$ $= Ab = 0$. All rate constants are related to used time scale and hav dimension h^{-1}.

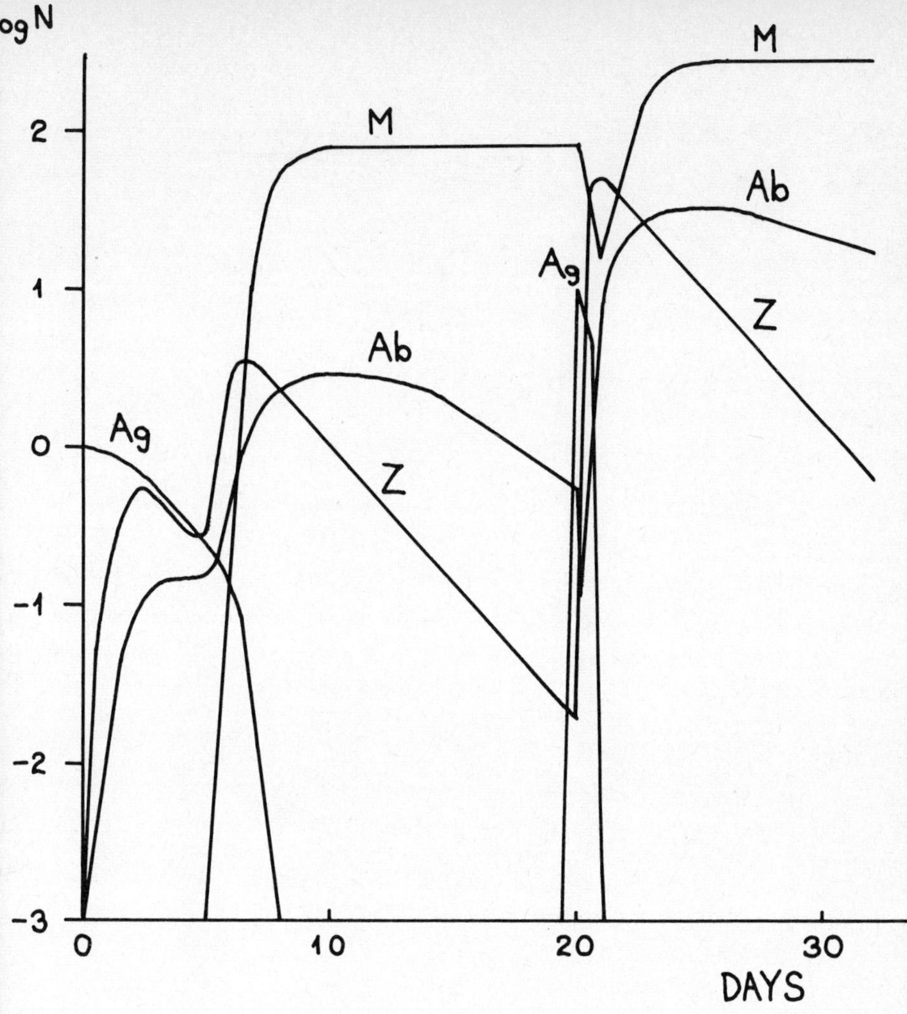

ig. 2. Primary and secondary responses. The simulated course of the number f antibody forming cells (Z), memory cells (M), amount (in arbitrary nits) of antigen (Ag) and antibody (Ab).

Another manifestation of the immune system is immunological toler-nce. Because the tolerance could be proved either by different mechan-sm than the immune response (e. g., suppression) or by the same arrange-ent but in particular conditions, we have tried whether it is possible o simulate tolerance in our model of the course of immune response. The esults are given in Fig. 3 (low dose tolerance) and Fig. 4 (high dose olerance).

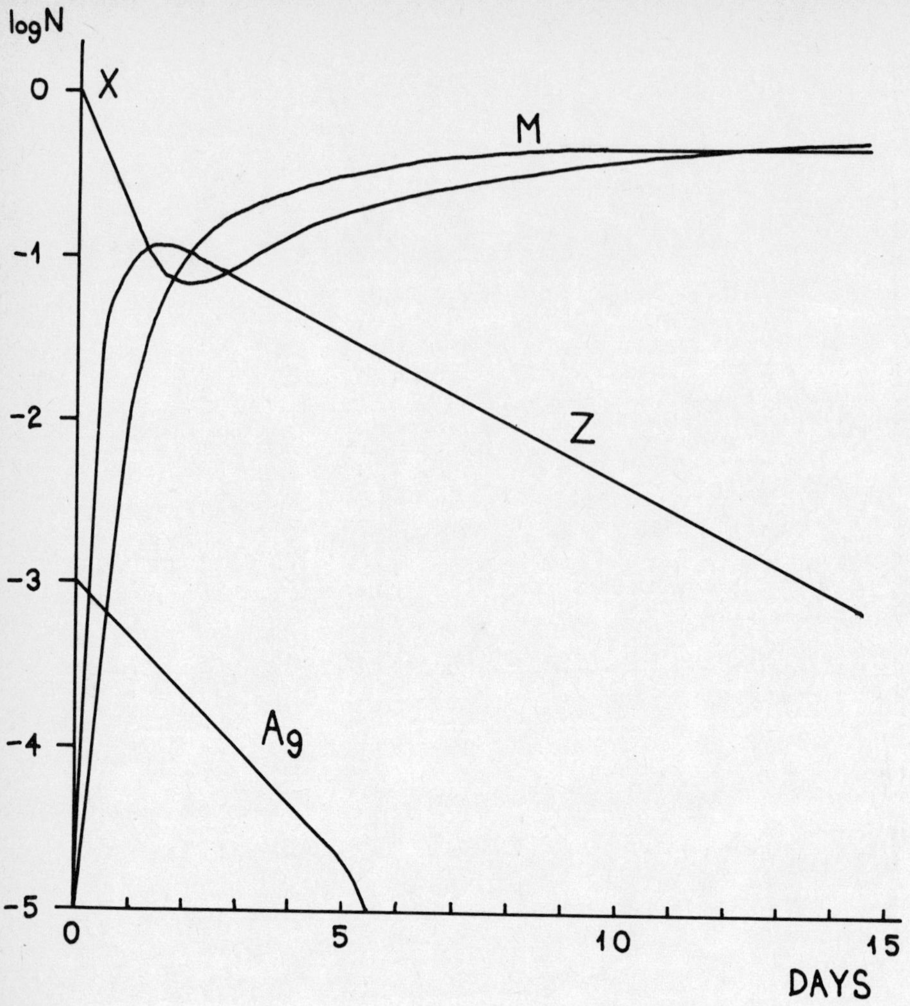

Fig. 3. Low dose tolerance. The simulated course of the number of precursors (X), antibody forming cells (Z), memory cells (M), and amount (in arbitrary units) of antigen (Ag_0 = 0.001; l_a = -0.005).

The results of computer simulation of this model indicate agreement with the present knowledge of the course of immune response. In a wide range of sets of parameters, during simulated immune response the antigen is eliminated, antibody forming cells and antibody are raised, and after primary response the memory cells remain in the system; the maximum of the secondary response is higher and is reached earlier than the maximum

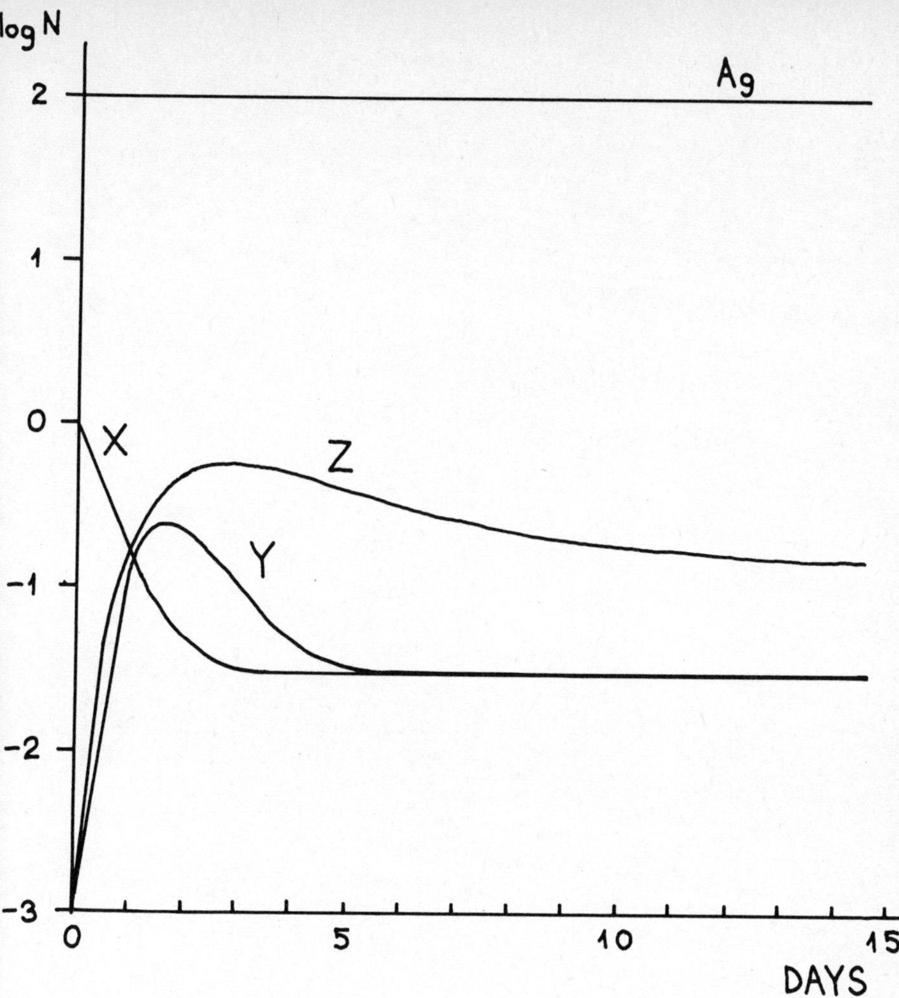

Fig. 4. High dose tolerance. The simulated course of the number of precursors (X), proliferating cells (Y), antibody forming cells (Z), and amount (in arbitrary units) of antigen (Ag_0 = 200; l_a = 0).

of the primary response. Furthermore, this mathematical model allows us to simulate low dose as well as high dose tolerance. These results indicate that special mechanisms (e. g., suppression mediated by suppressor cells) need not be the determining factor in immunological tolerance. (Similar conclusion results from the work of De Boer et al. 1985).

This model could serve, e. g., for testing the mode of influence an individual component might exert on other elements of the system as well as for desining experiments which could elucidate these interrelationships.

References

De Boer, R.J., Hogeweg, P., Dullens, H.F., De Weger, R.A., Den Otter, W.: J. Immunol. 134, 1985, 2748-2758

Jílek, M., Klein, P., in: Modelling and Optimization of Complex Systems. Springer-Verlag, Berlin 1979, 15-25

Jílek, M., Šterzl, J., in Developmental Aspects of Antibody Formation and Structure. Academia, Prague 1970, 963-981

Jílek, M., Šterzl, J., in: Morphological and Functional Aspects of Immunity. Plenum Publishing Comp., New York 1971, 333-349

Jílek, M., Šterzl, J., in: Trans. 6th Prague Conf. Information Theory, Statistical Decision Functions, Random Processes. Academia, Prague 1973, 275-289

Klein, P., Doležal, J., Šterzl, J., in: Optimization Techniques 1. Springer-Verlag, Berlin 1980, 535-545

Klein, P., Doležal, J., Šterzl, J.: J. Math. Biol. 13, 1981, 67-80

Přikrylová, D., Jílek, M., Doležal, J.: Kybernetika 20, 1984, 37-46

Přikrylová, D., Kůrka, P., in: Simulation of Systems in Biology and Medicine. ČSVTS, Prague 1984, 725/1-5

Sercarz, E., Coons, A.H., in: Mechanisms of Immunological Tolerance. Academia, Prague 1962, 73-83

Šterzl, J., in: Advances in Biological Science. Academia, Prague 1962, 149-173

FURTHER DEVELOPMENT OF THE MATHEMATICAL MODEL OF IMMUNOLOGICAL TOLERANCE

T. Hraba and J. Doležal

Institute of Molecular Genetics
Czechoslovak Academy of Sciences
142 20 Prague, Czechoslovakia

and

Institute of Information Theory and Automation
Czechoslovak Academy of Sciences
182 08 Prague, Czechoslovakia

1. Experimental Background and the First Mathematical Model

Our mathematical model of immunological tolerance to human serum albumin (HSA) in chickens [1, 2] was formulated on experimental evidence suggesting that the major mechanism underlying the inhibition of anti-HSA antibody production in tolerant chickens was B cell tolerance [3, 4]. The relevant experiments were carried out in chickens of homogeneous inbred lines and that made possible lymphoid cell transfers among the syngeneic experimental birds. The existence of suppressor cells induced in tolerant chickens was not proved by these cell transfers. This finding suggested a direct inhibition of immunocompetent cells (ICC) by the tolerizing administration of antigen. The inhibition was apparently irreversible, as escape from tolerance was not observed in the spleen cells of tolerant birds transferred to non-reactive recipients. In contrast to the situation in mammals tolerant to xenogeneic serum proteins, neonatal thymectomy did not detectably influence tolerance to HSA in chickens. On the other side, neonatal bursectomy increased and prolonged substantially the tolerance in chickens. From these and other findings we concluded that T cells do not play any substantial role in this tolerant state and that the major mechanism operating there is clonal deletion or irreversible inactivation of B lymphocytes.

The basic assumption for our mathematical model was that HSA injected early after hatching induced an irreversible inhibition of B cells and that the escape from tolerance was due to the spontaneous, antigen-independent maturation of new B lymphocytes from stem cells. However, the escape from tolerance calculated according to this mathematical model was much faster than the escape observed experimentally. At the time, when our mathematical model was formulated, we observed that anti-HSA antibody production induced in tolerant chickens by a cross-reactive antigen (bovine serum albumin - BSA) was much more intensive than after challenge with the tolerated antigen. The rate of the faster recovery from tolerance observed after BSA challenge agreed well with the calculated data. This finding suggested that also in chickens, the kinetics of B cell tolerance can be detected by immunization with cross-reactive antigens. There were a reasonable agreement between the calculated values of the duration of tolerance induced in chickens by different doses of HSA and the anti-HSA antibody production induced by BSA challenge in experiments carried out according to these predictions [5]. We also compared experimental data of other research groups on B cell tolerance kinetics in adult mice with the rates of recovery from tolerance calculated according to our model and we observed a good correspondence between them [6, 7].

2. Prevous Attempts to Improve the Model

Our experimental evidence did not support the T cell involvement in tolerance to HSA in chickens and it did not seem probable that some mechanism at the level of individual B cells could account for the different anti-HSA antibody production in tolerant chickens after challenge with HSA or BSA. Therefore, we suggested as possible explanation of this situation either interaction between B cells and macrophages or between B cells of different specifity reacting with HSA [4, 6]. However, our experimental data did not agree with the first explanation, because there was observed neither a lack of collaborative activity nor a suppressive activity of macrophages from tolerant birds. Furthermore, the rate of recovery from tolerance calculated according to our mathematical model under assumption that antibody production could occur only when two B cell clones reactive to different antigenic determinants of the tolerated antigen were present was still much faster than the recovery observed in the experiments [8]. In consequence we attempted to include T helper (T_h) cell tolerance in our mathematica model. The first version of this model was presented at the international symposium "Stromal and T Cell regulation of Haemopoietic Stem Cells" held in Moscow in March 1984, and later published in [8]. Here we present a more developed version of this model and discuss in greater detail its implications for the understanding of the mechanism(s) operating in chickens made tolerant by the injection of HSA on the day of hatching.

3. Present Modification of the Mathematical Model

In the present version of our model, two lymphocyte categories specifically reactive to HSA are considered:

(i) B lymphocytes, precursors of antibody producing cells;

(ii) T_h lymphocytes; their interaction with HSA specific B cells is considered a necessary condition of antibody production.

In both these cell categories two developmental compartments are anticipated:

i) the immature ICC compartment: I cells in the case of B lymphocytes and J cells in the case of T_h lymphocytes (immature T_h cells were not included in the previous version of our model [8]);

ii) the mature ICC compartment: X cells in the case of B, and U cells in the case of T_h cells (U cells were called Y cells in the previous version of our model).

There is ample evidence that immature B cells are more susceptible to tolerance induction than the mature ones, and a similar situation seems to exist also in T lymphocytes [9]. In our model we anticipate that the higher susceptibility of immature B and T_h cells (I and J cells) is responsible for the relatively easy induction of tolerance to HSA in newly hatched chickens. We assume that at the time of hatching only immature ICC - both B and T_h, i.e. I and J cells, are present in chickens and that mature ICC differentiate only after hatching. The presence of mature ICC, which are less susceptible to tolerance induction, is assumed to be the reason of the resistance to tolerance induction observed in older chickens. The transition from the immature to the mature cell compartment and the differentiation of immature lymphocytes from precursor cells lacking immunocompetence are spontaneous processes which are not dependent on action of antigen.

The sizes of I and X cell compartments of B cells are described by the following differential equations:

$$dI(t)/dt = t_I\,[\,I_E - I(t)] - M\,a(t)\,I(t), \tag{1}$$

$$dX(t)/dt = t_I\,I(t) - t_X\,X(t) - a(t)\,X(t), \tag{2}$$

where I(t) and X(t) are the numbers of I and X cells at time t, t_I and t_X are the rates of maturation of I into X cells and death of X cells, respectively. The quantity a(t) is the rate of irreversible inactivation of X cells by antigen and analogously Ma(t) that of I cells with $M > 1$; $a(t) = a_o \exp(-\lambda t)$, where a_o depends on the amount of antigen injected and λ is the rate constant of its non-immune elimination. From the steady-state considerations in the absence of antigen, i.e. $a_o = 0$, it simply follows that $t_I\,I_E = t_X\,X_E$ with index E denoting the steady-state values.

The following values of parameters were used during simulation runs (index 0 denotes the initial values): $I_0 = I_E = 50$, $X_0 = 0$, $X_E = 100$, $M = 5$, and $a_o = 2.4$, $\lambda = 0.72$, $t_I = 0.2$, $t_X = 0.1$ (all in days^{-1}). Denote $X_c(t)$ the number of X cells in the controls at time t, which is obtained as the solution of the model equations (1)-(2) with $a_o = 0$. Then

$$r_0(t) = 100[X(t)/X_c(t)] \tag{3}$$

is the percent measure of X cell recovery from tolerance.

The sizes of J and U cell compartments are quite analogously described by the following differential equations:

$$dJ(t)/dt = t_J\,[J_E - J(t)] - P\,a(t)\,J(t), \tag{4}$$

$$dU(t)/dt = t_J\,J(t) - t_U\,U(t) - N\,a(t)\,U(t), \tag{5}$$

where J(t) and U(t) are the numbers of J and U cells at time t, t_J and t_U are the rates of maturation of J into U cells and death of U cells, respectively. Again, in the steady-state one has $t_J\,J_E = t_U\,U_E$. Values of $J_0 = 100$, $U_0 = 0$, $U_E = 100$, $P = 50$, $N = 5$, and $t_J = 0.2$

and various t_U (both in $days^{-1}$) together with values of J_E correspond-ing to the steady state equation were used during simulation runs. The fairly high value of J_0 was assumed to describe the relatively fast maturation of T cell reactivity shortly after hatching. The percent recovery from tolerance was then measured as

$$r_1(t) = 100\,[X(t)/X_c(t)]\,[U(t)/U_c(t)], \tag{6}$$

where U_c is defined by equations (4)-(5) by setting $a_o = 0$.

Because the escape from tolerance of B cells is much faster than hat of T_h cells, the latter becomes the limiting factor in the reco-ery of immune reactivity to the tolerated antigen. When B cells scaped already from tolerance and T_h cells are not yet reactive to he tolerated antigen, the challenge of the tolerant animal with cross-reactive antigen can detect the recovered B cell reactivity. his is due to the fact that T_h cells reactive to epitopes of the ross-reactive antigen, which are different from those shared with the olerated one, can cooperate with B cells reactive to the tolerated ntigen and help them to produce antibodies.

The dynamics of tolerance computed according to the present model ere compared with the relative numbers of anti-HSA antibody forming ells in spleens of tolerant chickens challenged with HSA at the age f 2, 4, or 6 weeks. In these experiments, tolerance was induced by ne injection of 100 mg HSA administered on the day of hatching [10]. hese experimental values are compared with the computed curves of ecovery from tolerance for different T_h lifespans in Fig. 1. Curves , b, c, and d depict the r_1 time courses for U cell lifespans t_U = 0.02, 0.01, 0.007, and 0.004 ($days^{-1}$) and the corresponding values f J_E = 10, 5, 3.5, and 2. The experimental values (depicted as black ircles) agree best with the curve c for the U cell lifespan 145 days. his value, however, seems too high, especially for the young indivi-uals.

As there were described at least two types of antigen specific T_h ells collaborating with B cells in antibody production to the same ntigen [11], the mathematical model was further modified by the as-umption of the activity in anti-HSA antibody formation of two T_h cell opulations of the same size and lifespan. In this case the percent ecovery from tolerance is measured as

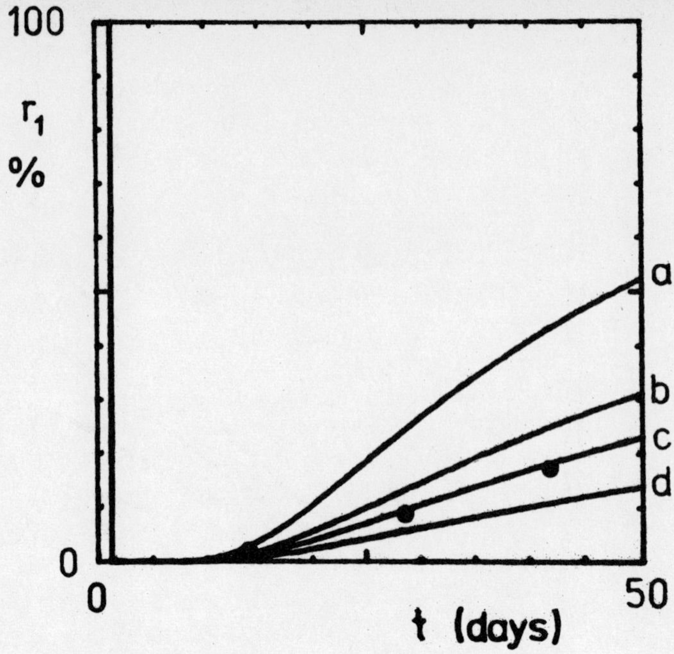

Fig. 1. Comparison of r_1 curves with experimental data

$$r_2(t) = 100\,[X(t)/X_c(t)]\,[U(t)/U_c(t)]\,[U(t)/U_c(t)]. \qquad (7)$$

The curves a, b, c, and d depicted in Fig. 2 give the r_2 time courses for U cell lifespans t_U = 0.03, 0.0225, 0.02, and 0.015 (days^{-1} and the corresponding values of J_E = 15, 11.25, 10, and 7.5. Recovery from tolerance computed according to this modification of the model was substantially slower than in the first one given by r_1. Experimental data fitted best the curve c for the U cell lifespan 45 days.

4. Discussion

There is a substantial difference between our model and most mathematical models of antibody production. These models simulate the proliferative and differentiative processes of antibody formation, they start with mature ICC, i.e. the stages corresponding to our X and U cell

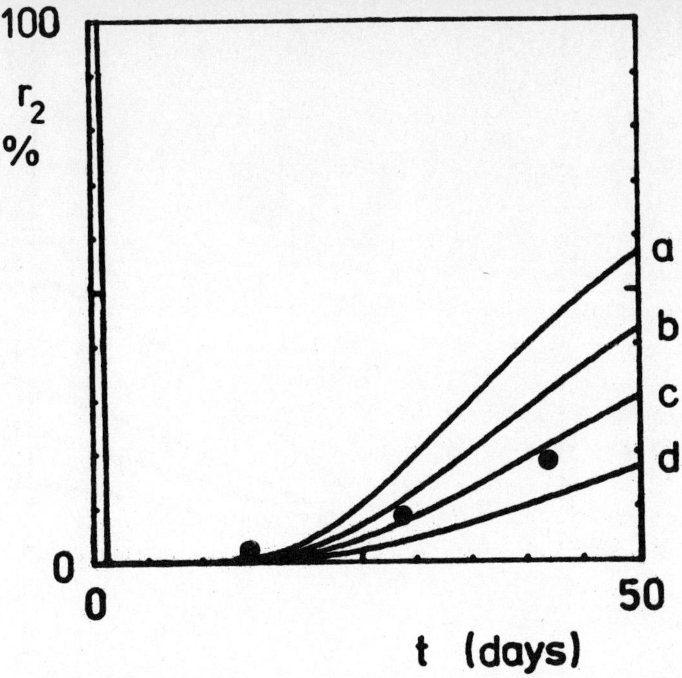

Fig. 2. Comparison of r_2 curves with experimental data

compartments, and they do not include the immature ICC and their antigen-independent maturation. Our model ends,where the models of antibody production start. It studies the recovery of immune reactivity in tolerant animals and assumes that X and U cells appearing in tolerant animals react to the tolerated antigen in the same way as the corresponding cells in normal animals do. Therefore, it is not necessary to model the process of antibody production after antigen challenge, as we can estimate from the relative intensity of antibody production in tolerant animals (compared with control animals) the relative number of mature ICC at time of challenge [7].

The advantage of our model is that it was developd in mutual interaction with experimental work. It was not only a valuable tool in the evaluation of hypotheses based on the obtained experimantal data, but it was also a source of suggestions for further experiments. The modified version, which includes T_h cells, seems to be able to explain the observed kinetics of tolerance to HSA in chickens satisfactorily, although the available data do not allow yet to choose one of the proposed situations as the probable one. This conclusion motivated us to reconsider experimental evidence for T cell involvement in antibody production to HSA in chickens and to look for some explanation of the absence of a detectable effect of thymectomy on tolerance to this antigen. Experiments are going on aimed to clarify these questions.

Our model assumes as the major mechanism of tolerance induction the direct inactivation of ICC by antigen. However, other mechanisms were observed to cause or participate in effecting the specific inhibition of immune reactions in immunological tolerance [12]. An important role seems to be played by suppressor cells. At present, there is also discussed a hypothesis attributing tolerance induction to an isolated antigen action on ICC, unaccompanied by the "second" signal, which is assumed to be interleukin-2 [13]. We intend to develop alternative models of tolerance which would include these and other possibilities.

References

[1] Klein, P., Doležal, J., Hraba, T.: Compartmental model of immunological tolerance to HSA in chickens. Folia biol. (Prague) 25: 345, 1979.

[2] Klein, P., Doležal, J., Hraba, T.: Compartmental models of immunological tolerance. Kybernetika 19: 285, 1980.

[3] Hraba, T., Karakoz, I., Madar, J.: Mechanisms of immunological tolerance to a xenogeneic serum protein in chickens. In: "Cellular and Molecular Mechanisms of Immunologic Tolerance" (Eds. T. Hraba and M. Hašek), Marcel Dekker, Inc., New York 1981, pp. 361-366.

[4] Hraba, T., Karakoz, I., Madar, J.: Immunological unresponsiveness to HSA in chickens. Ann. N.Y. Acad. Sci. 392: 47, 1982.

[5] Klein, P., Hraba, T., Doležal, J.: The use of immunological tolerance to investigate B cell replacement kinetics in chickens. J. Math. Biology 16: 131, 1983.

[6] Hraba, T., Klein, P., Doležal, J.: A simple mathematical model of immunological tolerance in chickens. In: "Mathematical Modelling in Immunology and Medicine" (Eds. G.I. Marchuk and L.N. Belykh), North-Holland Publishing Co., Amsterdam 1983, pp. 23-29.

[7] Klein, P., Hraba, T., Doležal, J.: Mathematical model of B lymphocyte replacement kinetics: its application to the recovery from tolerance in adult mice. Math.Biosci. 73: 228, 1985.

[8] Doležal, J., Hraba, T.: T helper cell inclusion into the mathematical model of immunological tolerance. Folia biol. (Prague) 30: 426, 1984.

[9] Scott, D.W.: Mechnisms in immune tolerance. CRC Crit. Rev. Immunol 5: 1, 1984.

[10] Hraba, T., Madar, J., Karakoz, I.: Antibody-producing cells in

chickens tolerant to human serum albumin. Folia biol. (Prague) 30: 281, 1984.

[11] Tada, T., Takemori, T., Okumura, K., Nonaka, M., Tokuhisa, T.: Two distinct types of helper T cells involved in the secondary antibody response. J. Exp. Med. 147: 446, 1978.

[12] Hašek, M., Hraba, T.: Active mechanisms of immunological tolerance. Survey Immunol. Res. 3: 253, 1984.

[13] Malkovský, M., Medawar, P.B.: Is immunological tolerance (non-responsiveness) a consequence of interleukin 2 deficit during the recognition of antigen? Immunology Today 5: 340, 1984.

PART III

INFECTIOUS DISEASE IMMUNITY, TUMOR IMMUNITY

MATHEMATICAL MODELLING OF INFECTIOUS DISEASES

G.I.Marchuk, A.L.Asachenkov,
L.N.Belykh and S.M.Zuev
Department of Numerical Mathematics
of the USSR Academy of Sciences
11 Gorky Str., 103905 Moscow, USSR

1. INTRODUCTION

At present the problems of immunity attract steady attention of the scientists from many countries. Such interest is not occasional. The proper functioning of the immune system is one of the necessary conditions of the viability of man. The functions of this system are numerous. It defends the organism from various infectious agents like bacteria and viruses, provides the destruction of mutant, in particular, cancer cells. Disturbances in the functioning of the immune system lead to various pathologies, for instance, the autoimmune and allergic diseases. It is also a well-known fact that immunity is one of the basic obstacles on the way of successful solution of the transplantation of the organs and tissues.

The human immune system can be represented as a collection of the lymphoid organs and tissues. With the help of the complex recognition mechanisms which distinguish "self" and "non-self" cells, the immune system produces cells and molecules that bind and destroy the "foreigner". The production of such a kind of defending cells and molecules called the immune response. In the realization of the immune response there take part at least three populations of the cells: T- and B-lymphocytes and macrophages. Each of those populations is specialized on the carrying out some particular functions.

The problems of mathematical modelling in immunology were considered at the IFIP International Conference in Würzburg, West Germany, 1977; at the Conference on Systems Theory in Immunology in Rome, Italy, 1978 at the Complex Systems Modelling Workshop in Novosibirsk, USSR, 1978; at the IFIP Conference on Optimization in Warsaw, Poland, 1979; at the conference on Mathematical Modelling in Immunology and Medicine in Moscow, USSR, 1982. All these evidently promoted the growth of popularity and prestige of this relatively new field of investigation.

Let us enumerate some problems in which, in our opinion, the international cooperation should be effective.

1. The development of the mathematical models of the immune processes various levels of detalization for more deep and more exact description of the immune and respective experimental approaches.
2. The investigation of the mathematical models for infectious diseases especially their chronic forms. Searching for more effective ways of treatment on the basis of immune processes control.
3. Detailed specification of the models of the separate parts and mechanisms of the immune response and respective experimental approaches, their comparison with experimental results and usage of these models for the design of experiments. This will economize time and materials, help to choose the most appropriate plan of the experiment and will guarantee the representativeness of the experimental data in a short time.
4. the development of methods for clinical and laboratory data processing and analysis as well as data from immunological experiment. For solution of particular problems such as evaluation of the effectiveness of the various methods of treatment, forecasting of disease dynamics. Development of the identification and parameter estimation techniques for the immunological process and infectious diseases based on the available experimental data.
5. Coordination of the efforts in the field of software development in order to save time and resources and facilitate the usage of the software for different groups of scientists.

2. INFECTIOUS DISEASE AND IMMUNE RESPONSE

In modern medical literature / 3 / the infectious disease is regarded as "mapping of interrelations between the members of biocenosis, one of which due to pathogenity mechanism is able to exist in another one, and the latter is able to contract to pathogenic action due to the defence mechanism".

It is known that it is immune system that is one of the main systems of body's defence from infection. The essense of immune response to the invasion of genetically different substances (antigen) including disease stimulants is to produce the specific material substances (antibody molecules or cell-killers) which are able to neutralize these antigens. More detailed, for antigen of given type (e.g., influenza or hepatitis viruses) in an organism there always exist so-called immunocompetent cells (small lymphocytes) which are able to recognize and react to the given antigen, this only. Thus, each concrete antigen is rigorously specific to its immunocompetent cells.

The interaction of an antigen with the receptors of such cell stimulates the latter to proliferation and differentiation. As the result, after 6-9 divisions there appears a population of plasma cells, the main function of which is to produce antibody molecules specific to the given antigen. Antibodies bind antigen that caused their formation and promote the further removing of antigen from the body.

We examined above a humoral immune response with responsibility of B-lymphocytes. The same scheme has a cellular immune response with responsibility of T-lymphocytes. Unlike humoral immune response, during cellular one there form cell-killers which are able to destroy the cells of their own organism damaged by antigen. Let us also note that T-lymphocytes can help B-lymphocytes in the development of humoral response. During infectious diseases, especially viral diseases, we can observe both forms of immune response, and what's more, antibodies neutralize antigen in blood and other liquids of organism, while killers destroy antigen in tissues of organ-target.

Thus, an infectious disease can be considered as a conflict between pathogenic antigen and immune system of an organism.

2.1. MATHEMATICAL MODEL OF INFECTIOUS DISEASE

Simplifying the above scheme of immune response, we can turn to the following system of equations which was suggested by G.I.Marchuk in 1975 / 13 / and was called the simplest mathematical model of infectious disease:

$$
\begin{aligned}
\frac{dV}{dt} &= (\beta - \gamma F)V, \\
\frac{dF}{dt} &= \rho C - \eta\gamma F, \\
\frac{dC}{dt} &= \xi(m)\alpha F(t-\tau)V(t-\tau) - \mu_c (C - C^*), \\
\frac{dm}{dt} &= \sigma V - \mu_m m,
\end{aligned}
\tag{1}
$$

with initial conditions at

$$V(0) = V^0 > 0,\ F(0) = F^0 \geqslant 0,\ C(0) = C^0 \geqslant 0,\ m(0) = m^0 \geqslant 0.$$

Here $V(t)$ - concentration (quantity) of antigen which is able to multiply and damage organ-target;

$F(t)$ - concentration (quantity) of antibodies. Antibodies are considered as material substrates of immune system (antibodies themselves, receptors of immunocompetent cells, etc.);

$C(t)$ - concentration (quantity) of plasma cells which are able to perceive antigenic stimulus and to produce antibodies in response to the latter;

$m(t)$ - relative characteristic of organ-target damage;

$\xi(m)$ - continuous non-increasing function which describes the disfunction of immune system due to considerable organ damage: $\xi(0)=1,\ 0\leq \xi(m)\leq 1,\ \xi(1)=0.$

In the frames of model (1) the disease process is described as follows. At some moment $t=t^0=0$ the initial doze of viruses penetrates into the body where it starts to multiply in the cells of organ-target and to injure the latter. Some part of viruses meets receptors of immunocompetent cells that leads to their stimulation. After time τ plasma cells appear in the organism. These cells produce antibodies which bind and neutralize viruses. If the organ was damaged seriously enough, then the total state of an organism aggravates that leads to the decreasing the effectiveness of immune response.

For the given model there have been proved the theorems of global existance and uniqueness of solution, its positive invariance. There have been also determined the conditions of asymptotic stability of stationary solutions of two types, one of which is interpreted as a healthy state of an organism, and another - as a chronic form of the disease.

The numerical experiments permitted distinguishing qualitatively different types of solutions which were interpreted as subclinical, acute with recovery, chronic and lethal forms of the disease.

The examination of the model solution properties leads to a number of biological conclusions. In particular, it occured that chronic forms of the disease appear in the process of weak stimulation of immune system, and one of the treatment methods is the disease aggravation (increase of virus concentration in an organism).The method causing such aggravation was suggested. It is injection of non-multiplying non-pathogenic antigen (biostimulant). On this basis the model of treatment was constructed / 13 /.

The different modifications of the model were used for the description of mixed infections, hypertoxic forms of disease, and temperature reaction of an organism during the immune response as well as for verifying the hypotheses for effect mechanism of stimulator of antibody production, for interpretation of clinical and laboratory data at some infectious diseases (viral hepatitis, influenza, etc.).

2.2. MATHEMATICAL MODEL OF ANTIVIRAL IMMUNE RESPONSE

Immune response to stimulants of viral infections in the organism, such as influenza, measles, poliomyelitis, viral hepatitis and others, includes two types: humoral response when the system of B-lymphocytes produces antibodies, and cellular response, when cytotoxic T-lymphocyte-effectors accumulate in the organism. It is cellular response that secures the defense of the organism. Antibodies neutralize viral particles circulating in blood but they are not capable of freeing the organism from infection since virions multiply inside the cells sensitive to the given virus. Antibodies do not penetrate inside the cells. Cytotoxic lymphocyte-effectors which have accumulated after the immune response, detect cells affected by the virus and kill them, in their role as killers of cells of the host organism. Thus antiviral immune response of the cellular type seems to be of autoimmune nature. This, however, is not to be confused with the real autoimmune reaction. The latter involves pathological reactions of the immune system against normal (unchanged) cells or normal cellular antigenic substances. By their antiviral immunity lymphocyte-killers destroy the cells of the host organism affected by the virus. Apparently, this is the only way to clean the organism from viruses.

Based on these facts and modern immunological knowledge of viral infection dynamics we distinguish the following main variables:

$V_f(t)$ - concentration of "free" viruses (viral particles freely circulating in the body) which are capable of multiplying in the cells of the organ sensitive to a given type of viruses;

$M_v(t)$ - concentration of stimulated macrophages which have interacted with free viruses;

$H_E(t)$ - concentration of T-lymphocyte-helpers, participating in a cellular type of immune response;

$E(t)$ - concentration of T-cell-effectors (killers);

$B(t)$ - concentration of immunocompetent B-lymphocytes capable of adopting the stimulation signal from stimulated macrophages and helpers (T-lymphocytes taking part in a humoral response);

$P(t)$ - concentration of plasma cells (antibody producents);

$F(t)$ - concentration of antibodies;

$C_v(t)$ - concentration of organ's cells infected with viruses;

$m(t)$ - non-functioning part of the organ damaged by viruses.

Now we introduce the following assumptions:

1. The quantities of "virgin" macrophages in the body M and of organ's cells C are considered constant and sufficiently large for the increase in stimulated macrophages M_V and in infected cells C_V to be proportional to the quantity of free viruses V_f .
2. The adoption of a stimulation signal by lymphocytes leads after a certain period of time necessary for their division and proliferation to the formation of the terminal cells' clone. To stimulate helpers a single signal from M_V is necessary and the double one (from M_V and a corresponding helper) for the stimulation of E and B cells.
3. Part of the formed clone of terminal cells can be stimulated to form a new clone under a corresponding signal. The remaining part executes other immune functions such as help at stimulation, killers' effect and antibody production.
4. The living cycle of the lymphocyte-helpers H_E and H_B is over after the interaction with lymphocytes E and B respectively (after helping E and B lymphocytes).
5. During a certain period of time infected cells C_V execute their normal function. Their death is due either to the development of irreversible viral infection or to their elimination by effectors E . The damaged mass of the organ is therefore the value of cells killed by viruses plus the value of cells killed by lymphocyte-effectors.

According to these assumptions we constructed /9/ the mathematical model of antiviral immune response which has the form:

$$dV_f/dt = \alpha_1 C_v E + \alpha_2 C_V - \alpha_3 M V_f - \alpha_4 V_f F - \alpha_5 V_f C_V ,$$

$$dM_V/dt = \alpha_6 M V_f - \alpha_7 M_V ,$$

$$dH_E/dt = \alpha_8 [\xi(m) P_1(t-\tau_H) - P_1(t)] - \alpha_9 P_2(t) - \alpha_{10} (H_E - H_E^*),$$

$$dH_B/dt = \alpha_{11} [\xi(m) P_3(t-\tau_{HB}) - P_3(t)] - \alpha_{12} P_4(t) - \alpha_{13} (H_B - H_B^*),$$

$$dE/dt = \alpha_{14} [\xi(m) \alpha_{15} P_2(t-\tau_E) - P_2(t)] - \alpha_{16} C_V E - \alpha_{17} (E - E^*), \tag{2}$$

$$dB/dt = \alpha_{18} [\xi(m) \alpha_{19} P_4(t-\tau_B) - P_4(t)] - \alpha_{20} (B - B^*),$$

$$dP/dt = \alpha_{21} [\xi(m) \alpha_{22} P_4(t-\tau_B)] - \alpha_{23} (P - P^*),$$

$$dF/dt = \alpha_{24} P - \alpha_{25} V_f F - \alpha_{26} F,$$

$$dC_v/dt = \alpha_{27} C V_f - \alpha_{28} C_v E - \alpha_{29} C_v,$$
$$dm/dt = \alpha_{30} C_v E + \alpha_{31} C_v - \alpha_{32} m,$$
$$P_1(t) = M_v H_E, \ P_2(t) = M_v H_E E, \ P_3(t) = M_v H_B, \ P_4(t) = M_v H_B B.$$

It can be easily seen that the stationary model solution corresponding to the healthy body state is the following:

$$V_f = M_v = C_v = m = 0, \quad H_E = H_E^*, \quad H_B = H_B^*,$$
$$E = E^*, \quad P = P^*, \quad B = B^*, \quad F = \alpha_{24} P^*/\alpha_{26} = F^*. \tag{3}$$

As before / 9 / we are interested in simulating the entirely natural situation - the infection of a healthy body with a small dose of free viruses V_f^0 at time $t = t^0 = 0$. This means that the system is in a stationary state (3) before infection, i.e. at $t < t^0$, but at $t = t^0$ the infection with a small dose $V_f(t^0) = V_f^0$ takes place. Other components at $t = t^0$ reserve their stationary values.

For the system (2) we have proved the theorems of global (i.e. for all $t \geq t^0$) existence of the unique solution and its non-negativity and have derived the stability condition for solution (3). A simple numerical analysis showed that this model reproduces the main forms of the disease, i.e. subclinical, acute with recovery, chronic and lethal forms. We use this model for simulating the disease course under the immunodeficiencies of different types. While the analysis of this model is not finished we are going to expand it introducing a specific organ (liver, lungs) rather than the abstract one as we have now and the local places (lymph nodes) where the immune response is developed. Thus our model will acquire the immuno-physiological meaning.

3. ESTIMATION OF THE MODEL COEFFICIENTS

Let us consider the model to be a system of ordinary differential equations

$$dx/dt = f(x(t), \alpha),$$
$$x(0) = x^0, \quad t \in [0, T]. \tag{4}$$

where $x(t) \in R^n$ is vector of state variables, $\alpha \in R^\ell$ is vector of coefficients or parameters. The peculiarity of model (4) is that it is linear with respect to α.

Let trajectory of the model variables be obtained by the experiments with animals or clinical observations. It means that there is a set of epochs of time

$$\Theta = \{ t_0, t_1, \dots, t_N \}, \quad 0 \leq t_0 < t_1 < \cdots < t_N \leq T.$$

and values of variables measured at these epochs are $X = \{ x_{t_0}, x_{t_1}, \dots, x_{t_N} \}$

If the experiment is carried out with a group of m animals, there is a group of trajectories $X_m = \{ x^i, \; i = 1, 2, \dots, m \}$ in which the trajectory $x^i = \{ x^i_{t_0}, x^i_{t_1}, \dots, x^i_{t_N} \}$ corresponds to the observation of the i-th animal. The experiments are carried out, of course, with animals of a single strain and therefore we can consider the set of trajectories X_ℓ as the result of l-times repeated experiment with one organism.

The result of experiment can be not a set of trajectories but a set of independent values of variables for $t \in \Theta$, i.e. $\hat{X} = \{ x^i_t, \; i = 1, 2, \dots, m, \; t \in \Theta \}$. This case takes place while performing the experiment in the following way. At the moment of time $t = 0$ a group of $m = \sum_{t \in \Theta} m_t$ animals receive the same quantity of antigen. At moment $t = t_0 > 0$ the model state variables on m_{t_0} animals are measured. As the animals die in consequence of the measurements, a group of $m - m_{t_0}$ survives. Then the measurements are repeated at the moments of time $t_1, t_2, \dots, t_N$.

3.1. APPLICATION OF ADJOINT EQUATIONS FOR ESTIMATING THE MODEL PARAMETERS

Let the model of the process under investigation be represented by the system of ordinary differential equations (4). Let $\bar{x} \equiv x_t(\bar{\alpha})$ denote the known solution of equation (4) with initial values $x(t^0) = x^0$. We shall call it an undisturbed solution of equation (4).

Assume that: - statistical errors in measuring have been removed and we deal with the preliminary processing data; - within the limits of the given accuracy

$$\hat{x}_t \cong x_t(\bar{\alpha} + \varepsilon \Delta \alpha), \qquad t \in \Theta,$$

where $\varepsilon > 0$ - a small parameter;

$x_t(\bar{\alpha}+\varepsilon\Delta\alpha)$ - a true or disturbed solution of equation (4) with initial values $x(t^o)=x^o$.

It is necessary to estimate model parameters so that

$$\| x_t(\bar{\alpha}+\varepsilon\Delta\alpha) - \hat{x}_t \|^2_{L_2} = \| J(\bar{\alpha}+\varepsilon\Delta\alpha)\|^2_{L_2} \to min \quad (5)$$

where

$$\| h(t) \|_{L_2} = \left(\int_0^T | h(t) |^2 dt \right)^{1/2},$$

Let us represent the disturbed solution in the following way:

$$x_t(\bar{\alpha}+\varepsilon\Delta\alpha) = x_t(\bar{\alpha}) + \varepsilon\Delta x_t(\bar{\alpha}) + \cdots \quad (6)$$

If we substitute (6) in (4), compare terms with identical degrees of the small parameter and limit oneself by the terms of only the first order we shall get:

$$d\,\delta x/dt - \frac{\partial f(\bar{x},\bar{\alpha})}{\partial x}\delta x = \frac{\partial f(\bar{x},\bar{\alpha})}{\partial \alpha}\delta\alpha, \quad (7)$$

$$\delta x(0)=0, \quad t\in[0,T], \quad \delta x \equiv \varepsilon\Delta x, \quad \delta\alpha \equiv \varepsilon\Delta\alpha.$$

The equation conjugated to (7) has the form:

$$d\,\delta y/dt + \frac{\partial f^T(\bar{x},\bar{\alpha})}{\partial x}\delta y = p(t), \quad (8)$$

$$\delta y(T) = 0.$$

The function $p(t)$ will be determined below.

Innerly multiplying (7) and (8) by δy and δx respectively, adding together and integrating the result with respect to time on $0 \le t \le T$ we obtain:

$$\langle \delta x, p \rangle = -\langle \delta y, \frac{\partial f(\bar{x},\bar{\alpha})}{\partial \alpha}\delta\alpha \rangle. \quad (9)$$

Let us choose $p(t)$ for $1 \le k \le n$ in the form of:

$$p_i(t) = \begin{cases} 0 & i \ne k, \\ \delta(t-\theta) & i = k, \quad i=1,\dots,n. \end{cases} \quad (10)$$

Then

$$\delta x_K(\theta) = -\left\langle \delta y^K, \frac{\partial f(\bar{x},\bar{\alpha})}{\partial \alpha}\delta\alpha \right\rangle = -\langle \delta\alpha, \Psi\rangle, \qquad (11)$$

where

$$\Psi = (\Psi_1, \dots, \Psi_\ell)^T,$$

$$\Psi_j = \int_0^T \sum_{i=1}^{n} \frac{\partial f_i(\bar{x},\bar{\alpha})}{\partial \alpha_j}\delta y_i^K\, dt, \quad j = 1, \dots, \ell.$$

We shall find the variation of coefficients $\delta\alpha_j$, $j = 1, \dots, \ell$ from the following condition:

$$\| \Lambda\,\delta\alpha - F \|^2 \Rightarrow min, \qquad (12)$$

where

$$F = (\delta\tilde{x}(\theta_1), \dots, \delta\tilde{x}(\theta_N))^T,$$

$$\delta\tilde{x}(\theta_r) = (\delta\tilde{x}_i(\theta_r) = x_{\theta_r}(\bar{\alpha}) - \hat{x}_{\theta_r}, \; i = 1, \dots, n, \; \theta_r \in \Theta),$$

$$\Lambda^{\theta_r} = \begin{bmatrix} \Psi_1^{1,\theta_r} & \dots & \Psi_\ell^{1,\theta_r} \\ \vdots & & \vdots \\ \Psi_1^{K,\theta_r} & \dots & \Psi_\ell^{K,\theta_r} \\ \vdots & & \\ \Psi^{n,\theta_r} & \dots & \Psi_\ell^{n,\theta_r} \end{bmatrix},$$

$$\Lambda = (\Lambda^{\theta_1}, \dots, \Lambda^{\theta_N})^T.$$

If undisturbed, real process state differs considerably from the true one, then the above algorithm could be considered as the first approximation to the solution of reverse problem. After finding the variation of coefficients $\delta\hat{\alpha}_j$, $j = 1, 2, \dots, \ell$ we can repeat the calculations having taken $\alpha_1 = \bar{\alpha} + \delta\hat{\alpha}$ as the vector of coefficients.

3.2. STOCHASTIC MODEL FOR THE DESCRIPTION OF DISTURBED MOTION

According to the idea given in section 3.1. let us consider undisturbed state to correspond to $x_t(\bar{\alpha}) \equiv x(t, \alpha)$ while the observed or disturbed one is realized in the model (4) with $\alpha = \bar{\alpha} + \delta\alpha(t)$

where $\delta\alpha(t) \equiv \delta\alpha_t \in R^l$ is a function of time. Considering i-th real trajectory we assume that

$$x_t^i = x_t(\bar{\alpha} + \delta\alpha_t^i), \quad t \in [0,T], \quad x_t^i \in R^n.$$

As $X^i = \{x_t^i, \ t \in \theta, \ i=1,2,\dots,m\}$ we consider the realization of random process given on the set θ , then the function set

$$\{\delta\alpha_t^i, \ t \in [0,T], \ i=1,2,\dots,l\}$$

is also a set of realizations of some random process $\delta\alpha$.
Thus we come to the following stochastic model for the description of disturbed state of the system:

$$dx/dt = f(x_t, \bar{\alpha} + \delta\alpha_t), \quad t \in [0,T]. \tag{13}$$

For all these let us consider, just like in section 3.1., the disturbances to be small. To underline this fact we should denote the disturbed motion as x_t^ε and rewrite the model (13) as follows:

$$dx^\varepsilon/dt = f(x_t^\varepsilon, \bar{\alpha} + \delta\alpha_t) = \varphi(\varepsilon, x_t^\varepsilon, \bar{\alpha}, \omega), \tag{14}$$

where x_0^ε is fixed, $\varepsilon > 0$ is a small parameter, $\omega \in \Omega$, Ω - a sample space of random process

$$\{x_t^\varepsilon(\omega), \ t \in [0,T], \ \omega \in \Omega\}.$$

Random disturbances in the right side of (14) we shall call small ones if with small $\varepsilon > 0$ x_t is close to $x_t(\bar{\alpha})$ with a high confidence level:

$$\lim_{\varepsilon \to 0} P\{\sup_{0 \le t \le T} |x_t^\varepsilon - x_t(\bar{\alpha})| > \delta\} = 0$$

for any $\delta > 0$.
This equality means that with small random disturbances the process (14) realizations with probability close to 1 are in the vicinity of undisturbed trajectory $x_t(\bar{\alpha})$. The equality can be interpreted as formal entry of assumption that observed trajectories have common law $x_t(\bar{\alpha})$. To construct the model (14) let us take into consideration the fact that random deviations $x_t - x_t(\bar{\alpha})$ are short-lived that means they are caused by fast random variable. Therefore in equation (13) assume

$$\delta\alpha_t = \xi_{t/\varepsilon}$$

where ξ_t is random process with values in R^l, $\varepsilon > 0$ is a small parameter. In this case

$$dx^\varepsilon/dt = f(x_t^\varepsilon, \bar{\alpha} + \xi_{t/\varepsilon}), \quad t \in [0,T]. \qquad (15)$$

Parameter ε in the right side of the model takes into account the division of variables into fast and slow. In fact, introduce a new variable

$$y_{t/\varepsilon}^\varepsilon = x_t^\varepsilon$$

to pass to a new time $s = t/\varepsilon$. Then from (15) we find that

$$dy_s^\varepsilon/dt = \varepsilon f(y_s^\varepsilon, \bar{\alpha} + \xi_s), \quad s \in [0, T/\varepsilon].$$

Multiplier ε in the right side of this system shows that the state variables are slow. The observed trajectories formerly assumed to be homogeneous. In the model (15) it means that the disturbances have unsystematic character, i.e. $\mathbf{E}\,\xi_t = 0$ for all t. Moreover, since random variable is fast let us consider that for arbitrary $T > 0$, $\delta > 0$ and $x \in R^n$ are uniformly on t

$$\lim_{\varepsilon \to 0} P\{|\int_t^{t+T} f(x, \bar{\alpha} + \xi_{s/\varepsilon})\,ds - Tf(x, \bar{\alpha})| > \delta\} = 0. \qquad (16)$$

In this case according to /18/ we can show that with $\sup_t E|f(x, \xi_t)|^2 < \infty$ for any $T > 0$, $\delta > 0$.

$$\lim_{\varepsilon \to 0} P\{\sup_{0 \le t \le T} |x_t^\varepsilon - x_t(\bar{\alpha})| > \delta\} = 0.$$

Thus, the model (15) describes small random deviations of disturbed state from undisturbed $x_t(\bar{\alpha})$.

The condition (16) is fulfilled, e.g., when at $\tau \to \infty$

$$cov\,(\xi_t, \xi_{t+\tau}) \to 0.$$

Such assumption is natural and it confirms with the fact that ξ_t is the fast variable. So, $cov\,(\xi_t, \xi_{t+\tau})$ subsides fast enough provided $\tau > T$ where T is a characteristic time of slow variable change. Strictly speaking, we can consider the process ξ_t to fulfil strong mixing condition /18/ with coefficient of mixing $\gamma(\tau)$ which subsides fast with growth of τ.

Then taking account of the assumptions concerning the right side of the model (4) and according to /18/ we can prove the following:

Theorem. Let components of vector-function $f(x, y)$ have continuous bounded through the whole space first and second partial derivatives. Assume that the random process ξ_t with values in R^l has with probability 1 the piece-wise continuous trajectories and fulfil strong mixing condition with coefficient $\gamma(\tau)$ such that

$$\int_0^\infty \tau [\gamma(\tau)]^{1/5} d\tau < \infty$$

and

$$\sup_{x,t} \mathbf{E} | f(x, \xi_t) |^3 < M < \infty .$$

Then the process

$$\zeta_t^\varepsilon = (x_t^\varepsilon - x_t(\bar{\alpha}))/\sqrt{\varepsilon}, \tag{17}$$

when $\varepsilon \to 0$ converges weakly on interval $[0, T]$ to Gaussian Markov process ζ_t^0 which satisfies the system of linear differential equations

$$d\zeta_t^0/dt = A(x_t(\bar{\alpha}), \bar{\alpha})\zeta_t^0 + \dot{w}_t^0, \quad \zeta_0^0 = 0, \tag{18}$$

where W_t^0 is Gaussian process with independent increments, zero mathematical expectation and covariance matrix K_t ,

$$K_t^{ij} = \mathrm{E}\, \omega_t^i \omega_t^j = \int_0^t Q^{ij}(x_s(\bar{\alpha}))\, ds, \tag{19}$$

$$Q^{ij}(x) = \lim_{T\to\infty} \frac{1}{T} \int_0^T\int_0^T Q_1^{ij}(x, s, t)\, ds\, dt,$$

$$Q_1^{ij}(x, s, t) = \mathbf{E} f^i(x, \xi_t) f^j(x, \xi_s), \quad i, j = 1, 2, \ldots, n,$$

$A(x, \alpha)$ is a square matrix.

$$A(x, \alpha) = (\partial f_i(x, \alpha) / \partial x_j)$$

where $f_i(x, \alpha)$ and x_j are the elements of vectors $f(x, \alpha)$ and x respectively.

Thus, assuming only division of variables in the system into fast and slaw we obtained that with essential difference of characteristic times of variable changes the process of deviations $x_t^\varepsilon - x_t(\alpha)$ can be considered as Gaussian Markov random process which satisfies equation

$$d(x_t^\varepsilon - x_t(\bar{\alpha}))/dt = A(x_t(\bar{\alpha}),\bar{\alpha})(x_t^\varepsilon - x_t(\bar{\alpha})) + \sqrt{\varepsilon}\, w_t^\circ. \quad (20)$$

Equation (20) determines correspondence between the set of real (random) trajectories of the model variables and the solution $x_t(\alpha)$. It allows to solve the problem of filtering the fast random variable ξ_t and to estimate the vector of the model parameters.

3.3. ESTIMATION OF THE MODEL PARAMETERS WITH MAXIMUM LIKELIHOOD METHOD

Using adduced results and according to /20/ let us examine the statistic estimation of the model parameters based on the principle of maximum likelihood.

So, we have the model as a system of ordinary differential equations

$$dx/dt = f(x_t, \alpha), \quad x(0) = q, \quad t \in [0,T] \quad (21)$$

where $x_t(\alpha)$ is a solution of the problem (21), $\alpha \in R^l$ is a vector of unknown parameters. The vector-function $f(x, \alpha)$ is linear with respect to α and its elements have continuous limited through the whole space first and second partial derivatives on $x \in R^n$.

As a result of experiment or clinical observations the ensemble X_m of real trajectories of the model state variables has been obtained. The ensemble X_m we consider as given on θ the set of realizations of random process $\{x_t^\varepsilon, \ t \in [0,T]\}$. It is assumed that vector $\bar{\alpha}$ exists such that

$$x_t(\bar{\alpha}) = E x_t^\varepsilon, \quad t \in [0,T].$$

The solution $x_t(\bar{\alpha})$ we consider as undisturbed motion, and the observed trajectories as the result of small random disturbances of the system (21), i.e.

$$dx^\varepsilon/dt = f(x_t^\varepsilon, \bar{\alpha} + \xi_{t/\varepsilon}), \quad x_0^\varepsilon = x_0, \quad t \in [0,T],$$

where ξ_t is random process with the values in R^l such that $\mathbf{E}\xi_t = 0$,

$$\lim_{T\to\infty} \frac{1}{T} \int_0^T\int_0^T \mathbf{E}\, \xi_t^i \xi_s^j \, ds\, dt = g^{ij},$$

where ξ_t^i is the i-th component of vector ξ_t and the values

g^{ij}, $i,j=1,2,\dots,\ell$ form a matrix of disturbances intensivities G.

Taking into account the results cited above we have the system of linear differential equations for deviation $\delta x_t = x_t^{\varepsilon} - x_t(\bar{\alpha})$:

$$d\delta x/dt = A(x_t(\bar{\alpha}),\bar{\alpha})\delta x_t + \dot{w}_t^{\circ}\sqrt{\varepsilon} \qquad (22)$$

To simplify, let us assume G to be diagonal. Then, taking into account linearity of the right side with respect to coefficients and the expression (21), we can write the model for deviations (22) as follows:

$$d\delta x/dt = A(x_t(\bar{\alpha}),\bar{\alpha})\delta x_t + B(x_t(\bar{\alpha}))\Gamma_1\dot{w}_t \qquad (23)$$

where Γ_1 is a matrix with elements $\sqrt{\varepsilon g^{ij}}$, $B(x)$ is such that

$$f(x,\alpha) = B(x)\alpha,$$

W_t is Winer process with increment covariation $I\,dt$, I - an indentity matrix.

Denote $M_t = E\delta x_t$, $R_t = \mathrm{cov}(\delta x_t, \delta x_t)$. Then using the technique cited in /11/ we can find that M_t and R_t satisfy equations:

$$dM_t/dt = A(x_t(\bar{\alpha}),\bar{\alpha})M_t,$$

$$dR_t/dt = A(x_t(\bar{\alpha}),\bar{\alpha})R_t + R_t A^T(x_t(\bar{\alpha}),\bar{\alpha}) + C(\bar{\alpha},\Gamma,t), \qquad (24)$$

where the matrix elements $C(\bar{\alpha},\Gamma,t)$ have the forms

$$C^{ij}(\alpha,\Gamma,t) = b^i(x_t(\alpha))\Gamma(b^j(x_t(\alpha)))^T, \quad \Gamma = \Gamma_1\Gamma_1$$

Here $b^i(x)$ is the i-th row of the matrix $B(x)$. To estimate the vector α and the matrix diagonal Γ at a set X_m write the density function

$$P(X_m \mid \alpha,\Gamma).$$

As the process δx_t is Markov one, then for a single trajectory we have

$$P(X_1 \mid \alpha,\Gamma) = \prod_{i=1}^{N} P(\delta x_{t_i} \mid \delta x_{t_{i-1}};\alpha,\Gamma).$$

And since we assume the trajectories to be independent, then

$$P(X_m \mid \alpha,\Gamma) = \prod_{i=1}^{m}\prod_{j=1}^{N} P(\delta x^i_{t_j} \mid \delta x^i_{t_{j-1}};\alpha,\Gamma),$$

where δx_t^i is a deviation vector of the i-th trajectory for the moment of time t. From equation (23) it follows that the conditional densities under the product sign are Gaussian ones:

$$P(\delta x^i_{t_j} \mid \delta x^i_{t_{j-1}}; \alpha, \Gamma) =$$
$$= \sqrt{(2\pi)^n \det(R_{t_j})}\, \exp\{-\tfrac{1}{2}(\delta x^i_{t_j} - M^i_{t_j})^T R^{-1}_{t_j} (\delta x^i_{t_j} - M^i_{t_j})\},$$

where $M^i_{t_j}$ and R_{t_j} are determined by equations (24) on interval $[t_{j-1}, t_j]$ with initial conditions

$$M^i_{t_{j-1}} = \delta x^i_{t_{j-1}} = x^i_{t_{j-1}} - x_{t_{j-1}}(\bar{\alpha}), \quad R_{t_{j-1}} = 0.$$

We can obtain parameters estimates from the condition minimum of the function /8/:

$$\Phi(\alpha, \Gamma) = -\ln P(X_m \mid \alpha, \Gamma).$$

If not a set of trajectories X_m is given, but a set of independent values X', then the problem becomes simple as far as for each epoch of time $t \in \theta$, M_t, R_t can be found from equations (24) at interval $[0, T]$ with initial conditions

$$M_0 = 0, \quad R_0 = 0$$

It means that $M_t = 0$ for all $t \in [0, T]$. In this case the estimates of parameters α, Γ minimize the following function

$$\tilde{\Phi}(\alpha, \Gamma) = \sum_{t \in \theta} \sum_{i=1}^{m_t} [\ln \det R_t + (x^i_t - x_t(\bar{\alpha}))^T R_t^{-1} (x^i_t - x_t(\alpha))] \qquad (25)$$

Now assume that the state variables are determined with an error, i.e. as the result of measurements we obtain a sum:

$$x_t = x^\varepsilon_t + \eta_t, \qquad t \in \theta,$$

where η_t is Gaussian white noise; $E\eta_t = 0$; $cov(\eta_t, \eta_t) = S_t$, where S_t is a diagonal matrix. In this case the matrix $R_t + S_t$ should be substituted in (25) instead of R_t. S_t can be independent on time. More often the measurements are such that the mean-square error σ^i_t of deviation of measurement of the i-th state variable constitutes several percent of the measuring value, i.e.

$$\sigma^i_t = \sqrt{s^{ii}_t} = k^i x^i_t(\bar{\alpha}), \quad i = 1, 2, \ldots, N,$$

where k^i 100% is a measurement error.

REFERENCES

1 Asachenkov A.L., Belykh L.N. Investigation of mathematical model of viral disease.- in: "Matematicheskie metody v klinicheskoi praktike". Novosibirsk, "Nauka", 1978.

2 Asachenkov A.L. The simplest model of temperature reaction influence on the immune response dynamics". - in: "Matematicheskoe modelirovanie v immunologii i meditsyne". Novosibirsk, "Nauka", 1982, p.40-44.

3 Baroyan O.V., Porter D.P. Internatinal and National Aspects of Modern Microbiology and Epidemiology.- Moscow, "Meditsyna", 1975, 520 p.

4 Marchuk G.I., Petrov R.V. Mathematical Model of Antiviral Immune response.- Moscow, Preprint of OVM AN SSSR, 1981, 22 p.

5 Marchuk G.I. Application of adjoint equations to the solutions of mathematical physics problems. - "Uspekhi mekhaniki", vol.4, No.1, 1981, p.3-27.

6 Petrov R.V. Immunology and Immunogenetics.- Moscow, "Meditsyna", 1976, 336p.

7 Balakrishnan A.V. Stochastic Differential Systems.- New York: Springer-Verlag, 1973.

8 Balakrishnan A.V. Kalman Filtering Theory.- Springer-Verlag, New York - Berlin - Heidelberg - Tokyo, 1984.

9 Belykh L.N., Zuev S.M., Marchuk G.I. On the mathematical modelling of disease.- Proc.of the IFIP TC-7 Conf. on Recent Advantages in System Modelling and Optimization, Hanoi, Vietnam, 1983, Springer-Verlag, 1983.

10 Belykh L.N. On the computational methods in disease models.- in: "Matematicheskoe modelirovanie v immunologii i meditsyne" (Eds.Marchuk G.I. and Belykh L.N.), North Holland, Amsterdam, 1983, p. 79-84.

11 Evlanov L.G., Konstantinov V.M. Systems with Random Parameters.- Moscow, "Nauka", 1976.

12 Lipster R.S., Shiryayev A.N. Statistics of Random Processes. Vols. 1 and II. New York - Heidelberg - Berlin: Springer-Verlag, 1977-78.

13 Marchuk G.I. Mathematical Models in Immunology.-Springer-Verlag, Berlin - Heidelberg - New York - Tokyo, 1983, 351 p.

14 Marchuk G.I. Methods of Computational Mathematics.- Moscow, "Nauka", 1980, 535 p.

15 Mathematical Modelling in Immunology and Medicine (Eds.Marchuk G.I.

and Belykh L.N.).- Amsterdam:North Holland Publish., 1983.

16 Mohler R.R., Kolodziej W.J. An overview of bilinear system theory and applications. Modelling and control in the biomedical sciences.- in: Lecture Notes in Biomathematics, vol.6, Berlin - Heidelberg - New York, Springer-Verlag, 1975.

17 Sage A.P., Melsa J.L. Estimation Theory with Applications to Communications and Control.- New York, McGraw Hill, 1971.

18 Venttsel A.O., Freidlin M.I. Fluctuations in Dynamical Systems by the Action of Small Random Disturbances.- Moscow, "Nauka", 1979, 424 p.

19 Zuev S.M. Statistical estimation of dynamics parameters of functional recovery process.- in: Matehmaticheskoe modelirovanie v immunologii i meditsyne", Novosibirsk, "Nauka", 1982, p. 93-100.

20 Zuev S.M. Statistical estimation of immune response mathematical model coefficients.- Proc. of the IFIP Conf.on Mathematical Modelling in Immunology and Medicine. Amsterdam: North Holland Publish., 1983.

COMPARISON OF STOCHASTIC MODELS FOR TUMOR ESCAPE

Seth Michelson
Department of Radiation Medicine and Biology Research
Rhode Island Hospital
593 Eddy Street
Providence, RI 02902 U.S.A.

In a previous presentation (Michelson, 1983), a stochastic compartment model describing antigenic modulation as an intragenerational tumor escape route was developed. In order to distinguish that model from a Darwinian selection mechanism, a second, intergenerational model has been developed.

Each model results in a single first-order, semi-linear, nonhomogeneous partial differential equation (PDE) for the time dependent bivariate probability generating function, G(s,z;t). From each PDE, two systems of ordinary differential equations (ODE's) describing the first and second order statistical moments for the random population sizes are derived.

Because of limitations in describing individual birth potentials as a time dependent deterministic function, solution of the ODE systems is hampered. A simulation system is therefore derived. The details of the system design are discussed, with the major emphasis directed toward modeling, realistically, the dynamics of cell population growth. Initial results depicting tumor growth in interferon treated melanoma patients are presented, and indicate that this simulation can effectively mimic the observed experimental data.

The theoretical aspects of the possible mechanisms for each model are discussed. The phenomena of modulatory "bounce" and early "sanctuary" are defined.

1.0 INTRODUCTION

In a classic study, Boyse and his colleagues (1967) discovered that certain antigenic structures can be modified by exposure to an active immune response *in vivo*. They experimented with congenic strains of mice, i.e., mice genetically identical except at one genetic locus. One such strain is termed TL-positive and the other is termed TL-negative, indicating the presence or absence of TL antigens on normal thymocytes and leukemia cells. Boyse was able to pass TL-positive thymocytes and leukemia cells through sensitized TL-negative hosts. The cells retrieved from the passages became "TL-negative like," i.e., the surface concentration of the TL antigen was decreased to imperceptible levels. Furthermore, the antigen was found to reappear if these cells were further passed back through their original hosts. Boyse has termed this phenomenon "modulation." The experimental results further show that the time required for the modulatory response would indicate that the mechanism is intragenerational.

In vitro experiments have been performed using T-cells as the immunogenic responders (Wolf *et al.*, 1977), and Old and colleagues (Old *et al.*, 1968) were able to induce modulation in the TL antigen system first used by Boyse by employing anti-TL antibody as the triggering agent *in vitro*.

In normal, resting cells TL antigens appear to be in an equilibrium state, undergoing metabolic turnover with a characteristic half-life (Liang and Cohen, 1977). In a series of experiments Liang and Cohen (1977) demonstrate that this half-life is significantly reduced by the presence of anti-TL antibody. They found through cytotoxicity assays, absorption assays, and immunofluorescence assays that the rate of antigen degradation increased, while the synthesis and shedding rates for the antigen remained approximately the same. Clearly, some resistance to lytic programming must exist, and this resistance may well be a characteristic of the particular cell line and a measure of line adaptability.

There is evidence that modulation acts as an active escape route in the therapeutic milieu as well. This may be especially true in the case of monoclonal antibody serotherapy (Levy and Miller, 1983). In particular, Ritz and his co-workers (1981) report on four patient histories in which monoclonal antibodies directed against common acute lymphoblastic leukemia antigen (CALLA) resulted in transitory therapeutic responses followed almost immediately by the emergence of a resistant subpopulation. The dynamics of the response preclude an intergenerational selection mechanism.

The data cited above are all indicative of intragenerational escape forms. However, other data exist that implicate an advantageous, stable genetic mutation (i.e., a Darwinian selection mechanism) as the escape route. MacDougall and his associates (1983) were able to develop an NK resistant subline of the K562 NK target cells by depleting the target population of effector-target conjugates; the resultant sublines could be cloned to establish partially resistant subclones. The resistant phenotype, which remained sensitive to antibody-complement lysis, ADCC, and effector T cells, remained NK resistant for over 1 year.

Kimber and Moore (1984) found similar results in their experiments selecting K562 targets. They observed that the cell clones maintained their resistance to NK recognition and lysis for over a full year in continuous culture. They concluded that one of two mechanisms must account for the acquired populational resistance. Either the NK cells are not able to recognize and conjugate with the surface target structures and are, therefore, unable to program the K562 target population for the lytic event, or the target cells are somehow resistant to the NK cytotoxic factors used in the programming stage. It is possible, then, for a cell to be recognized, but not programmed for either lysis or modulation. For the purposes of this research, we define "effective recognition" as the act of recognition, conjugation, and programming of target cells.

2.0 MODEL DEVELOPMENT

2.1 Assumptions

In the following theoretical development, a number of biological assumptions are made. Each of these assumptions carries with it implications for the mathematical development.

1. Each cell in the initial clone is equally nourished, and there does not exist any form of spatial hindrance to either the acquisition of nutrients or the access of immune effectors. Therefore, the lifelength, mutation rate, recognition probability, modulatory capacity, and death rate for each cell are independently and identically distributed probability distributions.

2. The lifelength of each cell is distributed in accordance with a gamma distribution (Harris, 1951).

3. The G_0 phase of the cell cycle is ignored in an initial clone and, furthermore, the recognition capacity of the immune effectors is not affected by the cycle state of the target cells.

4. The initial anti-tumor response can be described entirely as a phenomenological recognition function, representing the numbers, activity, efficiency, and specificity for target structures of the immune effector elements.

The first assumption sets the framework for the theoretical development of a stochastic model. Assumptions 2 and 3 are used in the development of a Monte Carlo simulation (Michelson, 1985). By ignoring G_0 and cycle specificity, and by assuming a gamma distribution for the lifelengths of the cells, a pipeline simulation is derived that represents both cell cycle kinetics and interactions between the targets and effector elements. The final assumption simplifies these interactions by circumventing immunologic feedback within the initial anti-tumor response.

2.2 Model Overview: Modulation

The model assumes two compartments. The first is the highly immunogenic compartment, and the second is the poorly immunogenic compartment. Cells in these compartments are considered homogeneous with respect to their target structure concentrations. They have randomly distributed lifelengths which are distributed in accordance with a gamma distribution (Harris, 1951). Cells divide and produce two daughters with the same immunogenic characteristics as the original parent.

Migration and death are specified as functions of immune recognition. However, cells may also die due to non-immune causes, and this is described by a constant hazard rate. It is assumed that these transition rates can be described as probabilities, conditioning upon the phenomenon of the immune response.

The model is presented schematically in Figure 1. Immunogenic migration is represented in the figure by α^+ and α^-. Death due to programming by the immune effectors is represented by the parameters μ^+ and μ^-. Death due to non-immunogenic hazards is represented by the parameters δ^+ and δ^-. The age dependent branching process is represented by the parameters ρ^+ and ρ^-. The hazard of immunogenic recognition is represented as the efferent interface between the immune system and the target tumor. The dashed line represents the immunologic feedback mechanism based on the afferent recognition of immunogenicity levels in the host. This section of the system dynamics is ignored (see Assumption 4 above).

2.3 Definition of Symbols and Terms: Modulation

Define:

$P_{n,m}(t)$ = Probability there are n immunogenic cells and m non-immunogenic cells at time t.

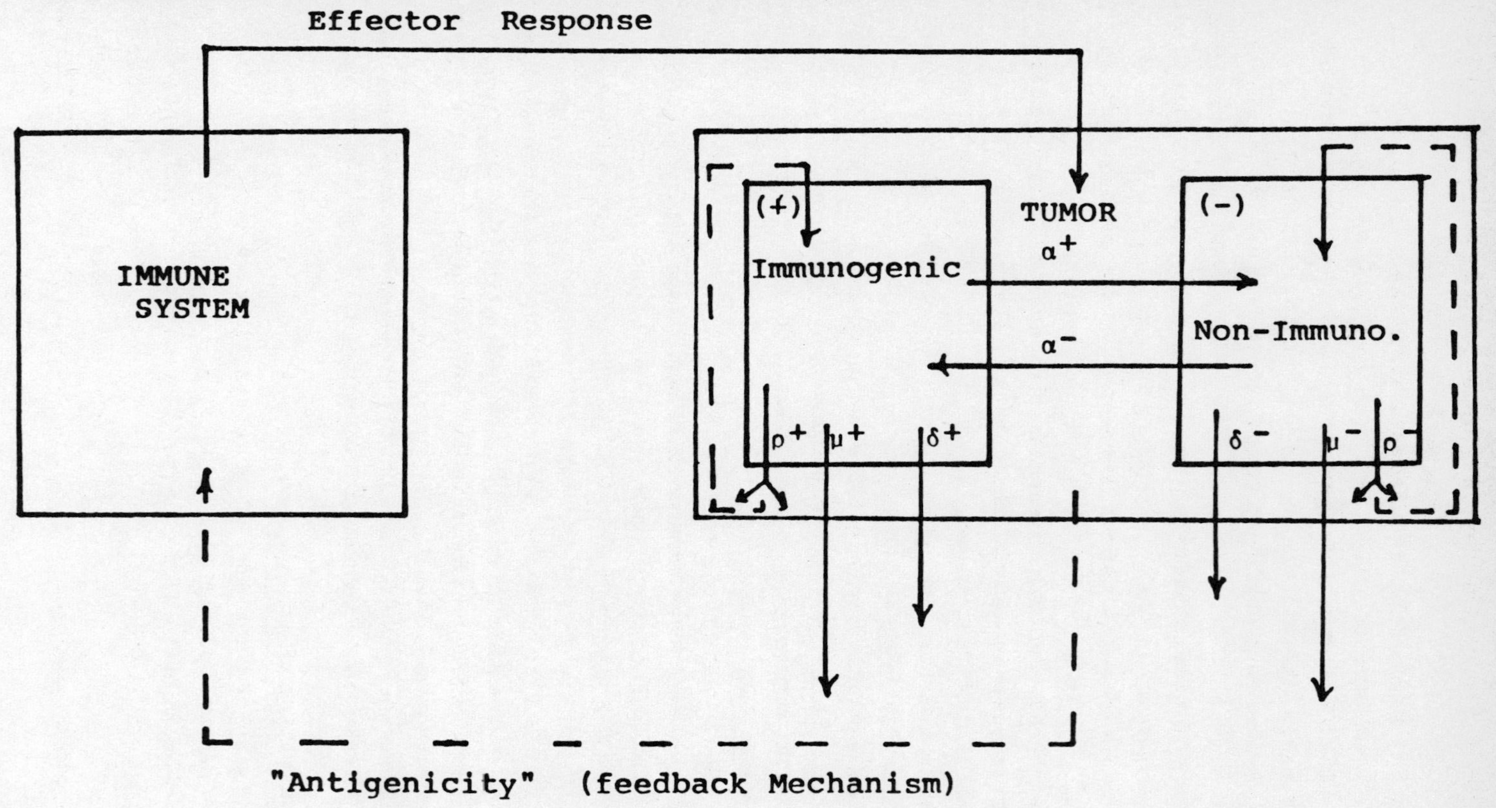

Figure 1 Modulation Model

$G(s,z;t)$ = Bivariate probability generating function for the joint populations.

$M^+(t)$ = The first factoral moment, i.e., the mean number of immunogenic cells at time t.

$M^-(t)$ = The first factorial moment, i.e., the mean number of non-immunogenic cells at time t.

$M_2^+(t)$ = The second factorial moment of the immunogenic compartment at time t.

$M_2^-(t)$ = The second factoral moment of the non-immunogenic compartment at time t.

$M_2^0(t)$ = The product moment between the two compartments at time t.

Ignoring terms of $o(\Delta t)$, the transition probabilities required for the theoretical development of this model are defined as:

$\alpha^+(t;t_0)$ t = Prob [immunogenic cell is recognized and emigrates to the non-immunogenic compartment (i.e., modulates) in the interval $(t,t + \Delta t)$ given a recognition event at time t_0].

$\mu^+(t;t_0)\Delta t$ = Prob [immunogenic cell is recognized and dies in the interval $(t,t + \Delta t)$, given a recognition event at time t_0].

$\delta^+\Delta t$ = Prob [immunogenic cell dies due to non-immunogenic causes in the interval $(t,t + \Delta t)$].

$\rho^+(t)\ \Delta t$ = Prob [immunogenic cell divides in the interval $(t,t + \Delta t)$ and produces two daughters, both of which are immunogenic].

$\alpha^-(t;t_0)\ \Delta t$ = Prob [non-immunogenic cell is not recognized and immigrates in the interval $(t,t + \Delta t)$, given a recognition event at time t_0].

$\mu^-(t;t_0)\Delta t$ = Prob [non-immunogenic cell is recognized and dies in the interval $(t,t + \Delta t)$, given a recognition event at time t_0].

$\delta^-\Delta t$ = Prob [immunogenic cell dies due to non-immunogenic causes in the interval $(t,t + \Delta t)$].

$\rho^-(t)\Delta t$ = Prob [non-immunogenic cell divides in the interval $(t,t + \Delta t)$ and produces two daughters, both of which are non-immunogenic].

2.4 Model Analysis: Modulation

The analysis of this type of model is based on the development of Kolmogorov-Chapman differential equations for the population probability function $P_{n,m}(t)$. It is similar to the analysis performed by Parasarathy and Mayilswami (1981). The birth-death approach of Kendall (1948) and Stephanopaulos and Fredrickson (1981) is used in this development, and the transition probabilities describe integer jumps in the joint population states. We assume for immunogenic cells that the probability of death due to immune recognition and programming, in a small interval $(t, t + \Delta t)$, is given by $\mu^{+}(t;t_0)\,\Delta t + o(\Delta t)$. We further assume that death due to non-immunogenic causes in the same small interval is given by $\delta^{+}\Delta t + o(\Delta t)$. We also assume that the probability of migration in a similarly small interval is given by $\alpha^{+}(t;t_0)\,\Delta t + o(\Delta t)$. The probability a cell divides in the same small interval is given by $\rho^{+}(t)\,\Delta t + o(\Delta t)$. We further assume that in a small Δt, the probability of two transitions occurring is exceedingly small, i.e., $o(\Delta t)$. We assume that similar transition probabilities exist for the non-immunogenic transitions also.

2.4.1 Typical Difference Equation

$$
\begin{aligned}
P_{n,m}(t+\Delta t) = {} & (n+1)P_{n+1,m}(t)\mu^{+}(t;t_0)\,\Delta t \;+ \\
& (n+1)P_{n+1,m-1}(t)\alpha^{+}(t;t_0)\,\Delta t \;+ \\
& (n-1)P_{n-1,m}(t)\rho^{+}(t)\,\Delta t \;+ \\
& (n+1)P_{n+1,m}(t)\delta^{+}\Delta t \;+ \\
& (m+1)P_{n,m+1}(t)\,\mu^{-}(t;t_0)\,\Delta t \;+ \\
& (m+1)P_{n-1,m+1}(t)\,\alpha^{-}(t;t_0)\,\Delta t \;+ \\
& (m-1)P_{n,m-1}(t)\rho^{-}(t)\,\Delta t \;+ \\
& (m+1)P_{n,m+1}(t)\delta^{-}\Delta t \;+ \\
& P_{n,m}(t)[1-(\,n[\,\mu^{+}(t;t_0)\;+ \\
& \alpha^{+}(t;t_0)+\rho^{+}(t)+\delta^{+}\,]\,\Delta t \;+ \\
& (\,m[\,\mu^{-}(t;t_0)\;+ \\
& \alpha^{-}(t;t_0)+\rho^{-}(t)+\delta^{-}]\,\Delta t)\,] \;+ o(\Delta t)
\end{aligned}
$$

Therefore,

$$dP_{n,m}(t)/dt = (n+1)[P_{n+1,m}(t)\ \mu^{+}(t;t_o) + P_{n+1,m}(t)\ \delta^{+} + P_{n+1,m-1}(t)\ \alpha^{+}(t;t_o)]$$
$$(n-1)P_{n-1,m}(t)\ \rho^{+}(t) + (m+1)[P_{n,m+1}(t)\ \mu^{-}(t;t_o) + P_{n,m+1}(t)\ \delta^{-} + P_{n-1,m+1}(t)\ \alpha^{-}(t;t_o)] +$$
$$(m-1)P_{n,m-1}(t)\ \rho^{-}(t) - P_{n,m}(t)[n(\mu^{+}(t;t_o) + \delta^{+} + \alpha^{+}(t;t_o) + \rho^{+}(t)) + m(\mu^{-}(t;t_o) + \delta^{-} + \alpha^{-}(t;t_o) + \rho^{-}(t))]$$

2.4.2 Bivariate Probability Generating Function (PGF)

Multiply $dP_{n,m}(t)/dt$ by the dummy variables s^n and z^m (where s and z take values between 0 and 1), and then sum the differential equations over the ranges n=0 to infinity and m=0 to infinity. If we define

$$G(s,z,t) = \sum_{o}^{\infty}\sum_{o}^{\infty} P_{n,m}(t)s^n z^m$$

we may then derive

$$\partial G(s,z,t)/\partial t = [(1-s)(\mu^{+}(t) + \delta^{+} - \rho^{+}(t)s) + (z-s)\ \alpha^{+}(t)]\ \partial G/\partial s + [(1-z)(\mu^{-}(t) + \delta^{-} - \rho^{-}(t)z) + (s-z)\ \alpha^{-}(t)]\ \partial G/\partial z.$$

It is possible from this partial differential equation to derive expressions for the first and second factorial moments in the form of ordinary differential equation systems.

2.5 Moments With Respect to Time

2.5.1 Mean

Define at s=1, z=1:

$M^{+}(t) = dG/ds$

$M^{-}(t) = dG/dz$

as the first factorial moments of the populations in the respective compartments. By definition, these are the expected values of the compartmental population sizes as functions of time. We may then derive:

$$dM^+(t)/dt = -(\mu^+(t) + \delta^+ + \alpha^+(t) - \rho^+(t))M^+(t) + \alpha^-(t)M^-(t)$$

$$dM^-(t)/dt = -(\mu^-(t) + \delta^- + \alpha^-(t) - \rho^-(t))M^-(t) + \alpha^+(t)M^+(t)$$

This forms a 2 X 2 Ordinary Differential Equation system, with the initial conditions

$M+ (0) = 1$

$M^- (0) = 0.$

These conditions correspond to the situation in which a single cell becomes malignant at an arbitrary time (which we call zero) and that it is initially immunogenic to the host.

2.5.2 Second Factorial Moments

Define at s=1 and z=1,

$$M_2^+(t) = d^2 [G(s,z,t)]/ds^2$$

$$M_2^-(t) = d^2 [G(s,z,t)]/dz^2$$

$$M_2^0(t) = d^2 [G(s,z,t)]/dsdz$$

as the second factorial moments of the two respective populations, and the product moment between the two populations.

Then it can be derived as above,

$$dM_2^+(t)/dt = \rho^+(t)M^+(t) - 2\beta^+(t)M_2^+(t) + \alpha^-(t)M_2^0(t)$$

$$dM_2^-(t)/dt = \rho^-(t)M^-(t) - 2\beta^-(t)M_2^-(t) + \alpha^+(t)M_2^0(t) \qquad (4)$$

$$dM_2^0(t)/dt = -[\beta^+(t) + \beta^-(t)]M_2^0(t) + \alpha^+(t)M_2^+(t) + \alpha^-(t)M_2^-(t)$$

where

$$\beta^+(t;t_0) = (\mu^+(t;t_0) + \delta^+ + \alpha^+(t;t_0) - \rho^+(t))$$

and similarly for $\beta^-(t;t_0)$

If we supply the initial conditions

$M_2^+ (0) = 0$

$M_2^- (0) = 0$

$M_2^0 (0) = 0$

then we have a well-defined 3 X 3 Ordinary Differential Equation System for the second factorial moments and the product moment as a function of time.

2.6 Model Overview: Darwinian Selection

If an intergenerational escape route were to exist, there must also exist some sort of mutation rate for surface target structure alteration during mitosis. The mutation rate is expressed as a probability that a cell resulting from mitosis has a different immunologic character than its parent. The change in character is assumed to be the result of some alteration in the concentration of the surface target structure. Because we assume these rates are very small, i.e., it is more likely that a cell remains like its parent than it changes, we specify these mutation rates in our model as $1 - \sigma^+$, and $1 - \sigma^-$. Here σ^+ is the probability that an immunogenic parent yields an immunogenic daughter at mitosis, and σ^- is the probability that a non-immunogenic parent yields a non-immunogenic daughter at mitosis.

The model is based upon essentially the same biological and mathematical assumptions described above. The only difference between the two models is the specification of intercompartmental communication. In this model, the only way a cell can enter the alternate compartment is if its surface structure, and hence its "immunogenicity," is altered as a result of mitosis. The essential points concerning death, immune recognition, cycle kinetics, etc., remain unchanged.

The model is then represented as in Figure 2. As described above, the interactions between the immune system and the tumor are through the effector elements of the system only. Therefore, the affector arm of the immune system is represented by a dashed line in Figure 2. Death, both from immune and non-immune causes is represented by the parameters

$\mu^+(t;t_0)$, δ^+, $\mu^-(t;t_0)$, and δ^-

as described above. Reproductive parameters $\rho^+(t)$ and $\rho^-(t)$ are also as described above. The intercompartment communications are now represented by the parameters σ^+ and σ^-.

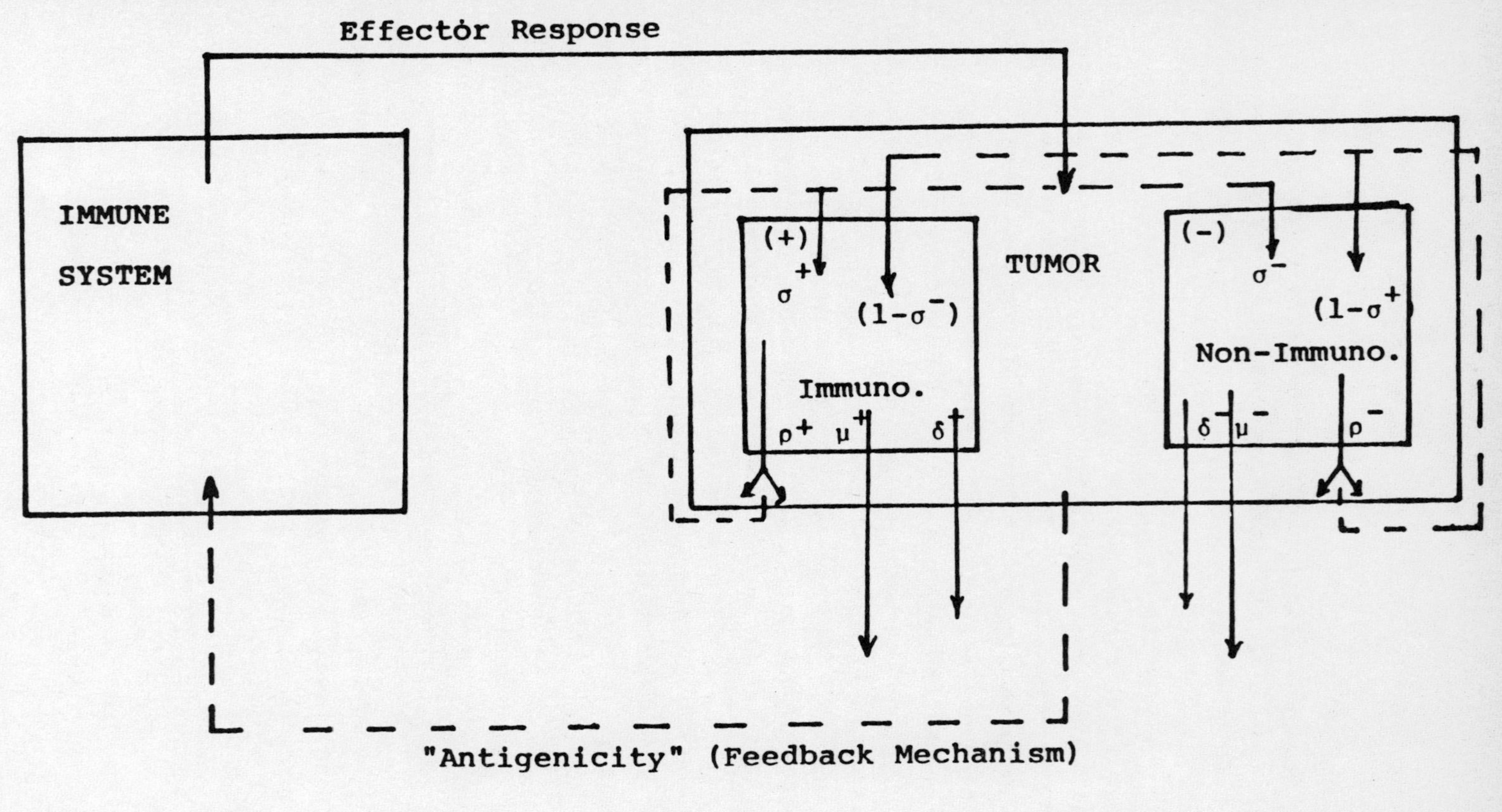

Figure 2 Darwinian Selection Model

2.7 Definition of Symbols and Terms: Darwinian Selection

To facilitate the understanding of the model and to allow for easy comparisons between the two escape routes, the mathematical notations and parameter definitions as defined above remain intact in this derivation. If we define:

$1-\sigma^+$ = Prob [dividing immunogenic cell produces one immunogenic offspring].

$1-\sigma^-$ = Prob [dividing non-immunogenic cell produces one non-immunogenic offspring].

The definitions are now complete for this derivation.

2.8 Model Analysis: Darwinian Selection

As in the previous case, the analysis of this type of model is based on the development of Kolmogorov-Chapman differential equations for the populational probability function $P_{n,m}(t)$. The same mathematical assumptions we employed above in the derivation of the intra-generational models, especially those used to define the transition probabilities, are assumed here.

2.8.1 Typical Difference Equation

$$
\begin{aligned}
P_{n,m}(t + \Delta t) \quad &= \\
&(n+1)P_{n+1,m}(t)\ \mu^+(t;t_0)\ \Delta t \quad + \\
&(n-1)P_{n-1,m}(t)\rho^+(t)(\sigma^+)^2\Delta t \quad + \\
&(n+1)P_{n+1,m}(t)\delta^+\Delta t \quad + \\
&(2n)P_{n,m-1}(t)\rho^+(t)(\sigma^+)(1 - \sigma^+)\ \Delta t \quad + \\
&(n+1)P_{n+1,m-2}(t)\rho^+(t)(1 - \sigma^+)^2\Delta t \quad + \\
&(m+1)P_{n,m+1}(t)\ \mu^-(t;t_0)\Delta t \quad + \\
&(m+1)P_{n,m+1}(t)\ \delta^-\Delta t \quad + \\
&(m-1)P_{n,m-1}(t)\rho^-(t)(\sigma^-)^2\ \Delta t \quad + \\
&(2m)P_{n-1,m}(t)\rho^-(t)(\sigma^-)(1 - \sigma^-)\ \Delta t \quad +
\end{aligned}
$$

$$(m+1)P_{n-2,m+1}(t)\rho^-(t)(1-\sigma^-)^2\Delta t \quad +$$

$$P_{n,m}(t)[1 - (n[\mu^+(t;t_0) + \rho^+(t) + \delta^+]\ \Delta t) +$$

$$(m[\mu^-(t;t_0) + \rho^-(t) + \delta^-]\ \Delta t)]$$

$$+ \quad o(\Delta t)$$

2.8.2 Bivariate Probability Generating Function (PGF)

Performing a similar analysis as that above provides us with our differential equations for each $P_{n,m}(t)$. Multiply $dP_{n,m}(t)/dt$ by the dummy variables s^n and z^m, where s and z are between 0 and 1 and, as above, derive the same double sum from n=0 to infinity and from m=0 to infinity. If we again define

$$G(s,z,t) = \sum_{0}^{\infty}\sum_{0}^{\infty} P_{n,m}(t)s^n z^m$$

we may then derive

$$\partial G(s,z,t)/\partial t \quad =$$

$$[(1-s)(\mu^+(t;t_0) + \delta^+) \quad +$$

$$\rho^+(t)(s^2(\sigma^+)^2 + 2sz(\sigma^+)(1-\sigma^+) +$$

$$z^2(1-\sigma^+)^2 \quad - s]\partial G/\partial s +$$

$$[(1-z)(\mu^-(t;t_0) + \delta^-) \quad +$$

$$\rho^-(t)(z^2(\sigma^-)^2 + 2sz(\sigma^-)(1-\sigma^-) +$$

$$s^2(1-\sigma^-)^2 \quad - z]\partial G/\partial z \ .$$

Note: $s^2(\sigma)^2 + 2sz(\sigma)(1-\sigma) + z^2(1-\sigma)^2 =$

$$(s(\sigma) + z(1-\sigma))^2$$

Therefore,

$$\partial G/\partial t = [(1-s)(\mu^{+}(t) + \delta^{+}) + \rho^{+}(t)((s(\sigma^{+}) + z(1-\sigma^{+}))^{2} - s)]\,\partial G/\partial s + [(1-z)(\mu^{-}(t) + \delta^{-}) + \rho^{-}(t)((z(\sigma^{-}) + s(1-\sigma^{-}))^{2} - z)]\,\partial G/\partial z.$$

It is possible from this partial differential equation to derive expressions for the first and second factorial moments in the form of ordinary differential equation systems for our intergenerational model.

2.9 Moments With Respect to Time

2.9.1 Mean

Define at s=1, z=1:

$M^{+}(t) = dG/ds$

$M^{-}(t) = dG/ds$

as the first factorial moments of the populations in the respective compartments. By definition, these are the expected values of the populational random variables as a function of time. Then,

$$dM^{+}(t)/dt = M^{+}(t)[-(\mu^{+}(t) + \delta^{+}) + \rho^{+}(t)(2(\sigma^{+}) - 1)] + M^{-}(t)\,2(1-\sigma^{-})\rho^{-}(t).$$

$$dM^{-}(t)/dt = M^{-}(t)[-(\mu^{-}(t) + \delta^{-}) + \rho^{-}(t)(2(\sigma^{-}) - 1)] + M^{+}(t)\,2(1-\sigma^{+})\rho^{+}(t).$$

This forms a 2 X 2 Ordinary Differential Equation system, with the initial conditions

$M^{+}(0) = 1$

$M^{-}(0) = 1$

These conditions correspond to the situation in which a single cell becomes malignant at an arbitrary time we call zero, and that it is initially immunogenic to the host.

2.9.2 Second Factorial Moments

Define at s=1 and z=1

$M_2^{+}(t) = d^2\,[G(s,z,t)]/ds^2$

$$M_2^- (t) = d^2 [G(s,z,t)]/dz^2$$

$$M_2^0 (t) = d \ [G(s,z,t)]/dsdz$$

as the second factorial moments of the two respective populations, and the product moment between the two populations.

Then it can be derived as above,

$$dM_2^+ /dt = \rho^+(t)2(\sigma^+)^2 M^+(t) + 2M_2^+ (t)[-(\mu^+(t) + \delta^+) + \rho^+(t)(2(\sigma^+) - 1)] + 4M_2^0 (t)(1 - (\sigma^-))\rho^-(t)$$

$$dM_2^- /dt = \rho^-(t)2(\sigma^-)^2 M^-(t) + 2M_2^- (t)[-(\mu^-(t) + \delta^-) + \rho^-(t)(2(\sigma^-) - 1)] + 4M_2^0 (t)(1 - (\sigma^+))\rho^+(t)$$

$$dM_2^0 (t)/dt = 2 \rho^+(t)(\sigma^+)(1 - \sigma^+)M^+(t) + 2\rho^-(t)(\sigma^-)(1 - \sigma^-)M^-(t) + 2(1 - \sigma^+) \rho^+(t)M_2^+ (t) + 2(1 - \sigma^-) \rho^-(t)M_2^- (t) + M_2^0 (t)[[-(\mu^+(t) + \delta^+) + \rho^+(t)(2(\sigma^+) - 1)] + [-(\mu^-(t) + \delta^-) + \rho^-(t)(2(\sigma^-) - 1)]]$$

If we supply the initial conditions

$$M_2^+ (0) = 0$$

$$M_2^- (0) = 0$$

$$M_2^0 (0) = 0$$

then we have a well-defined 3 X 3 Ordinary Differential Equation System for the second factorial moments and the product moment as functions of time.

2.10 Modulatory "Bounce" and Early Sanctuary

Modulation, by its very nature, is reversible. Individual cells which intragenerationally escape the anti-tumor response, will demodulate as a function of their recognition status. If a cell has been effectively recognized (i.e., been recognized, conjugated with, and programmed for modulation or lysis), it will react by either modulating or dying.

Clearly, recognition of a target cell by an immune effector is a function of the response level and the target's immunogenicity. If we assume that in the face of an overwhelming response (e.g., an *in vitro* modulation experiment), the loss of cells from the immunogenic compartment can be approximated by an exponential decay function, then, as a first approximation, we can assume that the hazard for recognition and modulation is a constant, K_1. Then, the conditional (transition) probability that a cell will be recognized and modulate, given a recognition probability, $f(t;t_0)$, is

$$K_1 f(t;t_0)\ \Delta t + o(\Delta t).$$

Similarly, a cell will begin demodulating once it has not been effectively recognized. The probability that it is not recognized is a function of the immune response levels, as well as the cell's "immunogenicity." Define the immunogenicity of any cell to be the percentage of its original surface concentration of target structures. We call that fractional scale S. If the loss of cells from the non-immunogenic compartment may also be approximated by an exponential decay function (with constant hazard rate, K_2), the probability that a cell demodulates in any small interval, Δt, is given by

$$K_2\ (1 - S\ f(t;t_0))\ \Delta t + o(\Delta t).$$

Given these expressions for the transition probabilities (see Figure 3), and assuming that immediate transitions exist between the compartments, there exists a point in time at which $f(t;t_0)$ assumes a value such that any cell which has modulated is as likely to demodulate as it is to remodulate. This value, $\hat{f}$, is given by the solution of

$$K_1 f(t;t_0)\ \Delta t + o(\Delta t) = K_2\ (1 - S\ f(t;t_0))\ \Delta t\ o(\Delta t)$$

or, ignoring terms of $o(\Delta t)$,

$$\hat{f}\ = K_2/(K_1 + S\ K_2)\ \Delta t.$$

We define modulatory "bounce" as the phenomenon of individual cells demodulating and remodulating to and from immune sanctuary. If the hazard for recognition achieves a level above $\hat{f}$, the system is said to be in a "modulatory" mode. By this we mean that on an individual level, a cell is more likely to be recognized and modulate than it is to be not recognized and demodulate. On the other hand, if the hazard of recognition does not achieve a level as great as $\hat{f}$, the system is said to be in a "demodulatory" mode.

The derivation of $\hat{f}$ has depended on the assumption that the transition from compartment to compartment is immediate, and that the cells do not traverse a spectrum of immunogenicity when demodulating. This supposition is addressed in a more complete discussion below. However, even in that more complete model, the transitioning, or "bouncing", from compartment to compartment is characteristically intragenerational. Cells escaping intergenerationally only alter their immunogenic character at mitosis; and, as discussed below, this

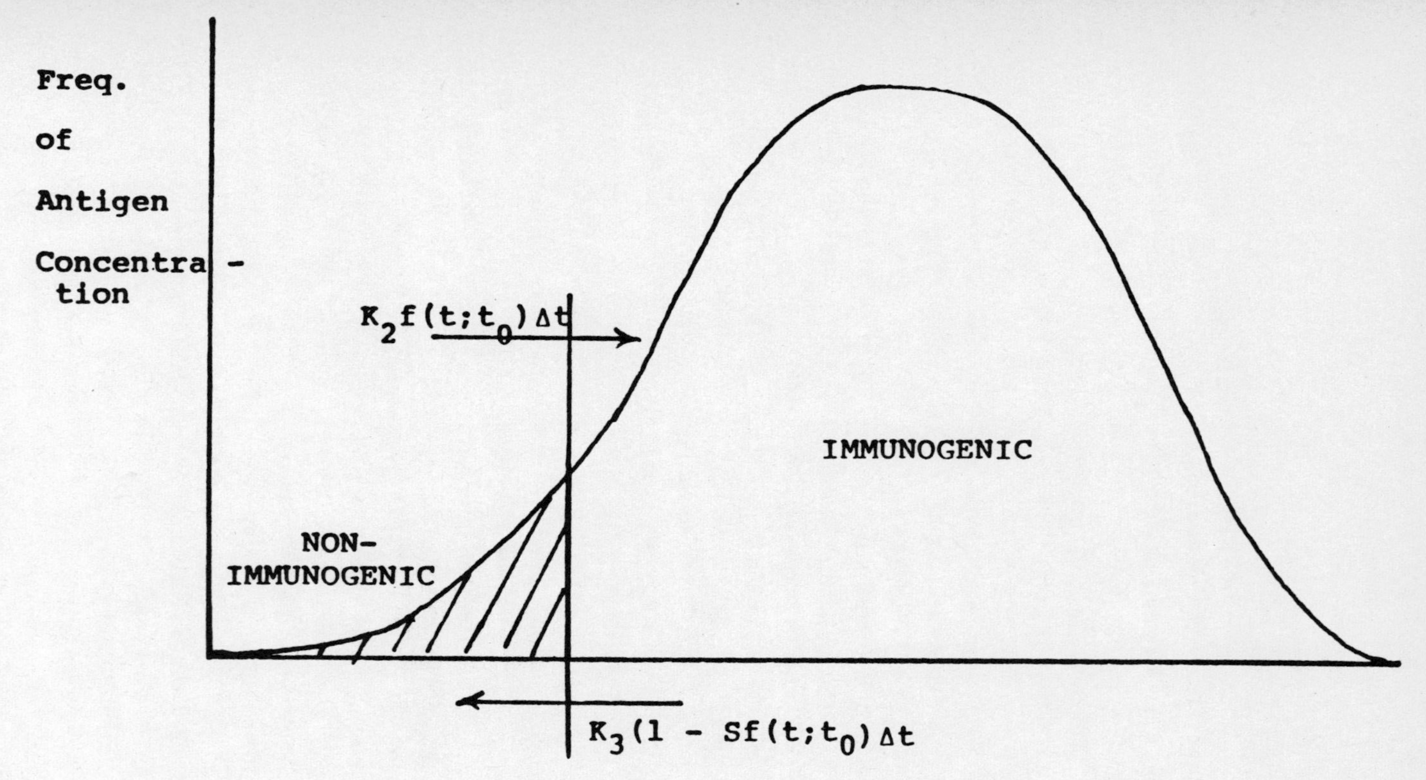

Figure 3 Stylized Distribution of Immunogenicity with Transition Probabilities for Modulation

type of transition must attain sanctuary early in the clonal evolution of the tumor.

3.0 DISCUSSION

3.1 Escape Profile

Our research has been based on two questions: How and why do tumor cells escape the immunogenic defenses in healthy animals? And, more specifically, Is there any observable difference in escaped tumors that we can exploit to give us some insight into the original escape mechanism employed by the tumor?

The early research of Boyse and his colleagues, Esmon and Little, Ritz and his co-workers, and Liang and Cohen, indicate that the modulating tumor cells, while kept under immunogenic pressures, are able to maintain their "non-immunogenic" character. As Liang and Cohen pointed out, these cells are not completely devoid of their surface (target) structures. But they do maintain surface concentrations so low that the probability of an immune effector element recognizing them as foreign is substantially decreased (i.e., they remain non-immunogenic). Fenyo and her colleagues (1968) observed in their virally induced tumors antigenic concentrations as low as 10% of normal. Young and Hakomori (1980), in their experiments, observed tumors with only 50% of the target antigen on their surfaces.

If the tumor cells escape by employing the intragenerational escape routes implicated in the Boyse type experiments, and _if_ they need escape from only an initial (i.e., primary) response wave, and _if_ the host does not mount a secondary immune response, then we may hypothesize that the initial transition to the non-immunogenic state is easily reversed when the immune response subsides. The resultant tumor, then, will emerge as an immunogenic clone. Why the host does not mount a secondary response or continue with some level of resistance in the primary response are matters for speculation beyond the scope of this research. However, if future research is pursued, these types of immune responses must be considered.

Suppose, on the other hand, that the escape route followed by the tumor is primarily intergenerational. In other words, a beneficial Darwinian style mutation occurs during some early mitosis. In our development, we have assumed that this type of mutation results in an alteration (decrease) in the concentration of the surface target structures. The result of this mutation is the development of "non-immunogenic" offspring. If we apply the same theoretical constraints to the immune response that we just mentioned, then one can expect that the initially escaping tumor cells are more likely to be non-immunogenic, and that safe and early sanctuary should result in a non-immunogenic tumor.

The details of the two escape mechanisms are discussed in greater detail below. However, it may prove instructive to study these two scenarios further.

Individual realizations from a series of simulations were plotted using the SASGRAPH facility at UCLA/OAC. Each plot is given as population size versus time. The actual population in each compartment in each realization was stored at the end of each simulated day. The results show that our simulations stopped in one of three states. The realizations either went extinct, escaped (according to our stopping rule), or the simulated time expired. The three classes are depicted throughout the plots (see Figures 4 to 15).

These curves were generated by the realizations which were generated in our simulation of interferon activation experiments conducted by Golub _et_ _al._ (1982a, 1982b). The levels of response and the dynamics of the various arms of the effector response are described elsewhere (Michelson, 1985). However, the main points for this discussion are included in the figures. Figures 4 to 9 represent intragenerational escape profiles. The tumor cells are escaping to the 10% immunogenicity level, and have an antigenic half-life of 12 hours.

In escaping populations, Figures 6 and 7 and even in populations that exceeded our simulation time limit, Figures 8 and 9, the tumors that eventually grew were immunogenic in character. The ability to "bounce" between the immunogenic and non-immunogenic compartments (see arrows on these figures) was fundamental to the escape. In populations that went extinct, Figures 4 and 5, even though transitory growth in the non-immunogenic compartment is observed, minimal modulatory "bounce" is still recognizable. Therefore, in intragenerationally escaping populations, with a single, primary, anti-tumor response wave, any tumor that does escape will eventually return to its immunogenic character. Furthermore, modulatory "bounce," while a necessary process for escape, is not a sufficient one.

Consider Figures 10 to 15. These figures represent the three classes of escape profile generated by realizations of simulations of intergenerationally escaping tumors.

In these instances, escaping populations, represented by Figures 12 and 13, result in essentially non-immunogenic tumors. The escape is facilitated by an early mutation to a non-immunogenic sanctuary.

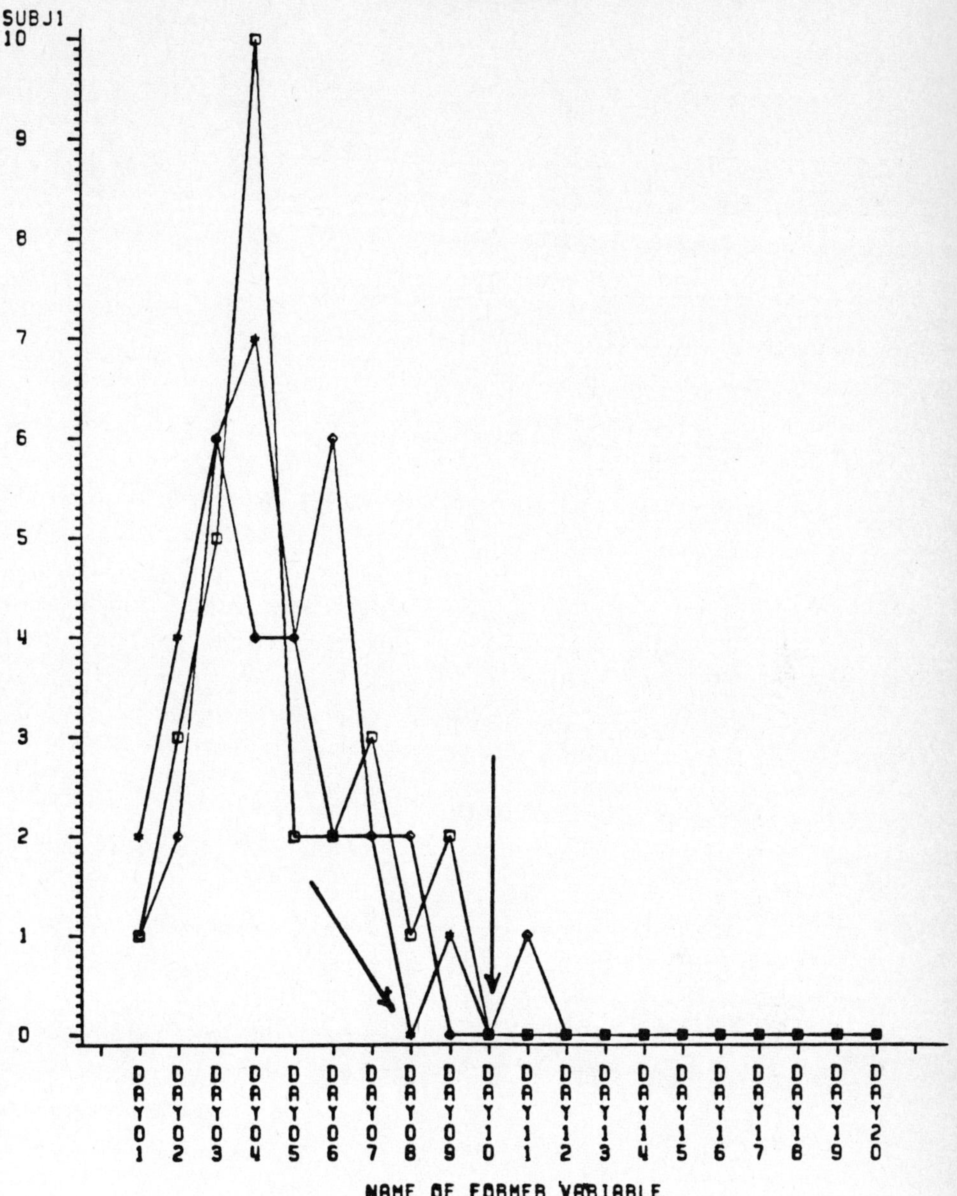
EXTINCTION -- IMMUNE COMPARTMENT
INTRAGENERATIONAL
SUBJ1
10
9
8
7
6
5
4
3
2
1
0
DAY01 DAY02 DAY03 DAY04 DAY05 DAY06 DAY07 DAY08 DAY09 DAY10 DAY11 DAY12 DAY13 DAY14 DAY15 DAY16 DAY17 DAY18 DAY19 DAY20
NAME OF FORMER VARIABLE
MODULATING (12HR HALFLIFE), ASCALE = 0.1

Figure 4

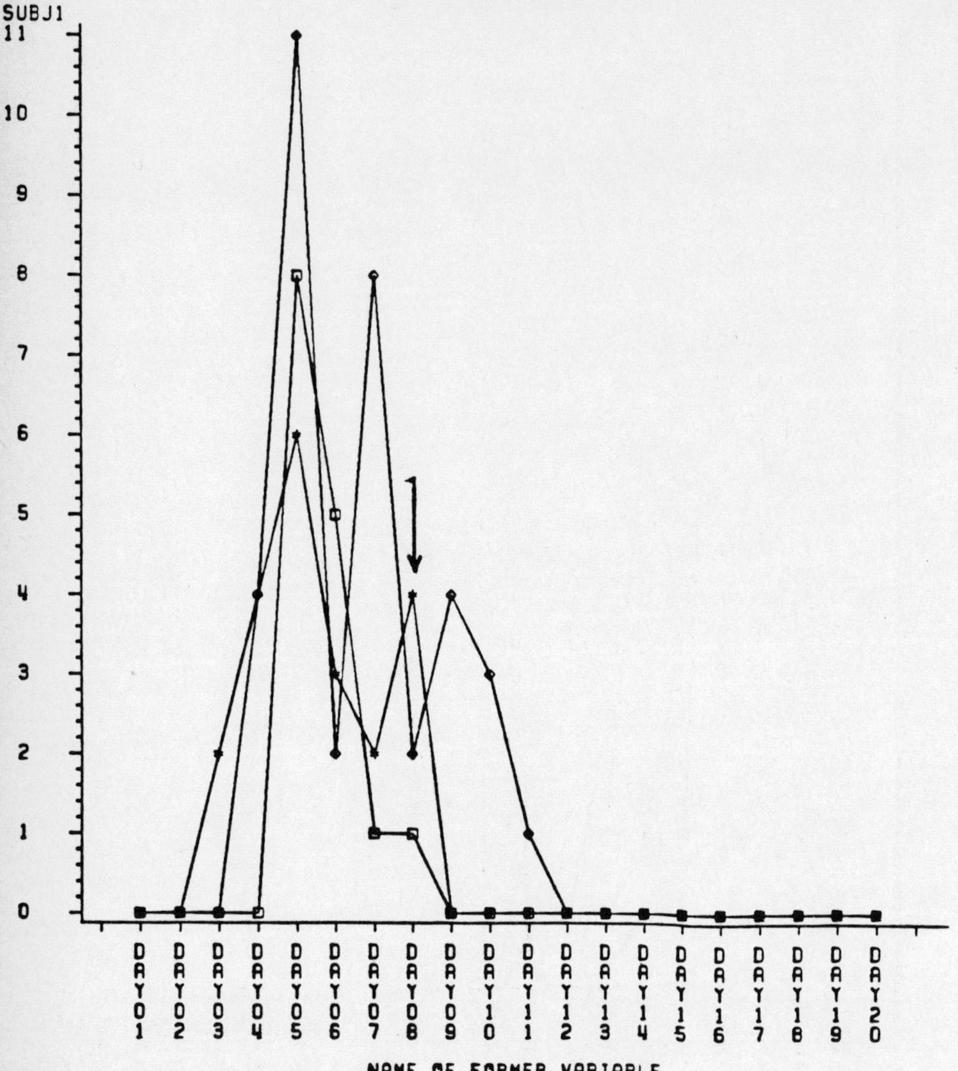
EXTINCTION -- NON-IMMUNE COMPARTMENT
INTRAGENERATIONAL
SUBJ1
11
10
9
8
7
6
5
4
3
2
1
0
DAY01
DAY02
DAY03
DAY04
DAY05
DAY06
DAY07
DAY08
DAY09
DAY10
DAY11
DAY12
DAY13
DAY14
DAY15
DAY16
DAY17
DAY18
DAY19
DAY20
NAME OF FORMER VARIABLE
MODULATING (12HR HALFLIFE), ASCALE = 0.1

Figure 5

ESCAPE -- IMMUNE COMPARTMENT

INTRAGENERATIONAL

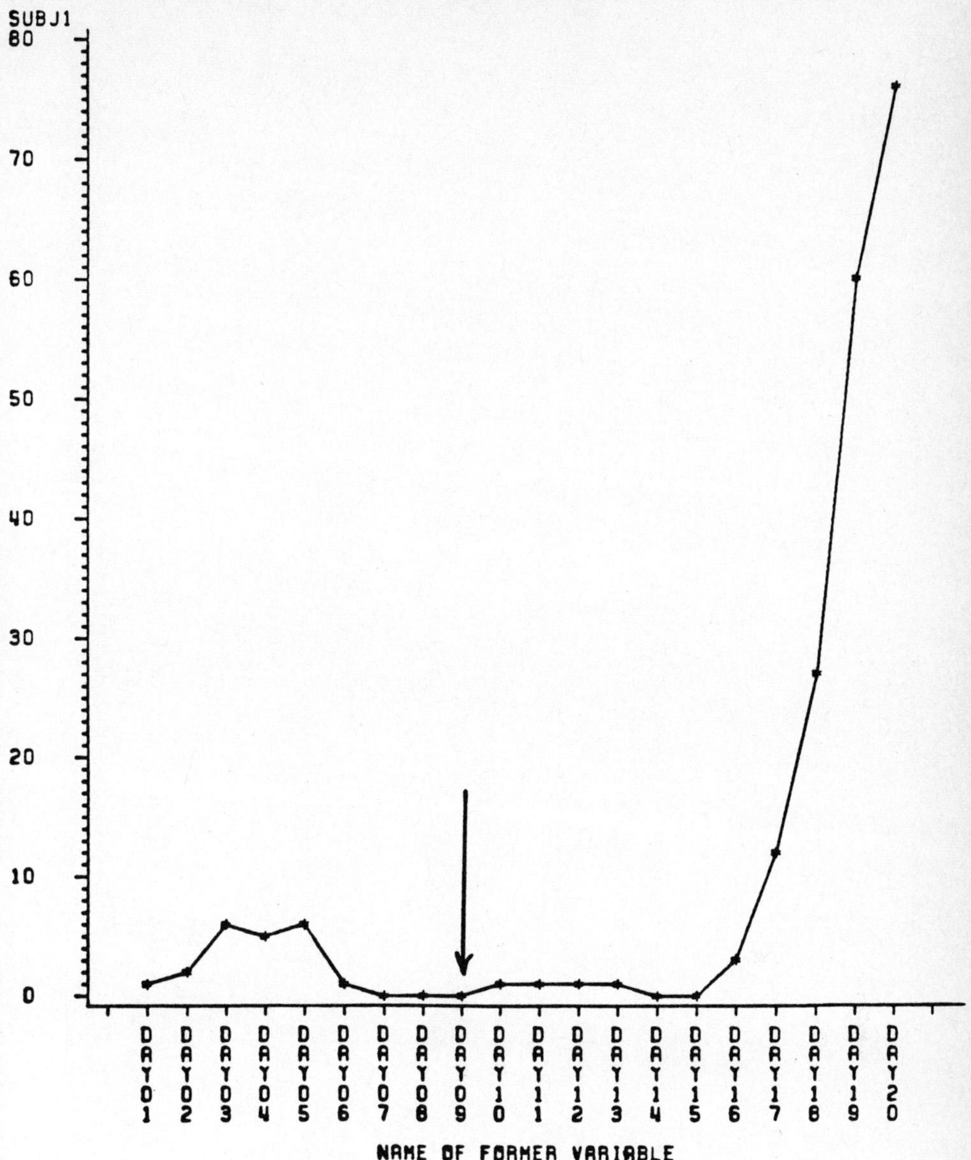

MODULATING (12HR HALFLIFE), ASCALE = 0.1

Figure 6

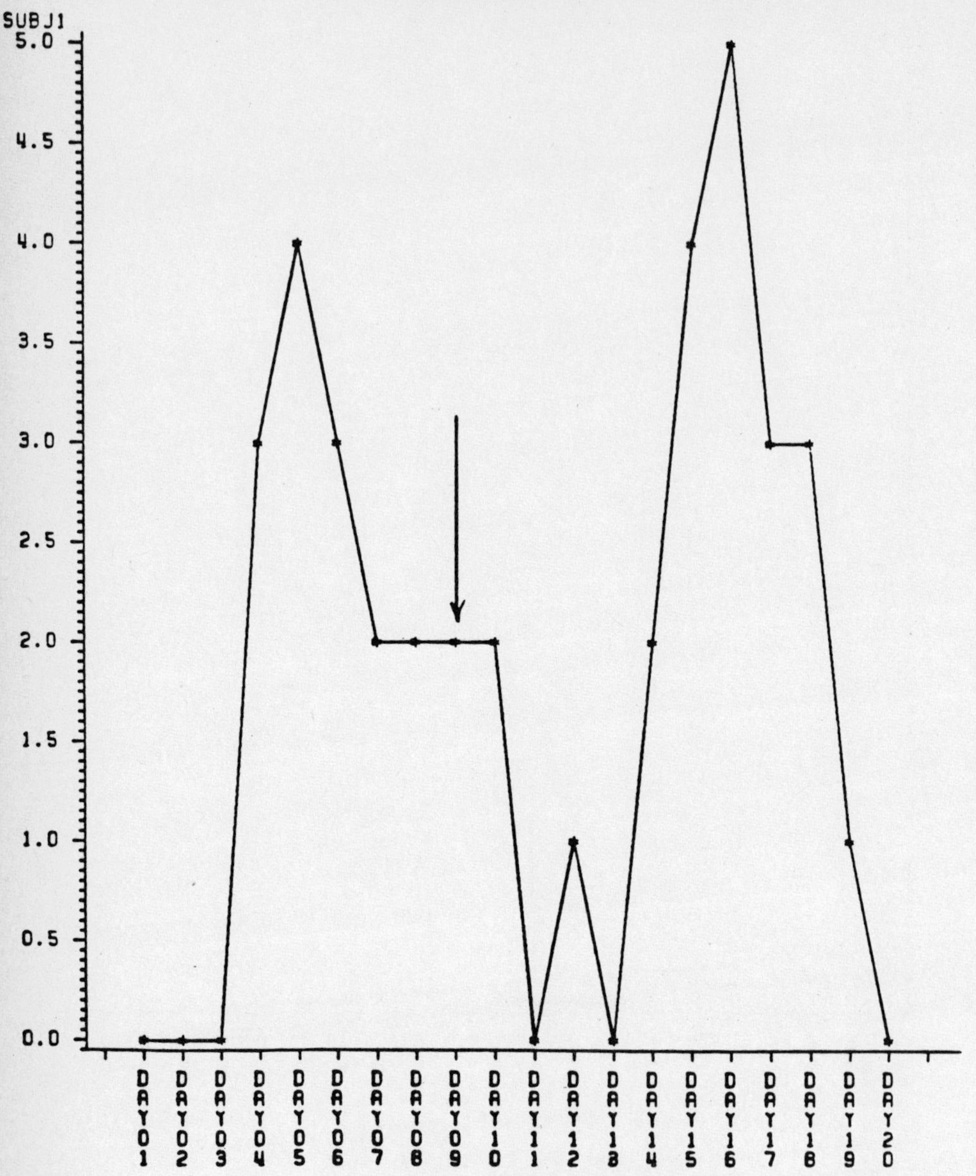
ESCAPE -- NON-IMMUNE COMPARTMENT
INTRAGENERATIONAL
SUBJ1
5.0
4.5
4.0
3.5
3.0
2.5
2.0
1.5
1.0
0.5
0.0
DAY01
DAY02
DAY03
DAY04
DAY05
DAY06
DAY07
DAY08
DAY09
DAY10
DAY11
DAY12
DAY13
DAY14
DAY15
DAY16
DAY17
DAY18
DAY19
DAY20
NAME OF FORMER VARIABLE
MODULATING (12HR HALFLIFE), ASCALE = 0.1

Figure 7

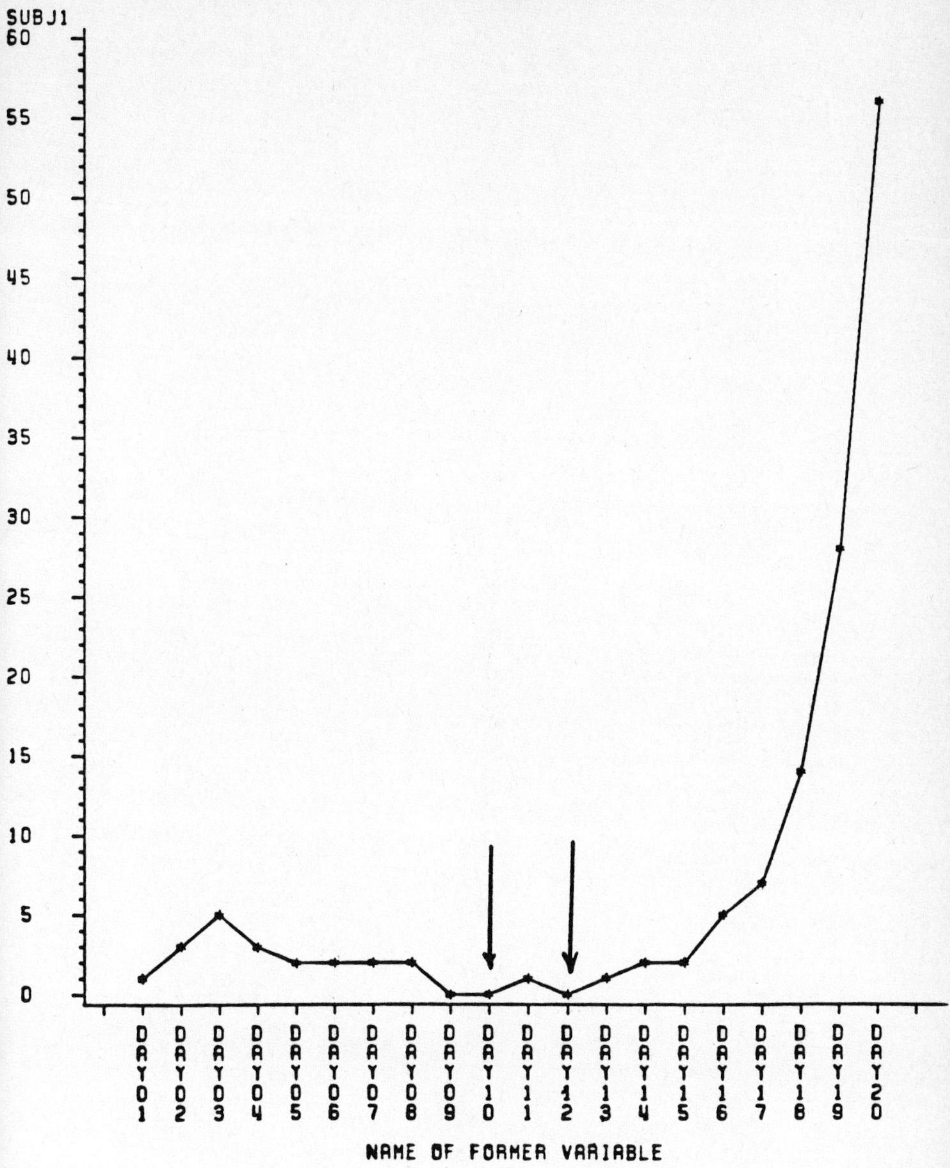
NEITHER -- IMMUNE COMPARTMENT
INTRAGENERATIONAL
SUBJ1
60
55
50
45
40
35
30
25
20
15
10
5
0
DAY01
DAY02
DAY03
DAY04
DAY05
DAY06
DAY07
DAY08
DAY09
DAY10
DAY11
DAY12
DAY13
DAY14
DAY15
DAY16
DAY17
DAY18
DAY19
DAY20
NAME OF FORMER VARIABLE
MODULATING (12HR HALFLIFE), ASCALE = 0.1

Figure 8

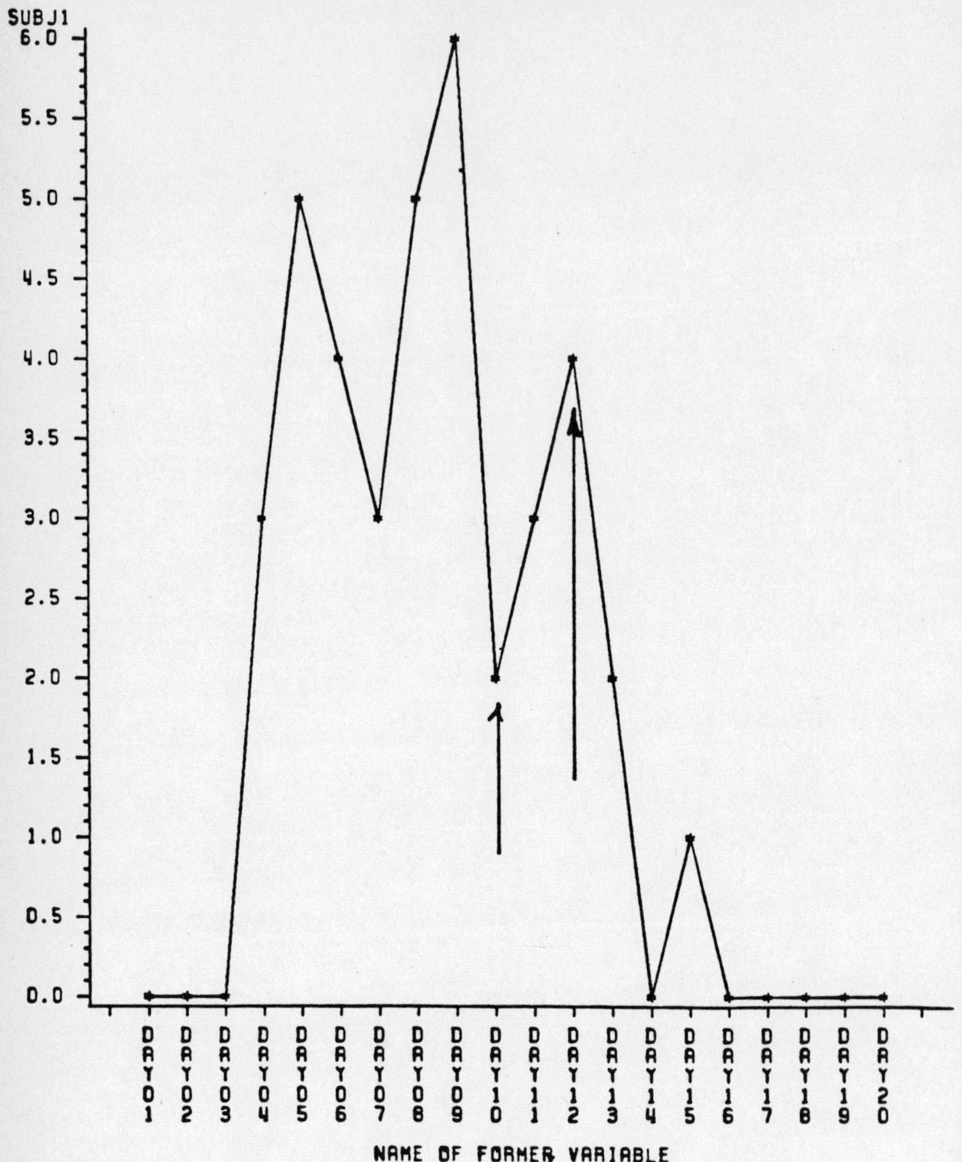

MODULATING (12HR HALFLIFE), ASCALE = 0.1

Figure 9

EXTINCTION -- IMMUNE COMPARTMENT

INTERGENERATIONAL

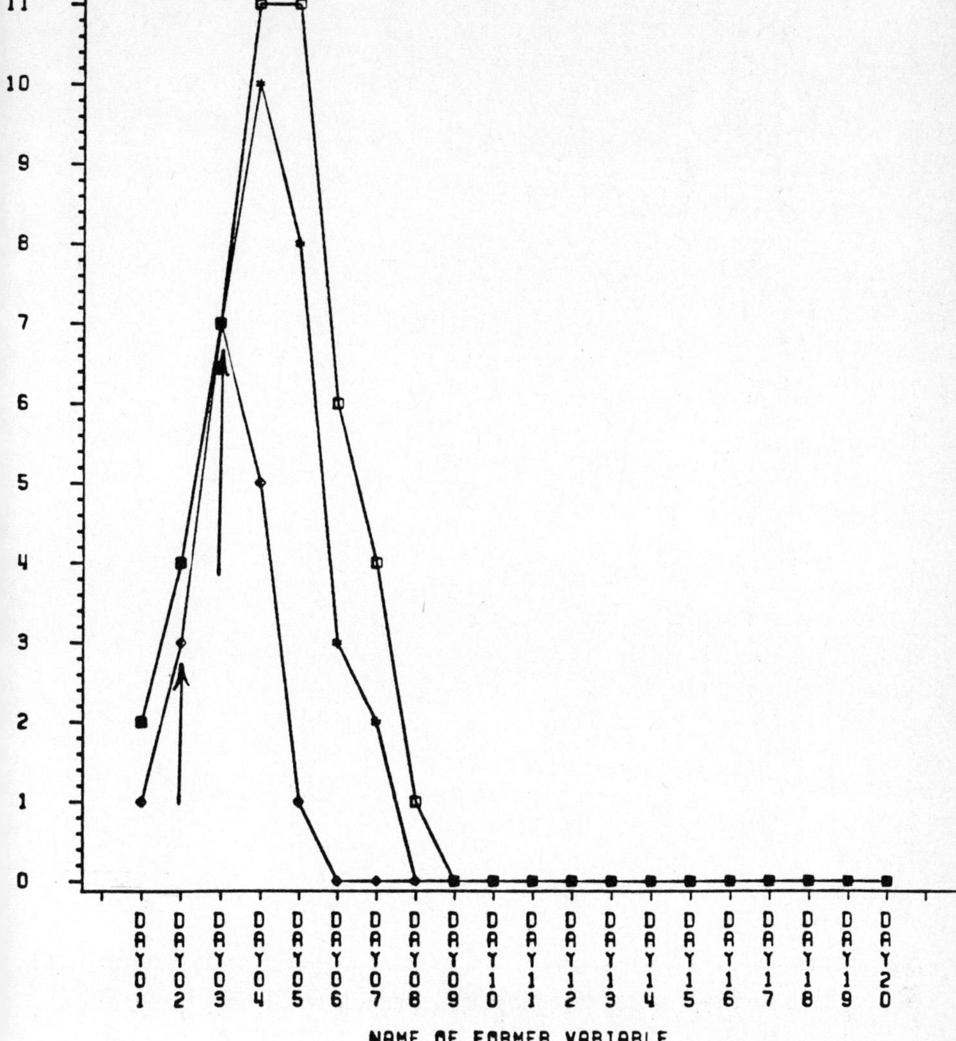

UNSTABLE SIGMA = 0.98 , ASCALE = 0.5

Figure 10

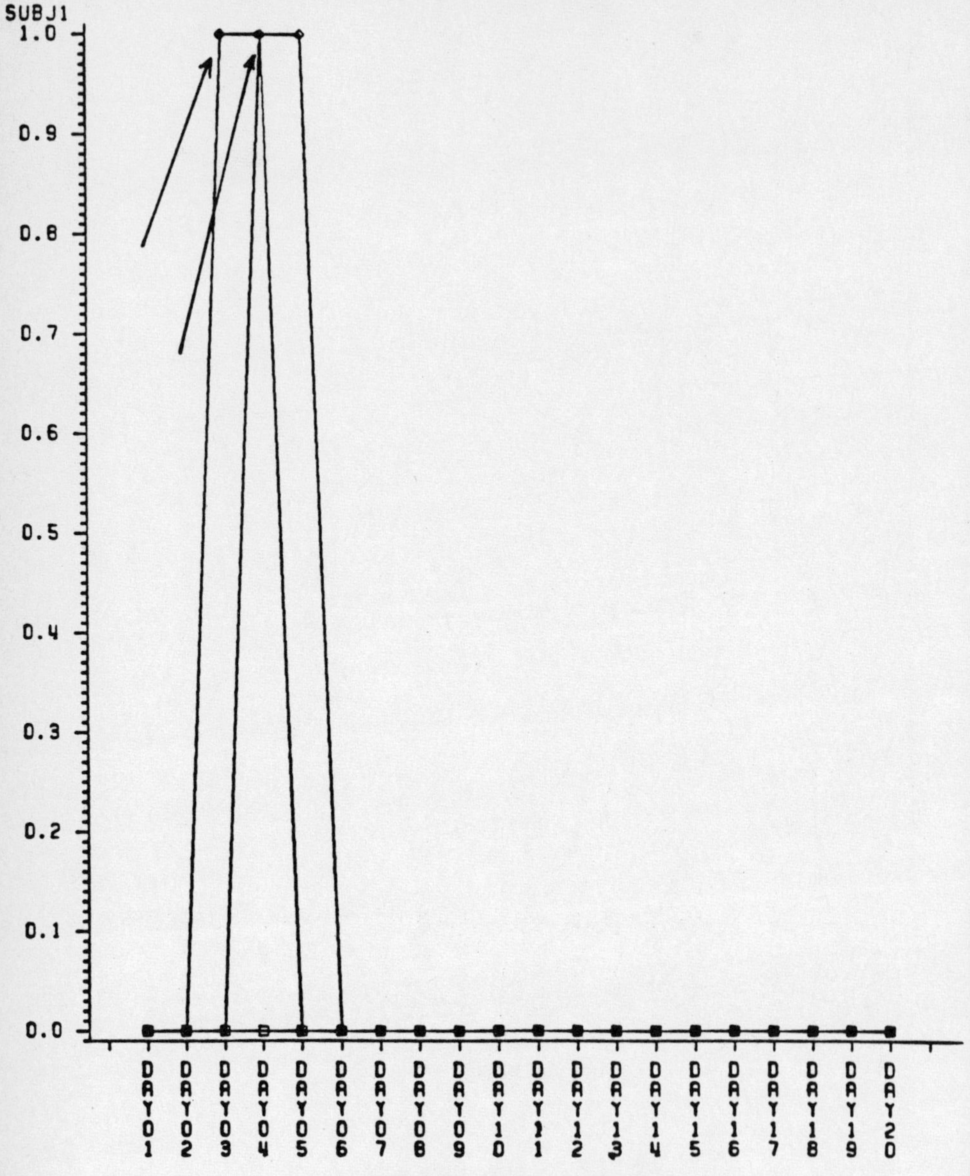

EXTINCTION -- NON-IMMUNE COMPARTMENT
INTERGENERATIONAL
SUBJ1
1.0
0.9
0.8
0.7
0.6
0.5
0.4
0.3
0.2
0.1
0.0
DAY01 DAY02 DAY03 DAY04 DAY05 DAY06 DAY07 DAY08 DAY09 DAY10 DAY11 DAY12 DAY13 DAY14 DAY15 DAY16 DAY17 DAY18 DAY19 DAY20
NAME OF FORMER VARIABLE
UNSTABLE SIGMA = 0.98 , ASCALE = 0.5

Figure 11

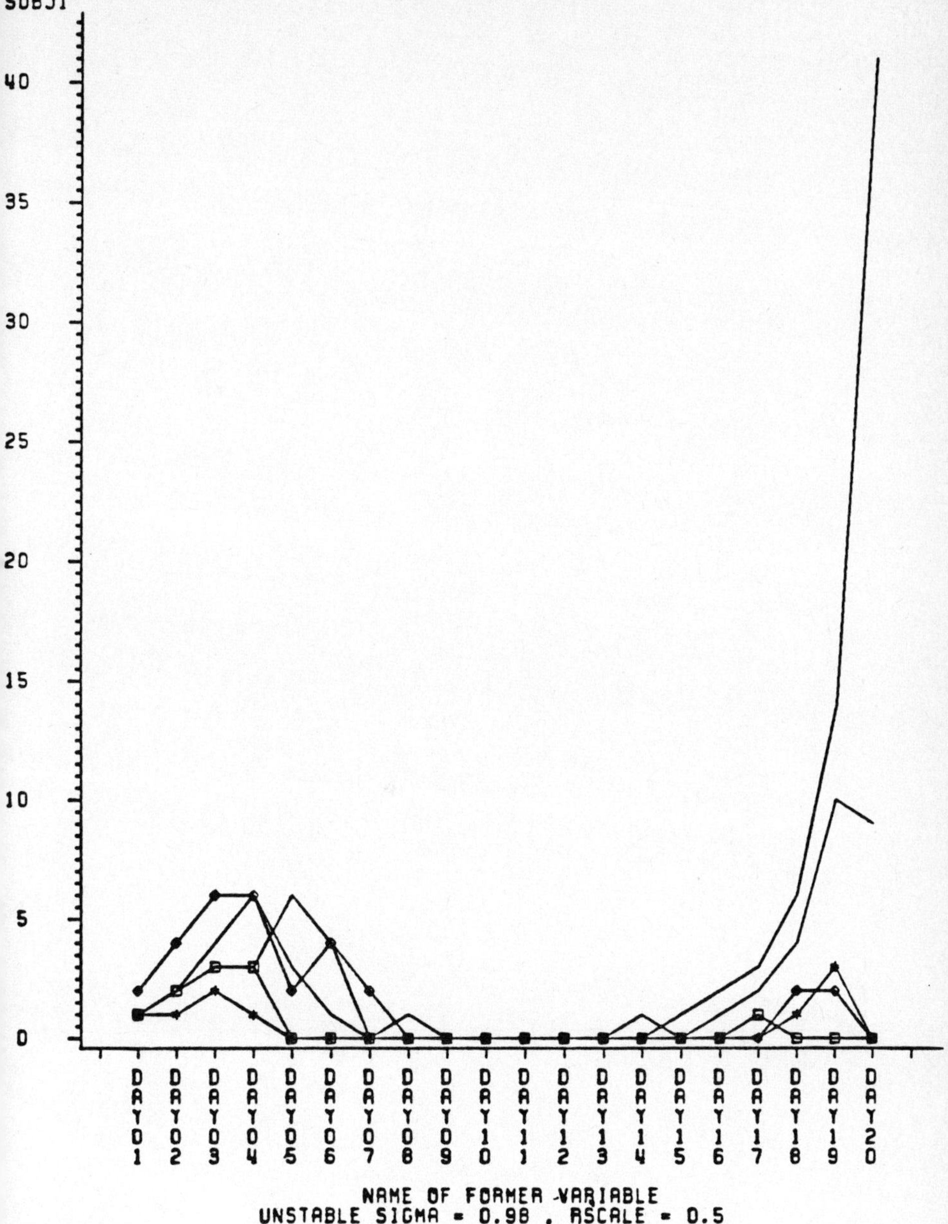
ESCAPE -- IMMUNE COMPARTMENT
INTERGENERATIONAL
SUBJ1
40
35
30
25
20
15
10
5
0
DAY01
DAY02
DAY03
DAY04
DAY05
DAY06
DAY07
DAY08
DAY09
DAY10
DAY11
DAY12
DAY13
DAY14
DAY15
DAY16
DAY17
DAY18
DAY19
DAY20
NAME OF FORMER VARIABLE
UNSTABLE SIGMA = 0.98 , ASCALE = 0.5

Figure 12

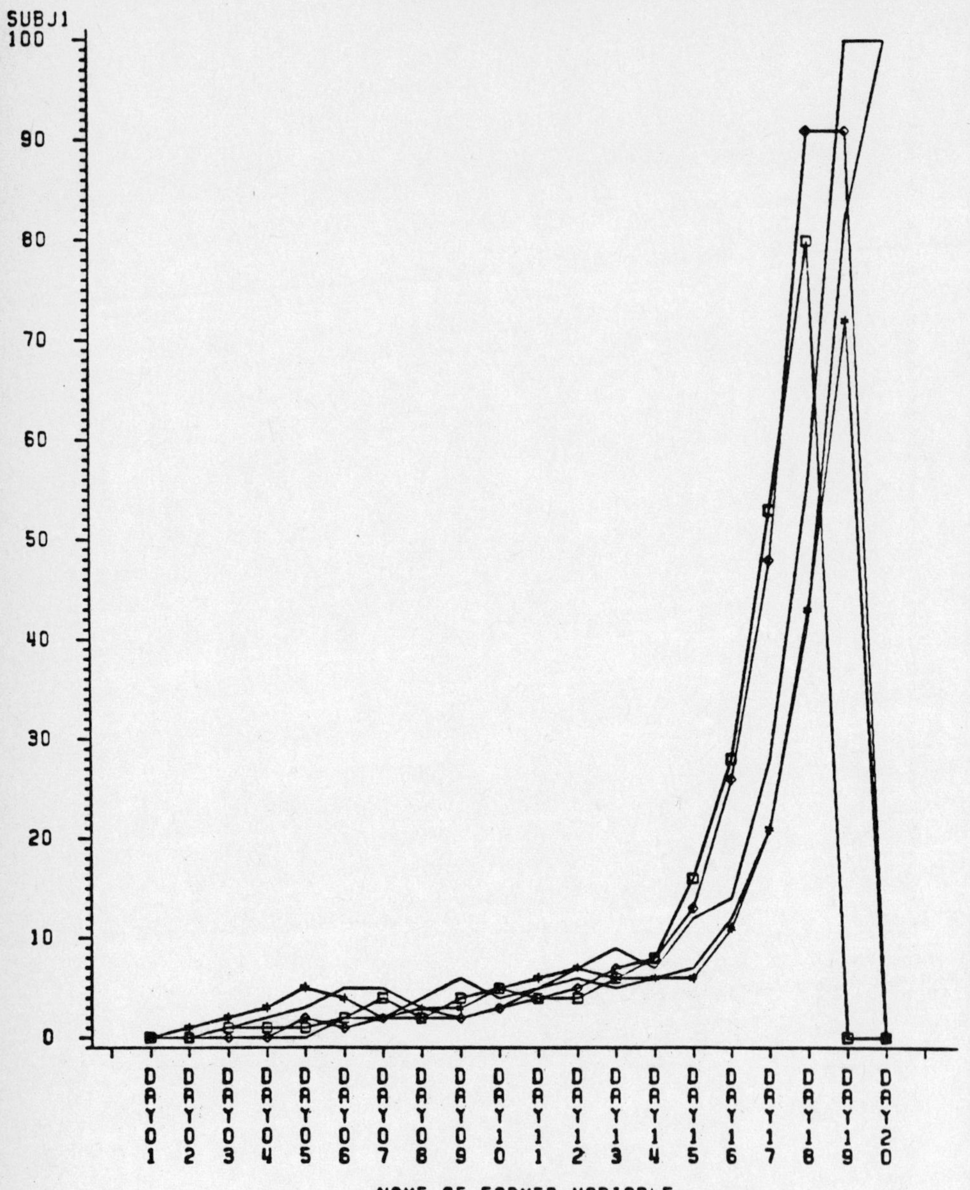
ESCAPE -- NON-IMMUNE COMPARTMENT
INTERGENERATIONAL
SUBJ1
100
90
80
70
60
50
40
30
20
10
0
DAY01
DAY02
DAY03
DAY04
DAY05
DAY06
DAY07
DAY08
DAY09
DAY10
DAY11
DAY12
DAY13
DAY14
DAY15
DAY16
DAY17
DAY18
DAY19
DAY20
NAME OF FORMER VARIABLE
UNSTABLE SIGMA = 0.98 , ASCALE = 0.5

Figure 13

NEITHER -- IMMUNE COMPARTMENT

INTERGENERATIONAL

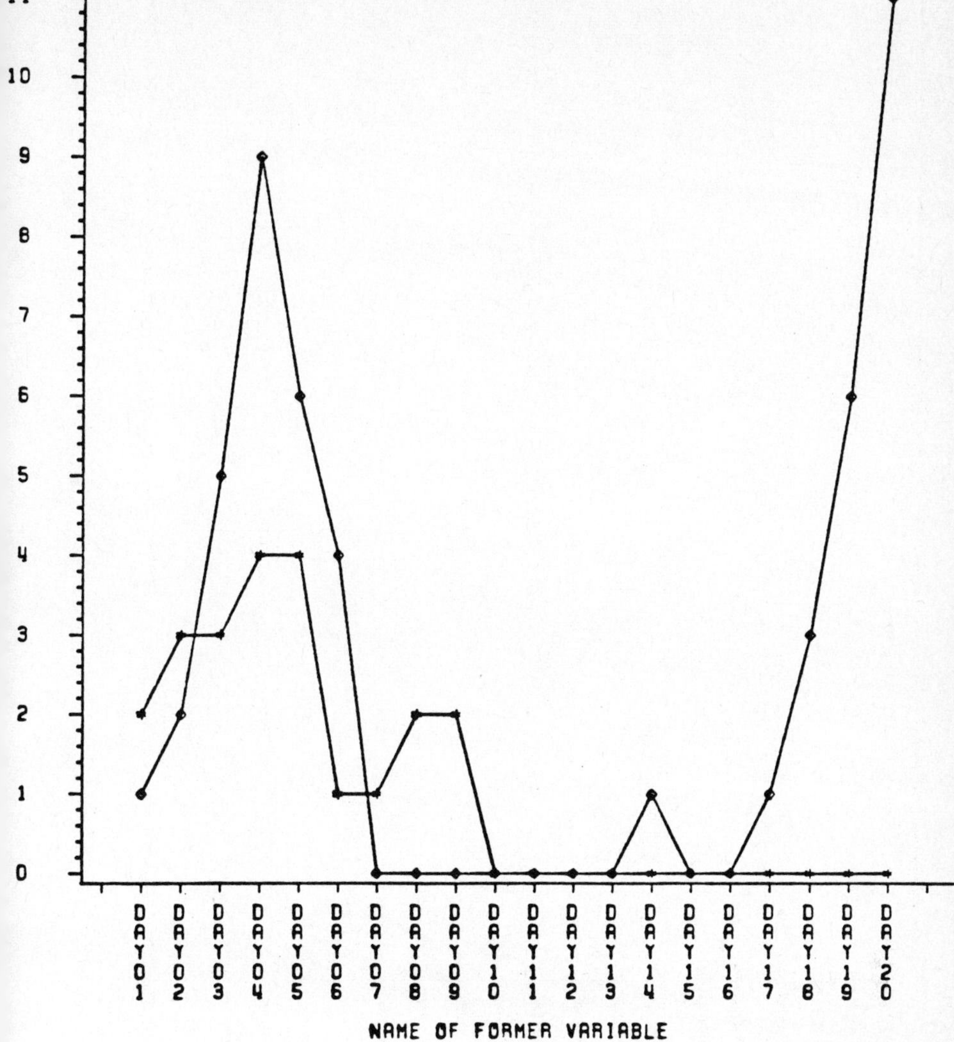

UNSTABLE SIGMA = 0.98 , ASCALE = 0.5

Figure 14

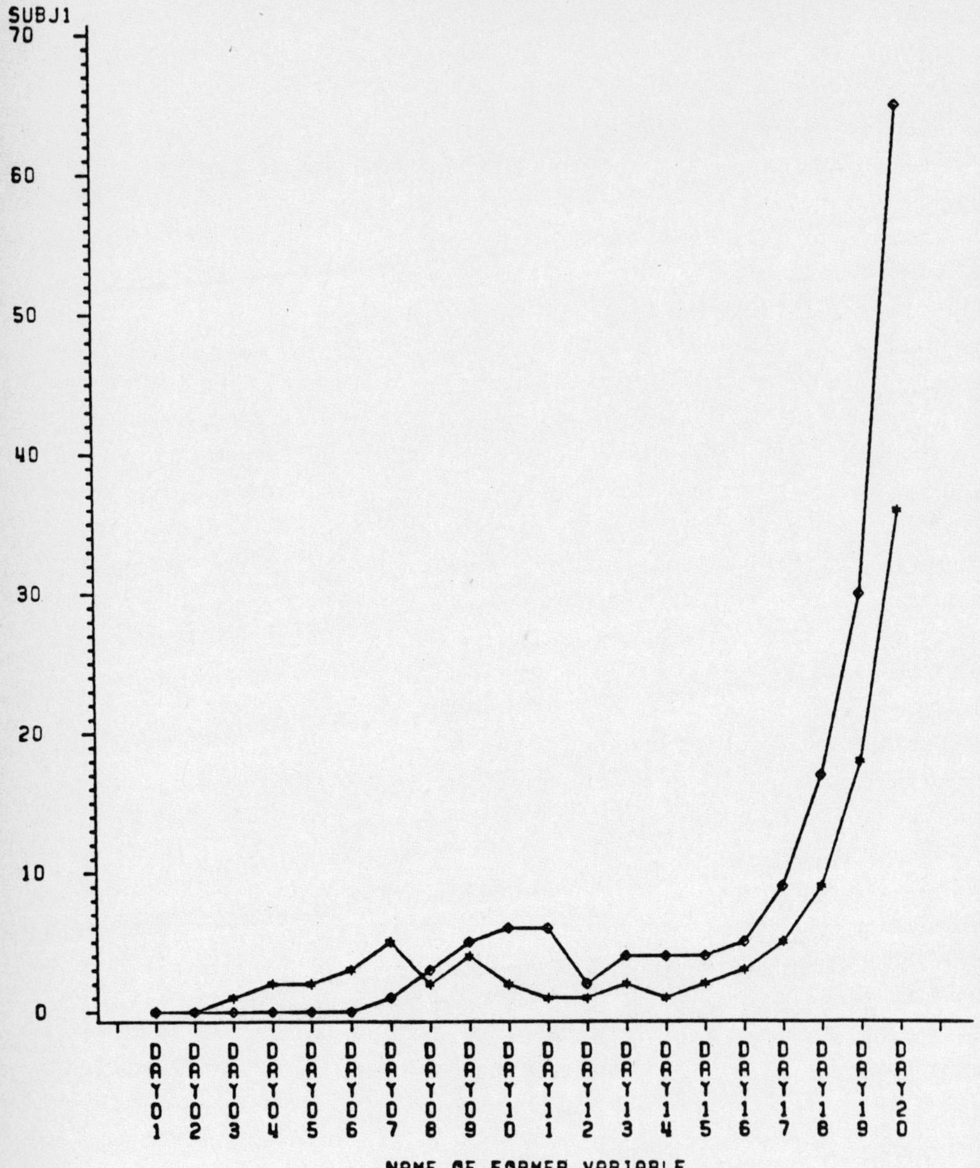

NEITHER -- IMMUNE COMPARTMENT
INTERGENERATIONAL
SUBJ1
70
60
50
40
30
20
10
0
DAY01
DAY02
DAY03
DAY04
DAY05
DAY06
DAY07
DAY08
DAY09
DAY10
DAY11
DAY12
DAY13
DAY14
DAY15
DAY16
DAY17
DAY18
DAY19
DAY20
NAME OF FORMER VARIABLE
UNSTABLE SIGMA = 0.98 , RSCALE = 0.5

Figure 15

However, as in the case of modulatory "bounce," this escape route proved to be necessary but not sufficient for escape (see arrows in Figures 10 and 11). The concomitant growth of an immunogenic subpopulation in the escaping tumors is the result of a late mutation suffered by a dividing non-immunogenic parent. Early reversion to an immunogenic character, one which might have occurred during the height of the immune response, is less likely to establish a flourishing immunogenic colony within the tumor.

Clearly, these experiments are simplistic. However, if we know something of a tumor's escape mechanism, these results can give us some insight into type of tumor we can expect to observe.

Before we discuss the implications of modulatory "bounce" and "early sanctuary," it may be instructive to speculate upon the types of tumors we should expect to see under more realistic circumstances.

Suppose that rather than assuming these cells grow in an uninhibited spatial conglomeration, we assume that the tumor takes on a spherical shape, so that access to the core cells is sterically hindered. Then, in an intragenerationally escaping tumor, we would expect that those cells freed of immune interactions would revert to their original immunogenic character. We should expect that a cross section of the tumor would be "immunogenically anular." Non-immunogenic cells should occupy the outer shell, while the core would be mostly made up of immunogenic cells. However, there may also exist isolated foci of non-immunogenic cells occupying the spaces around any angiogenically induced blood supply points.

Cells that escape intergenerationally should present a more complete mosaic of cellular distribution. Selective pressures should insure that non-immunogenic cells will continue to make up the outer shell of the solid tumor. However, a conglomerate of immunogenic and non-immunogenic cells should make up the tumor core. Because early escape was probably based in the non-immunogenic compartment, the interior should be composed, on the most part, of non-immunogenic cells. Within this non-immunogenic volume, a random (Poisson) distribution of immunogenic foci should exist. The intensity of the random mutation process should correspond to the distribution of immunogenic foci.

In and of themselves, these theoretical results are intellectually stimulating. But consider them within the context of autograft experiments which date back to the late 1950's (Grace and Kondo, 1958). A number of experiments were conducted in which tumor grafts from terminally ill patients were re-implanted into the patient at sites distant from the original resection (Nadler and Moore, 1965; Kioke, et al., 1963; Grace, et al., 1961). The motivation for these studies was the observation that surgery could inadvertently spread fragments of the primary or metastatic lesions within the patient, resulting in new, malignant foci. The investigators wondered whether this dispersion could account for an actual relapse to the disease state.

What they found is that even in patients with actively growing disease, either autografts of solid tumor fragments, or saline-based innocula were usually rejected. The rejection rates ranged from 87.5% (14/16) to 86.6% (71/82). Additionally, in autologous graft experiments, Kioke and his colleagues found that tumor takes occurred only when solid fragments were used as the graft. Tumor homogenates were routinely rejected.

Suppose we consider these data within the context of our theoretical results. Suppose that the tumor grafts were derived from an intergenerationally escaping clone. If our suppositions about the three dimensional structure of the solid tumor are correct, then any solid graft to a remote site should present a stable, non-immunogenic surface to the host defenses. However, unless the mutation rate is rather high (e.g., 5%), the tumor innocula should also be stably non-immunogenic.

Now, suppose that the tumor grafts were originally derived from an intragenerationally escaping clone. Then the surface of any solid tumor graft, while not stably non-immunogenic, will remain non-immunogenic as long as an adequate immune pressure is maintained. However, an immunogenic face might be part of the graft. This face could either revert to the non-immunogenic state, or cause a rejection of the graft. Secondly, when tumor cells are extracted, minced, and resuspended in a saline innoculum, cells of the immunogenic center become accessible to the elements of the immune system. Further, it is not clear whether these experimental manipulations affect the non-immunogenic character of the surface cells. It is possible that they can cause some demodulation as well.

The fact that both innocula and solid grafts were routinely rejected, and that no case of innocula-based transfer ever resulted in a tumor take, would seem to imply that these tumors originally escaped intragenerationally. However, it might also be true that local immunosuppressive agents (e.g., the T-suppressors as observed by Kripke and Fisher [1982], and Gransten et al. [1984]) are actively protecting the tumor cells at their original site. Further study into this possibility should be pursued.

3.2 Escape Mechanisms

We have just described two types of escaping populations and their immunogenic escape profiles. In this section, we will discuss the actual escape mechanisms employed by these populations and the potential clinical ramifications they may post.

Recall that we defined the phenomenon of modulatory "bounce" above. The "bounce" resulted from the fact that a modulated cell is less immunogenic than it was originally. Therefore, the probability that it will be recognized in any small interval, of length Δt, is proportionately decreased. As a first approximation, we used a linear proportionality constant that represented the decreased concentration of surface target structures. By assuming that an instantaneous transition between the immunogenic and non-immunogenic states existed, we were able to derive a value for the recognition probability level, $\hat{f}$, at which a single cell was as likely to modulate as it was to demodulate. Recall that the value of $\hat{f}$ was given by

$$\hat{f} = K_2 / (K_1 + S K_2)$$

From this definition, we defined two modes of activity for intragenerationally escaping cells. The first, the modulatory mode, was observed when the probability of recognition attained a level greater than $\hat{f}$ during any similar interval.

Because we assumed that K_1, K_2, and S were inherently defined as characteristics of our tumor populations, we were able to derive a single theoretical value for $\hat{f}$. However, suppose the demodulatory process is a gradual renewal of target structure concentrations. Then for cells to return to their original status, they must traverse a spectrum of increasing immunogenicity (much like our simulated cells do in the parallel pipe model [Michelson, 1985]). Then, at any point during the return journey, we can associate a unique surface concentration parameter (between 0 and 1) with each individual cell.

As a function of these surface concentrations, then, cells that are less likely to be recognized for a given level of $f(t;t_0)$ are in a demodulatory mode. The more immunogenic cells, however, may be in a modulatory mode. Therefore, cells may "bounce" back and forth between these modes as the recognition function and surface concentrations traverse their respective spectra.

In the entire discussion above, we have completely ignored the inherent capacity of each cell to survive in a hostile environment. If we define "adaptability," ν, to be the ratio of the probability that a cell, once recognized, will modulate versus the probability it will die, our simulation results showed that the more adaptable a tumor clone is, the more likely it is to survive and escape.

These two phenomena, working together, determine whether an intragenerationally escaping tumor clone will avoid the immune response, develop an active, growing tumor, and display the three-dimensional characteristics hypothesized above.

For intergenerationally escaping tumors, the escape mechanism is much simpler to describe. If a cell, early in the tumor's evolution, can attain immunologic sanctuary, then the tumor is more likely to escape the host defenses. And, except for random foci of immunogenic character, the escaping clone will be predominantly non-immunogenic.

The way a tumor escapes may eventually impact the effectivity of various immunotherapeutics. Consider, first, intragenerationally escaping tumors. If a tumor clone is small enough so that we can ignore any stereo-geometric sanctuary, then it is possible for a clinical regimen to be designed so that we may take advantage of the modulatory "bounce" phenomenon.

Two therapeutic options present themselves. Firstly, treatments could be timed and dosed so that the level of recognition activity at the tumor site (as a function of effector numbers, specificity, etc.) is maintained at levels just below our theoretical threshold $\hat{f}$ for extended periods of time. This strategy attempts to maintain a continuous demodulatory mode for the individual cells, forcing them to bouhce back to their immunogenic state once they have modulated. At each subsequent recognition, the cells would again be forced to either modulate or die.

The second therapeutic option also takes advantage of modulatory "bounce." In this scenario, the active immunological agents are infused in bolus doses at pre-determined time points. The periods for these injections are determined so that they coincide with the peak "bounce back" times of the non-immunogenic cells. Again, the population as a whole will be forced to remodulate or die.

Adaptability may be a determining factor in the choice of the eventual course of treatment. If a clone appears to be very adaptable (i.e., $\nu \ll 1.0$), then we would probably want to "hit" the cells as many times as possible during the treatment period. Then the cells, which have only a small chance of dying on each "hit," will be "hit" so often that, by sheer numbers alone, they will eventually lyse. The best way to accomplish this would be to maintain the recognition levels just below our theoretical threshold, $\hat{f}$. In other words, we would want to employ the first treatment strategy.

On the other hand, if the cells prove less adaptable (i.e., $\nu > 1.0$), the second therapeutic option may prove to be the therapy of choice. In this scenario, if cells are not modulating as often as they are being killed, many large, single doses of the anti-tumor, or immunoactivating, agent may be a more efficient treatment schedule.

Consider, now, tumors which escape intergenerationally. Clearly, cells attaining immunologic sanctuary during the tumor's evolution can not be given any respite from the hostile immunologic pressures. Furthermore, as discussed in greater detail below, an intergenerationally escaping tumor clone must be "hit" hard and "hit" early. Once a cell has escaped to the (stable) non-immunogenic state, the chances of completely destroying the tumor are poor.

Therefore, if cells escaping intergenerationally are to be treated, it must be assumed that they are stably non-immunogenic. Even therapeutic strategies which are designed to prophylactically guard against the spread of metastases should be designed with this consideration in mind. And because of these obvious constraints, immunotherapy directed against these types of tumors may prove to be wholly ineffective.

REFERENCES

Boyse, E.A., E. Stockert, and L. Old. 1967. Modification of the Structure of the Cell Membrane by Thymus Leukemia (TL) Antibody. PNAS 58:954

Esmon, N.I. and J.R. Little. 1976. Different Mechanisms for the Modulation of TL Antigens on Murine Lymphoid Cells. J. Immunol. 117:919

Fenyo, E.M., E. Klein, G. Klein, and K. Sweich. 1968. Selection of an Immunoresistant Maloney Subline with Decreased Concentration of Tumor Specific Surface Antigens. JNCI 40:69

Fisher, M.S. and M.L. Kripke. 1982. Suppressor T Lymphocytes Control the Development of Primary Skin Cancers in Ultraviolet-Irradiated Mice. Science 216:1133-1134

Golub, S.H., F. Dorey, D. Hara, D.L. Morton, and M.W. Burk. 1982a. Systemic Administration of Human Leukocyte Interferon to Melanoma Patients I. Effects on Natural Killer Function and Cell Populations. JNCI 68:703-710

Golub, S.H., P. D'Amore, and M. Rainey. 1982b. Systemic Administration of Human Leukocyte Interferon to Melanoma Patients II. Cellular Events Associated with Changes in Natural Killer Cell Cytotoxicity. JNCI 68:711-717

Grace, J.T. Jr. 1964. Clinical Aspects of Immunity in Untreated Cancer. Ann. N.Y. Acad. Sci. 114:736-746

Grace, J.T. Jr. and T. Kondo. 1958. Investigations of Host Resistance in Cancer Patients. Ann. Surgery 148:633-641

Grace, J.T. Jr., D.M. Perese, R.S. Metzger, T. Sasabe, and B. Holedrige. 1961. Tumor Autograft Responses in Patients with Glioblastoma Multiforme. J. Neurosurg. 18:159-167

Gransten, R.D., J.A. Parrish, D.J. McAuliffe, C. Waltenburg, and M.I. Greene. 1984. Immunologic Inhibition of Ultraviolet Radiation-induced Tumor Suppressor Cell Activity. Science 224:615-617

Kendall, D.G. 1948a. On the Generalized "Birth-and-Death" Process. Ann. Math. Stat. 19:1

Kendall, D.G. 1948b. On the Role of a Variable Generation Time in the Development of a Stochastic Birth Process. Biometrika 35:316

Kimber, I. and M. Moore. 1984. Clonal Variation of NK Sensitivity Among K562 Lines. In: Natural Killer Activity and Its Regulation. Proc. Int'l. Sympos. on Natural Killer Activity and Its Regulation. (Ed. T. Hoshino, H.S. Koren, and A. Uchida) Excerpt Medica. 308-312

Kioke, A., G.E. Moore, C.B. Mendoza, and A.J. Watne. 1963. Heterologous, Homologous, and Autologous Transplantation of Human Tumors. Cancer 16:1065-1071

Levy, R. and R.A. Miller. 1983. Tumor Therapy with Monoclonal Antibodies. Proc. 66th Annual Meeting, Fed. of American Soc. Expt. Biol. New Orleans, LA. Apr. 16, 1982. 2650-2656

Liang, W. and E.P. Cohen. 1977. Detection of Thymus Leukemia Antigen on the Surface Membranes of Murine Leukemia Cells Resistant to Thymus Leukemia Antibodies and Guinea Pig Complement. JNCI 58:1079

MacDougall, S.L., C. Shustik, and A.K. Sullivan. 1983. Target Cell Specificity of Human Natural Killer (NK) Cells. I. Development of an NK-Resistant Subline of K562. Cellular Immun. 76:39-48

Michelson, S. 1983. A Two Compartment Stochastic Model for Antigenic Modulation. Presentation. Eleventh IFIP Conference on System Modeling and Optimization, Copenhagen, Denmark.

Michelson, S. 1985. (to be published) Stochastic Compartment Models for Tumor Escape. Ph.D. Dissertation. Univ. of California, Los Angeles, CA.

Nadler, S.H. and G.E. Moore. 1965. Autotransplantation of Human Cancer. JAMA 191:105-106

Parthasarathy, P.R. and P. Mayilswami. 1981. Stochastic Compartmental Models with Branching Particles. Bull. Math. Biol. 43:347

Ritz, J., J.M. Pesando, S.E. Sallan, L.A. Clavell, J. Notis-McConarty, P. Rosenthal, and S.F. Schlossman. 1981. Serotherapy of Acute Lymphoblastic Leukemia with Monoclonal Antibody. Blood 58:141-152

Stephanopaulos, G. and A.G. Fredrickson. 1981. Extinction Probabilities in Microbial Predation: A Birth-Death Approach. Bull. Math. Biol. 43:165

Wolf, J.E., R.B. Fanes, and Y.S. Choi. 1977. Antigenic Changes of DBA/2J Mastocytoma Cells When Grown in BALB/C Mouse. JNCI 58:1407

Young, W.W. and S. Hakomari. 1980. Therapy of Mouse Lymphoma with Monoclonal Antibodies to Glycolipids: Selection of Low Antigenic Variants In Vivo. Science 212:487

IMPLICATIONS OF MACROPHAGE T-LYMPHOCYTE INTERACTIONS FOR TUMOR REJECTABILITY

Rob J. de Boer and Pauline Hogeweg
BIOINFORMATICS GROUP
University of Utrecht
Padualaan 8, 3584 CH Utrecht
The Netherlands

ABSTRACT

A relatively detailed model of experimentally described macrophage T-lymphocyte interactions has been developed. In this model we investigate the immune response to tumors that differ in antigenicity and/or in initial size. Having deliberately omitted from the model tumor escape mechanisms (e.g. suppression, antigenic modulation or heterogeneity), we study the circumstances that nevertheless lead to progressive tumor growth.

The model behavior shows that: (1) tumor antigenicity can best be defined in terms of helper T cell reactivity; (2) small differences in the availability of HTL (*) markedly influence tumor rejectability; (3) compared with the impact of macrophages, the impact of CTL increases more with increasing tumor antigenicity; and (4) sneaking through and tolerance are intrinsic to this model.

HTL have a large impact on the model behavior (i.e. the immune response) because there are self-reinforcements in the HTL activation and proliferation process. Interestingly, unresponsiveness (tolerance) evolves in this model, despite the presence of these self-reinforcements and the absence of negative interactions (e.g. suppression). Tolerance is caused by a proliferation threshold that comes into existence when T-lymphocyte effectors are made short-lived. We discuss the advantages of using numerical integration combined with numerical phase state analysis. Stable steady states in this model do exist but are of minor importance.

ABBREVIATIONS: ANGRY cytotoxic macrophage(s), APC antigen presenting cell(s), CTL cytotoxic T-lymphocyte(s), CTLP CTL-precursor(s), HTL helper T-lymphocyte(s), HTLP HTL-precursor(s), IFN interferon, IL 2 interleukin 2, MAF macrophage activating factor, MPH normal macrophage(s), NK natural killer cell(s).

INTRODUCTION

Immune reactions usually involve interactions between a large number of cell types. Mathematical models in immunology are however normally simplifications, representing only part of the available immunological data. Two types of model simplifications should be distinguished: those imposed by the modelling formalism (and the method of analysing the model) and those imposed for reasons of informatic minimalization. In order to obtain insight into the dynamics of complex systems, the former type of simplification should be minimized, whereas the latter type should be maximized.

Models that incorporate only part of the data, i.e. cell-interactions experimentally known to exist, exhibit behavior that corresponds to experimentally known phenomena. The investigation of the relationships between the set of incorporated interactions (i.e. the micro level) and the model behavior (i.e. the macro level) [1] provides insight into the role of the various processes that are involved in immune reactions. Moreover, it is possible to pinpoint the "key interactions" responsible for generating a specific phenomenon if all redundant interactions are removed, i.e. a model is simplified (e.g. [2]).

Here we investigate immune responses to tumors, i.e. antigens capable of endless replication. Many different effector cells are known to play a role in the immune resistance to tumors: e.g. NK cells, B cells, helper T cells, cytotoxic T cells and macrophages [3]. Our model specifies only a subset of these cells (i.e. helper and cytotoxic T cells and macrophages), and only one compartment is taken into consideration. The interactions between the incorporated cell types are however specified in a relatively "knowledge oriented" way. Interestingly, the behavior of the model is diverse, and corresponds to a number of phenomena described experimentally.

We have incorporated the following data in the model (see Table 1 and Fig. 1): a) small tumors grow exponentially [4], large ones linearly; b) T-lymphocytes and macrophages can become cytotoxic towards tumor cells [3]; c) macrophages process tumor cell debris (which accumulates upon normal tumor cell death and upon tumor cell lysis), and present the processed tumor associated antigens in an antigenic form [5]; d) HTLP activation requires antigen presentation, whereas CTLP activation does not [6]; e) CTL and HTL are capable of proliferation (in response to IL2) [7, 8], whereas macrophages are not [9]; f) CTLP maturation into the CTL stage requires the presence

Table 1. FORMAL REPRESENTATION OF THE MODEL

```
APC     = (MPH + ANGRY)*DEBRIS/(KMD + DEBRIS)
FACTOR = HTL*APC/(KMP + APC)
INFLAM = H*FACTOR/(KMF + FACTOR)
dCTLP/dt = I1 + I1*INFLAM - A*CTLP*TUMOR - EL*CTLP
dHTLP/dt = I2 + I2*INFLAM - A*HTLP*APC    - EL*HTLP
dMPH/dt  = I3 + I3*INFLAM - A*MPH*FACTOR - EM*MPH
dPCTLP/dt= A*CTLP*TUMOR - A*PCTLP*FACTOR - EL*PCTLP
dCTL/dt  = A*PCTLP*FACTOR + P*CTL*FACTOR/(KMF + FACTOR) - DL*CTL
dHTL/dt  = A*HTLP*APC     + P*HTL*FACTOR/(KMF + FACTOR) - DL*HTL
dANGRY/dt= A*MPH*FACTOR - DM*FACTOR
dTUMOR/dt= R*TUMOR/(1+TUMOR/KR) - KILL*(ANGRY+CTL)*TUMOR/(KMK + TUMOR)
dDEBRIS/dt=-ED*DEBRIS + D*TUMOR + KILL*(ANGRY+CTL)*TUMOR/(KMK + TUMOR)
```

Table 1. The cell interactions specified by the model. Tumor cell killing is effected by two effector cells: cytotoxic T-lymphocytes (CTL) and cytotoxic macrophages (ANGRY). CTL precursors (CTLP) require both activation by antigen (TUMOR) and stimulation by lymphoid factor (FACTOR) before they transform into cytotoxic effector cells, which are capable of proliferation. Transformation of macrophages (MPH) into their cytotoxic effectors (ANGRY) is caused by lymphoid factors (FACTOR) released by activated helper T cells (HTL) upon restimulation of the latter by antigen presenting cells (APC). Only HTL produce lymphoid factors; the different factors are assumed to be kinetically identical and are combined into one variable (FACTOR). HTL precursors (HTLP) become activated (effectors) upon interaction with APC. Effector T-lymphocytes (CTL, HTL) proliferate in response to interleukin 2 (FACTOR); effector macrophages on the other hand can only be formed from their precursors. The influx of precursors is increased with INFLAM during an inflammation reaction. The intensity of the inflammation reaction depends on the concentration of lymphoid factors (FACTOR). Effector restimulation (KMP), proliferation stimulation (KMF) and tumor cell killing (KMK) [49] follow conventional Michaelis-Menten kinetics.

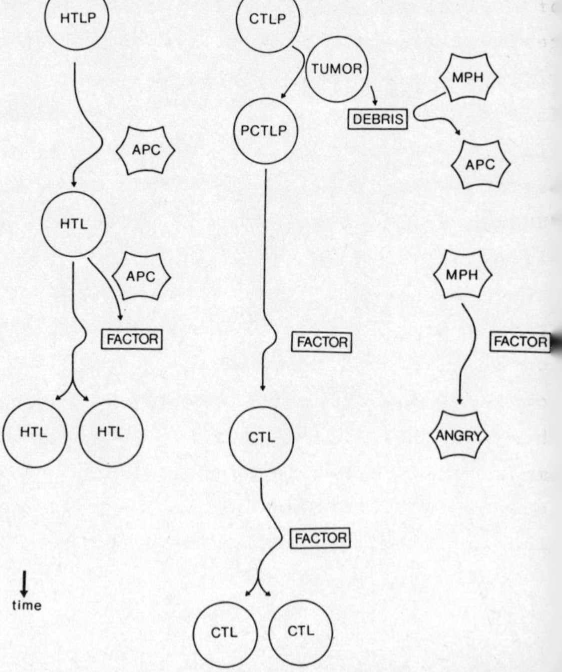

Figure 1. The interactions incorporated in the model.

Table 2. PARAMETER SETTING OF THE MODEL

A	10^{-3}	activation rate	per cell per day
D	0.1	DEBRIS generation rate	units per cell per day
DL	0.02 or 0.2	lymphocyte effector decay	per day
DM	1.0	cytotoxic macrophage decay	per day
ED	2.0	debris decay	per day
EL	0.02	lymphocyte precursor efflux	per day
EM	0.05	normal macrophage efflux	per day
H	9.0	inflammation constant	
I1	1.0 or 200	CTLP influx	cells per day
I2	0.01 to 1000	HTLP influx	cells per day
I3	125000	macrophage influx	cells per day
KILL	10.0	killing capacity	cells per cell per day
KMD	10^7	presentation saturation	units
KMF	50.0	factor saturation	units
KMK	10^5	killing saturation	cells
KMP	10^3	restimulation saturation	cells
KR	10^9	growth rate saturation	cells
P	1.0	proliferation rate	cells per cell per day
R	1.0	tumor growth rate	cells per cell per day

Table 2. The parameter setting of the model is based upon experimental data concerning the immune resistance of DBA/2 mice to the SL2 tumor after the tumor has been injected into the peritoneal cavity of the mice [20]. The parameter values were discussed previously in more detail [14]. The degree of tumor antigenicity is defined as the number of lymphocyte precursors that can be activated upon introduction of the tumor, i.e. antigenicity corresponds to T-lymphocyte influx (I1 and I2). In order to represent different tumors I1 and I2 are varied. We study the effect of T-lymphocyte effector longevity (DL) by changing it 10-fold.

of a lymphoid differentiation factor [10, 11]; and g) upon antigenic restimulation HTL produce lymphoid factors: T cell growth factor (IL2) [7, 8], T cell differentiation factor [10, 11], macrophage activating factor (MAF, IFN) [12], and factors inducing an inflammation reaction [13]. This model is an extension of models described in more detail previously [14, 15]. Here HTL are restimulated by APC (instead of by TUMOR) and CTL induction requires the presence of HTL-derived differentiation factors.

For the informatic minimalization reasons mentioned above, only stimulating (positive) interactions have been incorporated in our model. Suppressor cells (of T cell or of macrophage origin [16, 17]) however "down regulate" anti-tumor immune responses (i.e. influence them negatively). In order to investigate whether the failure of immune responses hinges upon suppression and/or other tumor escape mechanisms (e.g. antigenic heterogeneity [18] or modulation [19, Michelson: this volume]) we have omitted these mechanisms.

The experimental system upon which this model and its parameter setting (Table 2) are based on the ascitic growth of the SL2 tumor in the peritoneal cavity of DBA/2 mice [20, 21]. In this paper we describe (theoretical) experiments with tumors that differ in antigenicity. To this end we define the degree of antigenicity as the initial sizes of the T-lymphocyte precursor populations that can be activated upon introduction of that antigen.

It turns out that (minimal differences in) tumor antigenicity can determine whether rejection or progressive tumor growth occurs (Fig. 4), i.e. can determine the failure of the response. Progressive tumor growth can either be accompanied by an ever increasing T-lymphocyte response (Fig. 3 and 8c) or by a constant and very limited reaction (Fig. 8a). Suppression, which is absent, is thus redundant for the failure of the response.

METHODS

We investigate our model by introducing tumors of varying antigenicity and/or tumors in various initial doses. These model immune systems provide a more advantageous environment for experimenting than do wet immune systems because a) all variables are easily observable, and b) the system structure can be manipulated easily (i.e. the impact of different processes can be studied through their incorporation or omittance).

The model is formulated in ordinary differential equations. APC, FACTOR and the inflammation reaction are incorporated in the form of quasi steady state variables. The model is studied by means of numerical integration (i.e. by simulation). Analytical methods would put more severe constraints on the complexity of the model immune system. Furthermore analytical methods usually concentrate on the existence of steady states, which are not necessarily of prime interest.

The power of the simulation method is augmented by static analysis of the state space. We obtain insight into the qualitative differences in the model behaviour by static (graphical) analysis. We reduce the 9-D state space of the model (there are 9 variables) to various 3-D or 2-D state spaces by making quasi steady state assumptions for the other (6 or 7) variables. It turns out that such state spaces with 0-isoclines provide a valuable tool for the interpretation of the model behavior. For instance, specific phenomena can be related to specific forms (folds) of the 0-isocline planes.

The model is investigated by means of GRIND [22]. GRIND performs numerical searches for 0-isoclines; it integrates by means of ROW4A [23], which is a robust integrator for the analysis of stiff systems of ordinary differential equations.

RESULTS AND CONCLUSIONS

antigenicity. In Fig. 2 the model immune system is challenged with a tumor consisting of one cell and having an antigenicity corresponding to I1=1.0 (CTLP=50) and I2=0.2 (HTLP=10). In Fig. 3 the same system is challenged with a tumor of equal size but which is slightly less antigenic (i.e. I1=1.0 and I2=0.1 (HTLP=5)). The former tumor (Fig. 2) is rejected, whereas the latter (Fig. 3) grows in an uncontrolled manner. We therefore conclude that minimal differences in HTLP reactivity (here 5 cells, see Fig. 4) can markedly influence tumor rejectability.

The immune reactions to these two tumors are very similar up till day 10. At day 10, the CTLP have been transformed into PCTLP by activation, the PCTLP remain constant (the availability of differentiation factor limits their maturation into the CTL stage), some DEBRIS has accumulated, HTL induction has just started, and a few hundred ANGRY macrophages have been induced. In comparison to the "progressive growth" case (Fig. 2), the TUMOR is 1% smaller in the rejection case (Fig. 3), DEBRIS is 6% larger, ANGRY and HTL are about twice as large, and PCTLP is roughly equal. Note that the initial (at day zero) HTLP populations also differ by a factor two. HTL proliferation is a self-reinforcing process because these cells produce their own growth factor (IL2). The difference in the HTL numbers of the two immune reactions therefore increases (up till day 15, when the tumor is rejected). Moreover, HTL activation is also self-reinforcing: HTLP activation requires the accumulation of DEBRIS, the HTL thus generated induce ANGRY macrophages, which in turn increase the accumulation of DEBRIS by lysing tumor cells. In addition, the production of IL2 and MAF (FACTOR) increases upon an increase in DEBRIS, since HTL depend on antigen presentation for restimulation. These self-reinforcements in the HTL dynamics explain why minor changes in HTLP reactivity have a major impact on tumor rejectability.

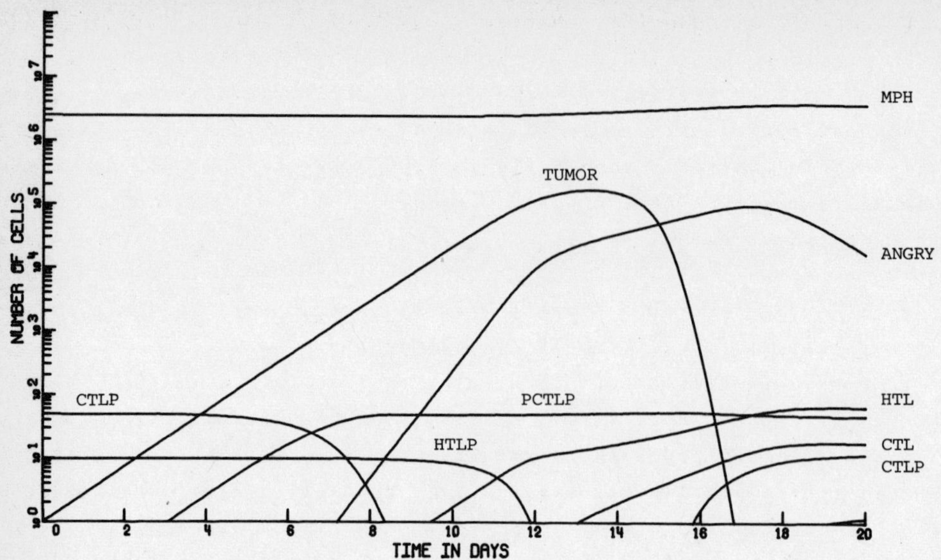

Figure 2. The rejection of a tumor of an antigenicity correponding to I1=1.0 (CTLP=50) and I2=0.2 (HTLP=10) introduced as a single cell into a non-immunized system (day 0). Parameters as in Table 2, DL=0.02.

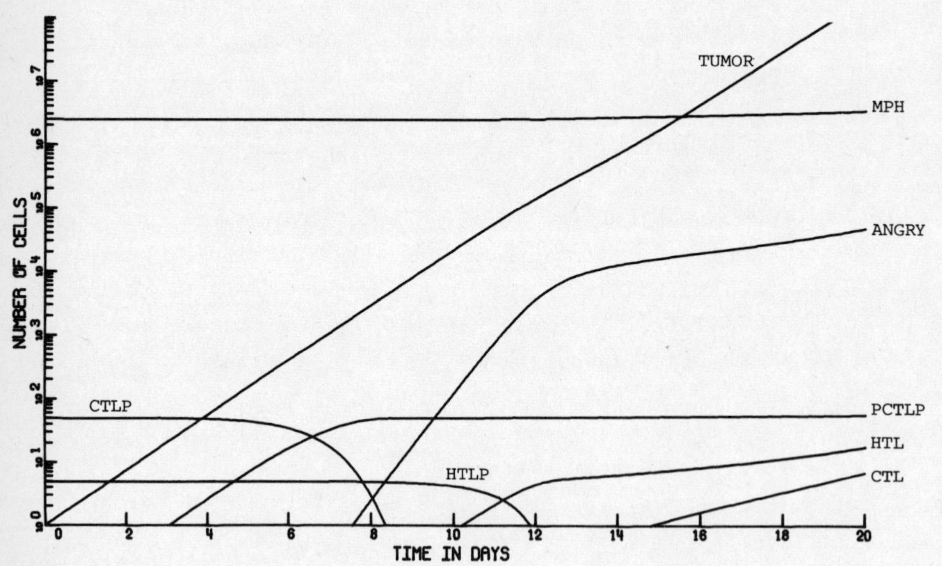

Figure 3. The progressive growth of a tumor corresponding to I1=1.0 (CTLP=50) and I2=0.1 (HTLP=5) introduced as a single cell at day 0. Parameters as in Table 2, DL=0.02.

The general relation between antigenicity and rejectability is depicted in Fig. 4. The figure shows that weakly antigenic tumors cannot be rejected whatever their initial size, whereas tumors that are slightly more antigenic can be rejected even if they are introduced in a large dose. Hundred-fold variations in CTLP reactivity do not change the form and position of the graph in Fig. 4. As was concluded before for our previous models [14], tumor antigenicity can thus best be defined as helper T cell reactivity. Experimentally tumor antigenicity is usually defined as the size of the largest rejectable tumor, which is in our analysis a very insensitive parameter.

Weakly antigenic tumors that escape (e.g. Fig. 3) do not however evoke weaker immune reactions. At day 24 of the simulation shown in Fig. 3 all effector populations are larger than the maximum populations reached in the rejection case (Fig. 2). However, because the tumor is large (>10^9 cells) at that time these effectors have little effect. These results are in close correpondance with the data of Lannin et al. [24], who show that the T-lymphocyte response to a fibrosarcoma is "too little and too slow" for tumor rejection.

Helper T cells play a crucial role in the immune reaction of the model. Helper reactivity for instance determines tumor rejectability (Fig. 4). Moreover, otherwise lethal tumors can be rejected when the

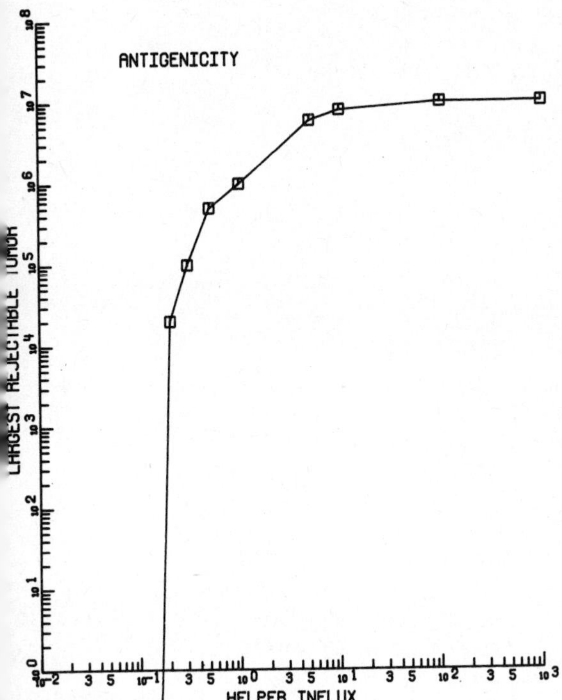

Figure 4. The relation between tumor rejectability (i.e. the size of the largest rejectable tumor) and tumor antigenicity (i.e. HTLP reactivity). The tumors range in antigenicity from I2=0.01 (HTLP=0.5) to I2=1000 (HTLP=50,000). Parameters as in Table 2, DL=0.02.

model is previously immunized with that tumor, due to an increase in HTL numbers [14]. In addition, adoptive transfer of 5 HTL at day zero enables the current model to reject the lethal tumor of Fig. 3. The effect that HTL have on the model behavior is depicted in Fig. 5. At low HTL numbers (i.e. at the back of the cube) the ANGRY isocline lies entirely below the TUMOR´=0 isocline, whereas at high HTL numbers (at the front) the largest part of the ANGRY isocline lies above the TUMOR

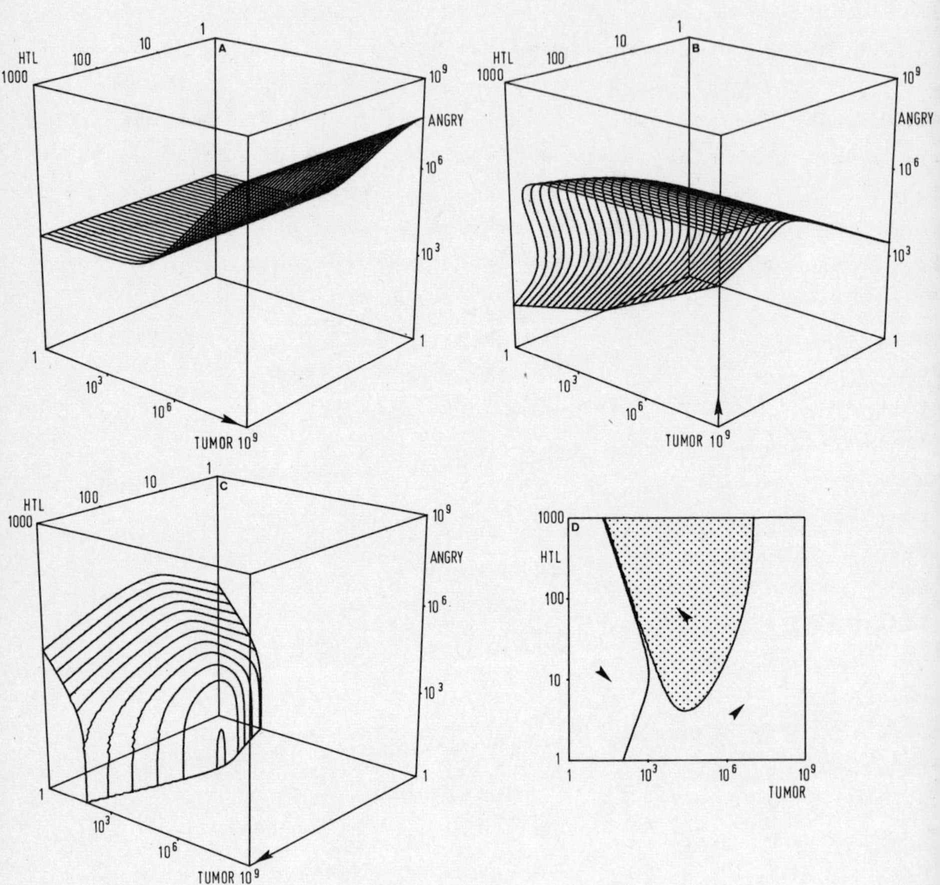

Figure 5. Phase portrait of the model challenged with the tumor of Fig. 3 (rejection). Assuming CTLP, HTLP, MPH, PCTLP, CTL and DEBRIS at their respective (positive) quasi steady state values, we depict the TUMOR´=0 (A), the ANGRY´=0 (B) and the HTL´=0 (C) isocline planes. The arrows indicate the local direction of trajectories. In Fg. 5d ANGRY is also in quasi steady state, the region corresponding to TUMOR´<0 (tumor regression) is shaded in that figure. Parameters as in Table 2, I1=1.0, I2=0.2, DL=0.02.

isocline. Therefore, at the front there is a large region in which TUMOR decreases and ANGRY increases (which corresponds to tumor regression). At the back however trajectories never ascend into the TUMOR´<0 region because ANGRY numbers cannot become large enough there. Tumor rejection is hence impossible at low HTL numbers. In the 2-D phase portrait (Fig. 5d), where ANGRY is at quasi steady state, it is evident that tumor regression (i.e. the shaded region) is only possible at high HTL numbers. The figure (5b, d) also shows that the macrophage response cannot grow infinitely large, so large tumors always increase (large tumor trajectories move to the right along the horizontal part of the ANGRY isocline (Fig. 5b)).

effector switch. In contrast to the "precursor bound" macrophage response [2] the T-lymphocyte response is "proliferative" [15] because it can become infinitely large by repeated T-lymphocyte proliferation. Tumors that are too large to be rejected by macrophages can therefore be rejected by the CTL population if the latter proliferates (provided the tumor population does not have a faster per capita growth rate than the CTL population). However, for the tumor depicted in Fig. 3, CTL proliferation into a large effector population takes such a long time that the tumor meanwhile has killed the mouse. (Since mice die from tumors of about 10^8 cells [25], we stop the simulations around that size). Highly antigenic tumors on the other hand correspond, by definition, to large T-lymphocyte precursor populations, which require fewer cell divisions (i.e. less time) to reach the size required for tumor rejection. In Fig. 6 we show such a case. Note that smaller doses of this highly antigenic tumor (i.e. I1=200, I2=10) would easily be rejected by the ANGRY macrophages.

About 10^8 CTL and 10^7 HTL are present at the time of tumor rejection (day 10). For both populations this roughly corresponds to a 10,000-fold increase (T-lymphocyte populations are reported to be able to expand to this extent [26]). After the rejection of the tumor, proliferation however continues because a large amount of DEBRIS has accumulated; DEBRIS is removed relatively slowly. The removal of DEBRIS upon phagocytosis by macrophages has been omitted from this model for simplicity. Moreover, we have ignored absorption of IL2 by the proliferating cells; if IL2 absorbtion were incorporated the IL2 concentration would decrease faster after tumor rejection. Prolonged proliferation after tumor rejection is probably unrealistic.

In general however, this result (i.e. the predominance of CTL in reactions to large highly antigenic tumors) does correspond to the experimental data. Ishii et al. [27] show that the T-lymphocyte infiltrate of methylcholanthrene-induced sarcomas increases with

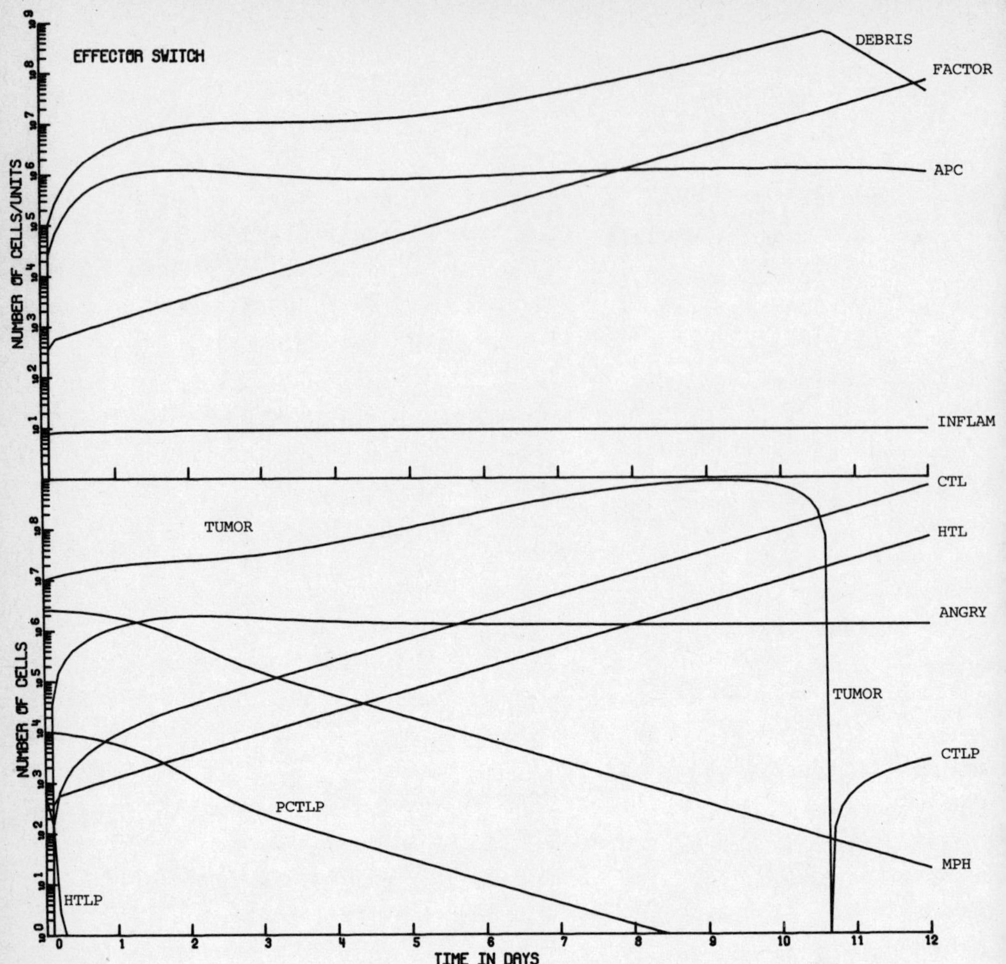

Figure 6. The rejection of an highly antigenic tumor, i.e. I1=200 (CTLP=10^4) and I2=10 (HTLP=500). A large graft of this tumor (10^7 cells) is introduced at day 0 into a non-immunized system (a smaller dose would be rejected by macrophages). Parameters as in Table 2, DL=0.02.

increasing antigenicity of the tumor, whereas the macrophage infiltrate remains grossly equal. CTL are reported to play a significant role in the immune resistance to virus-induced, i.e. highly antigenic, tumors [3]. The current model also accounts for the experimental fact that immunization mainly increases the T-lymphocyte part of the anti-tumor immune response [28]. Immunization increases the number of T-lymphocytes, which consequently require fewer cell divisions (i.e. less time) to become abundant.

Fig. 7 shows the TUMOR′=0 isocline plane in a TUMOR, HTL, and

Figure 7. Phase portrait of the model. In a TUMOR, CTL, HTL state space we depict the TUMOR′=0 isocline plane. CTLP, HTLP, MPH, PCTLP, ANGRY and DEBRIS are assumed to be in (positive) quasi steady state. The arrows indicate the local direction of trajectories. The form and the position of this plane are independent of tumor antigenicity (i.e. I1 and I2) because both T lymphocyte effectors (HTL and CTL) are part of the state space. The figure thus represents all tumors studied hitherto. Parameters as in Table 2, DL=0.02.

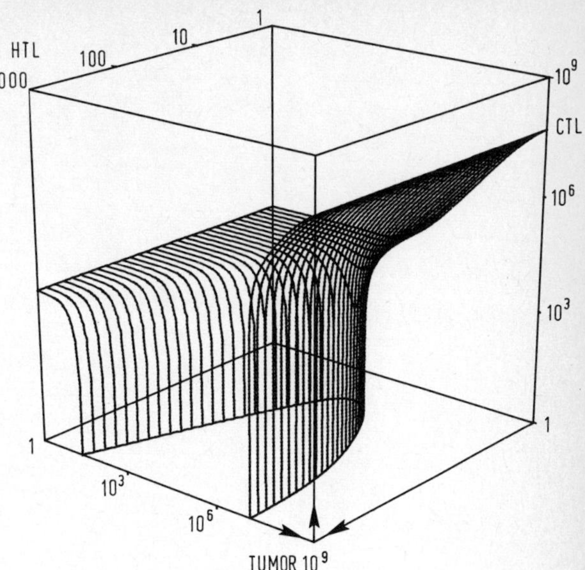

CTL state space (ANGRY and all other variables are in quasi steady state). At high HTL numbers (and hence high ANGRY numbers) intermediate sized tumors regress (i.e. in the central valley), larger tumors however only decrease at high CTL numbers (i.e. above the plane).

<u>sneaking through and low zone tolerance</u>. Although most of the parameters of the model were taken from the literature, see Ref. [14], several had to be filled in arbitrarily. The lifespans of the activated T-lymphocytes (HTL, CTl, PCTLP) are amongst the parameters that were chosen arbitrarily. Experimentally these cells are known to be short-lived as effector cells but they are also known to be long-lived as "memory" cells. The processes that determine T-lymphocyte longevity are largely unknown [29]. In the previous simulations (Fig. 2-7) the rate of T-lymphocyte effector decay was (simply) chosen identical to that of their precursors (i.e. 50 days). In this section however we choose to make the T-lymphocyte effectors (HTL, CTL) short-lived (5 days); all other parameters are left the same.

The longevity of T-lymphocyte effectors has a profound effect on the model behavior. An example is illustrated in Fig. 8. This tumor (having an antigenicity corresponding to I1=1.0, I2=0.3) grows progressively (i.e. sneaks through) when it is introduced in a small dose (e.g. 1 cell, Fig. 8a), it is rejected when introduced in intermediate doses (e.g. 10^4 cells, Fig. 8b), and it grows

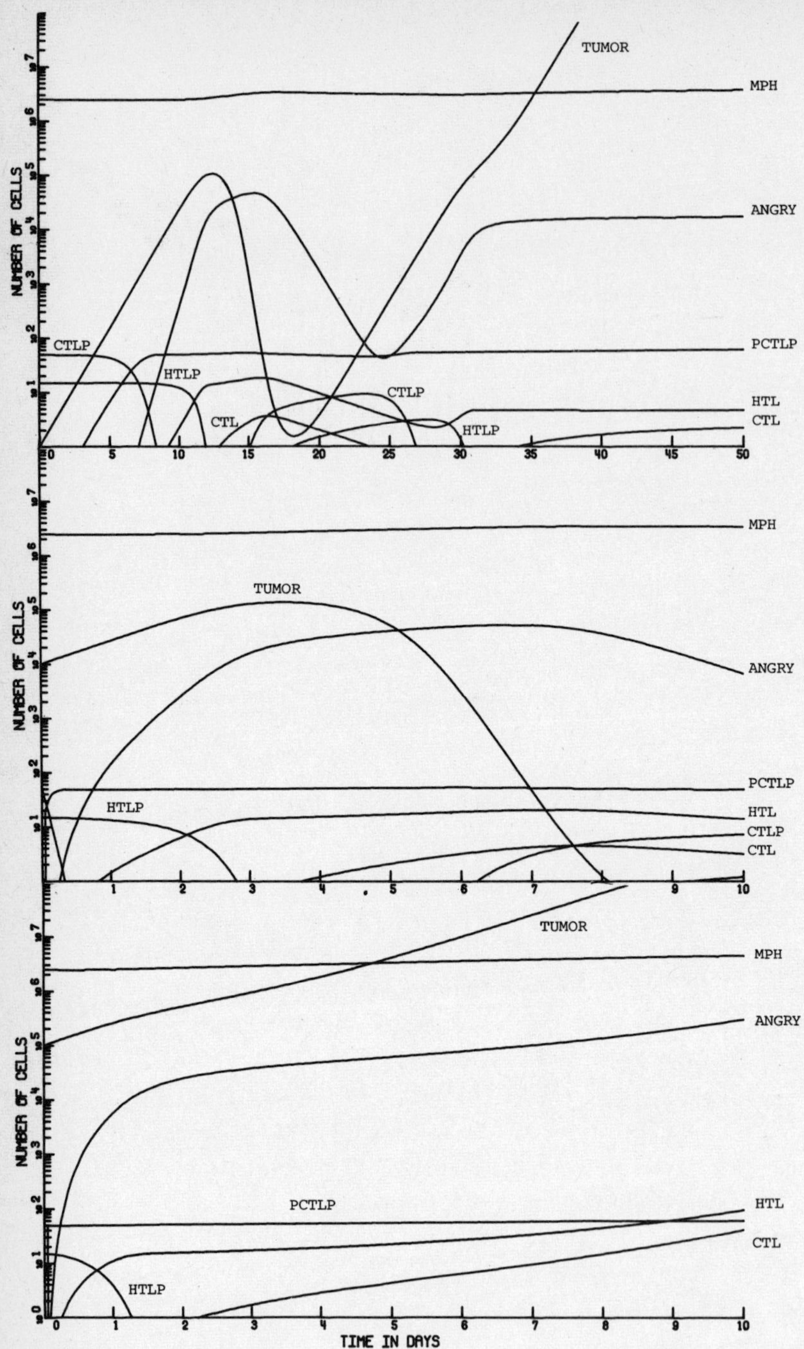

Figure 8. The sneaking through phenomenon. A tumor corresponding to I1=1.0 and I2=0.3 is introduced as a single cell (A), in a dose of 10^4 cells (B), and in a dose of 10^5 cells (C). Only the intermediate sized tumor can be rejected (B). Parameters as in Table 2, DL=0.2.

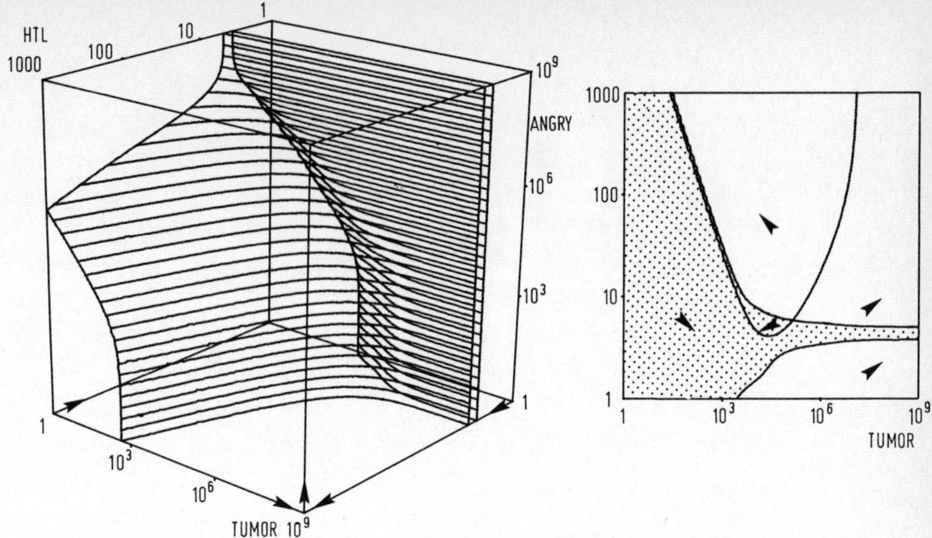

Figure 9. Phase portrait of the sneaking through phenomenon. All variables not depicted in the figure are assumed to be at quasi steady state. The HTL′=0 isocline separates the state space into distinct regions of HTL increase; the HTL′<0 region is shaded in Fig. 9b. The arrows indicate the local direction of trajectories.

progressively again (i.e. breaks through) when it is introduced in a large dose (e.g. 10^5 cells, Fig. 8c). Such behavior is known experimentally as the sneaking through phenomenon: the progressive growth of initially small tumors in circumstances where larger tumors are rejected [30]. Immunization with the same tumor enhances the sneaking through behavior of the model (i.e. increases the range of tumor doses in which sneaking through occurs) [15], which is in agreement with the experimental data [31].

The progressive growth of the tumor introduced in a large dose (Fig. 8c) is accompanied by an ever increasing immune reaction involving extensive T-lymphocyte proliferation. The progressive growth phase of the initially small tumor (Fig. 8a) by contrast, corresponds to a constant response of limited magnitude. Expansion of the antigen (the tumor) does not result in an increase of the immune response. This is known experimentally as tolerance or unresponsiveness. In this model sneaking through thus corresponds to low zone tolerance, i.e. tolerance arising upon the introduction of very small doses of antigen [32, 33]. Prehn [30] argued that sneaking through could not be due to (low zone) tolerance because experimentally it was known to be enhanced by immunization [31]. The present form of sneaking through however is enhanced by immunization and does correspond to low zone tolerance.

The process whereby sneaking through (tolerance) evolves in this model can be revealed by examination of the phase plots in Fig. 9. The figure shows that HTL populations increase when they are small, decrease at intermediate HTL numbers (shaded in 9b), and increase again at large HTL numbers. Thus although the HTL population is capable of infinite growth it first has to bridge a region in which it decreases. We define the minimum size of the HTL population required for continuous increase by proliferation as the proliferation threshold. The proliferation threshold corresponds to the HTL′=0 isocline that is situated at high HTL numbers. If effector cells are long-lived, the proliferation threshold, and hence sneaking through behavior, is absent (Fig. 5c, d).

HTL proliferation depends on the IL2 concentration (i.e. depends on the size of the HTL populations), and is thus a self-reinforcing process. HTL decay however is independent of the presence of other HTL. It is therefore evident (if the maximum proliferation rate exceeds the decay rate) that large (stimulated) HTL populations increase. Small HTL populations, on the other hand, produce only a little IL2, and, as a consequence, proliferate slowly. If these cells are short-lived, the slow proliferation rate will be outweighed by the decay rate. This corresponds to population decrease.

In this model tolerance is thus intrinsic to the kinetics of IL2 production. Small doses of antigen induce low IL2 concentrations because few effectors are activated. As a consequence these effectors decay without much proliferation. By the time the antigen has grown large enough to be able to activate a large number of precursors concomittantly (i.e. large enough to induce high IL2 concentrations), the precursor population has been reduced considerably due to the previous activations. If activation of the remaining precursor population is insufficient to generate an effector population larger than the proliferation threshold, the system is unresponsive (tolerant). Precursor depletion (here by activation) thus disables the system to such an extent that it is never again able to mount immune responses to that antigen. Precursor depletion was previously shown to be responsible for sneaking through in precursor bound models (i.e. systems that specify proliferation as a "once only" occurence) [2]. The proliferation threshold makes the current proliferative T-lymphocyte system precursor bound when it is slowly activated.

These results are in close correspondence with recent experimental data [34, 35], which show that immunological activation in the absence of IL2 results in tolerance. In fact, it has been repeatedly shown that antigenic stimulation (signal 1) in the absence of helper T cell factors (signal 2) results in tolerance [36, 37, 38]. We show here that the absence of signal 2 (FACTOR) can be caused by slow activation, and, moreover, that a high turnover rate of effector cells suffices for the generation of tolerance.

DISCUSSION

methodology. In this paper we have concentrated on the dynamic behavior of the model, and not on the existence of steady states. We have shown that small differences in the model's initial state can markedly influence the dynamic behavior. For instance, the (artificial) introduction of 5 HTL at day zero (i.e. adoptive transfer) changes the progressive tumor-growth behavior into tumor rejection behavior. In addition, the results on sneaking through show that the initial antigen dose can be of crucial importance for the outcome of the immune response (this is in fact one of the most interesting results).

Furthermore it is dynamically important that we stop the simulations whenever the tumor becomes smaller than one cell (i.e. tumor rejection) and whenever it grows too large (which corresponds to death of the host). For instance, the immune reactions to the tumors of Fig. 2 and 3 have a stable equilibrium at CTL=7050, ANGRY=2950, and HTL=4876, TUMOR=1.3 and HTL=2551, TUMOR=2.5 respectively. Both steady states are however only reached (a) after an unrealistically long time (>100,000 years), and (b) either via extremely small (Fig. 2, after "tumor rejection") or via extremely large (Fig. 3, after day 20) tumor sizes. These steady states are very similar (they differ by a factor two in HTL and TUMOR numbers upon a 2-fold change in antigenicity), but the corresponding dynamic behavior of the model is very different (i.e. rejection versus progressive tumor growth). It thus turns out that biologically meaningful results could only be obtained by studying the dynamic behavior; the steady states of these models are of minor (biological) importance.

Numerical integration (simulation) is the only tool available for this sort of "dynamical" analysis of complex models. One of the disadvantages of numerical integration is the large parameter and state space that have to be investigated. The (numerical) steady state analysis that we perform (by means of 0-isoclines) however structurizes this large search space. Moreover, we show that the number of dimensions of state spaces can be reduced (by making quasi steady state assumptions) with preservation of an interpretable correspondance of the 0-isocline plot to the model behavior. Thus, the combination of numerical integration and graphical analysis of 0-isoclines enables us to study the interesting (dynamical) properties of relatively large models without "getting lost" in confusingly large parameter and state spaces.

compartimentalization. In this model we consider only one compartment, i.e. the peritoneal cavity of a DBA/2 mouse. For macrophages this is a reasonable assumption because these cells probably do not recirculate. Macrophages enter the tissue compartment (e.g. the peritoneal cavity) from the blood compartment, and they are reported to die (although this remains uncertain) in the lymph node draining the tissue compartment [39]. T-lymphocytes on the other hand do recirculate, and moreover they do so rapidly [40]. However, because T-lymphocytes recirculate rapidly the populations in the model can also be considered to represent the total T-lymphocyte populations (i.e. those of the whole body), since all T-lymphocytes then travel through the peritoneal cavity often. If T-lymphocytes do indeed recirculate rapidly, increased T-lymphocyte influx (i.e. inflammation) becomes of minor importance. INFLAM in that case however incorporates the increased production of T-lymphocyte precursor cells after an antigenic stimulation [41].

antigenicity. The relationship between tumor rejectability and tumor antigenicity, as depicted in Fig. 4, remains similar if effectors are made short-lived. For instance, a tumor corresponding to I2=0.2 cannot be rejected whatever its size (if DL=0.2), whereas the tumor of Fig. 8 (I2=0.3) can be rejected when it is large. If introduced in small doses the latter tumor will however sneak through (Fig. 8a). Thus, although the form of the curve of the largest rejectable tumor (Fig. 4) remains the same, it is no longer true that tumors that are smaller than the largest rejectable tumor are also rejected.

It is important to note that the ascitic SL2 tumor grows fast (about one division every 16 hours) [20]. The fact that the model's immune response is "too slow" for tumor rejection may therefore depend on a fast growth rate of the tumor. The form of the relation between tumor rejectability and tumor antigenicity however remains the same for slow growing (e.g. R=0.1) tumors. The curve is shifted to the left, i.e. to tumors with a lower degree of antigenicity. However small doses of slow growing tumors, which can be rejected in large doses, rapidly reach a stable equilibrium (i.e. exhibit tumor dormancy [42]). This occurs independently of T-lymphocyte longevity. Sneaking through of slow growing tumors is thus absent for this particular parameter setting; however it does occur for other parameter values. CTL are more important in the reaction to slow growing tumors that to fast growing tumors because they have more time for proliferation.

implications of interactions. This model deviates from a related model investigated previously [14, 15] in two interactions: here (1) HTL restimulation depends on APC (formerly on TUMOR), and (2) CTLP differentiation depends on HTL (formerly independent). We have studied both models using an almost identical parameter setting. The study of various models for a fixed set of parameters (i.e. the multi-model fixed-parameter approach [2]), provides insight into the role of the interactions that are varied. Alternatively, a set of different models can be studied for "externally equivalent" parameter values, see Refs. [43, 44]. The behavior of the current model differs from that of the previous model in that it shows the continued T-lymphocyte proliferation after tumor rejection. This is due to the incorporation of HTL restimulation by APC instead of by TUMOR. The incorporation of HTL factors required for the differentiation of CTLP seems to have little effect.

CTL proliferation is incorporated at the effector stage. We have also studied models that incorporate CTL proliferation at the intermediate non-cytotoxic stage. These proliferating cells mature (terminally) into the cytotoxic effector stage upon the release of HTL-derived differentiation factors [45]. The incorporation of these interactions influences the system behavior markedly: CTL populations no longer grow infinitely large because they mature into non-dividing effectors at some stage of the immune response. This can lead to "exhaustive terminal differentiation" [46] which corresponds to the theoretically described "overmaturation" [47, 48]; this results in reduced immune responses in the case of high doses of antigen. Low zone tolerance (e.g. sneaking through) however remains unaffected by the incorporation of terminal differentiation [45].

tolerance. We have shown above that in this proliferative model, in which no negative (e.g. suppressive) interactions were incorporated, unresponsiveness evolves when T-lymphocyte precursor cells become depleted. In the case of tumors this generates the sneaking through phenomenon. In the case of antigens that do not expand infinitely (e.g. an allogenic organ graft) this corresponds to a stable equilibrium between the organ at its normal size and an immune reaction of very limited magnitude [45]. Such a tolerance state evolves in low zone circumstances (like sneaking through evolves here) and in "neonatal" circumstances, i.e. in immature immune systems. Depletion of helper T cell precursors and the course of IL2 production determine whether tolerance or a vigorous immune reaction develops.

ACKNOWLEDGEMENTS

We are grateful to Prof. Rudy Ballieux for his enthusiastic support. The participants of the workshop are thanked for their helpful criticism; which we have tried to incorporate in the present paper. We thank Miss S.M. McNab for linguistic advice.

REFERENCES

1. Hogeweg, P. and B. Hesper. 1981. Two predators and one prey in a patchy environment: an application of MICMAC modelling. J. Theor. Biol. 93:411.
2. De Boer, R.J. and P. Hogeweg. 1985. Tumor escape from immune elimination: simplified precursor bound cytotoxicity models. J. Theor. Biol. 113:719.
3. Herberman, R.B. 1983. Lymphoid cells in immune surveillance against malignant transformation. In: Adv. in Host Defense Mechanisms, Vol. 2. Eds. J.I. Gallin and A.S. Fauci. Raven Press, New York P. 241.
4. Steel, G.G. 1977. Growth kinetics of tumours. Clarendon Press, Oxford.
5. Unanue, E.R. 1984. Antigen-presenting function of the macrophage. Ann. Rev. Immunol. 2:395.
6. Czitrom, A.A., G.H. Sunshine, T. Reme, R. Ceredig, A.L. Glasebrook, A. Kelso, and H.R. McDonald. 1983. Stimulator cell requirements for allospecific T cell subsets: specialized accessory cells are required to activate helper but not cytolytic T-lymphocyte precursors. J. Immunol. 130:2.
7. Wagner, H., C. Hardt, K. Heeg, K. Pfizenmaier, W. Solbach, R. Bartlett, H. Stockinger, and M. Röllinghoff. 1980. T-T cell interactions during CTL response: T cell derived helper factors (interleukin 2) as a probe to analyse CTL responsiveness and thymic maturation of CTL progenitors. Immunol. Rev. 51:215.
8. Mizel, S.B. 1982. Interleukin 1 and T cell activation. Immunol. Rev. 63:51.
9. Van Furth, R. and D. Blusse Van Oud Alblas. 1982. The current view on the origin of pulmonary macrophages. Pathol. Res. Pract. 175:38.
10. Wagner, H., C. Hardt, B.T. Rouse, M. Röllinghoff, P. Scheurlich, and K. Pfizenmaier. 1982. Dissection of the proliferative and differentiative signals controlling murine cytotoxic T-lymphocyte responses. J. Exp. Med. 155:1876.

11. Falk, W., D.N. Männel, and W. Dröge. 1983. Activation of cytotoxic T-lymphocytes requires at least two spleen cell-derived helper factors besides interleukin 2. J. Immunol. 130:2214.
12. Kelso, A. and A.L. Glasebrook. 1984. Secretion of interleukin 2, macrophage-activating factor, interferon, and colony-stimulating factor by alloreactive T-lymphocyte clones. J. Immunol. 132:2924.
13. Van Loveren, H., K. Kato, R. Meade, D.R. Green, M. Horowitz, W. Ptak, and P.W. Askenase. 1984. Characterization of two different Ly-1^{+}T cell populations that mediate delayed-type hypersensitivity. J. Immunol. 133:2402.
14. De Boer, R.J., P. Hogeweg, H.F.J. Dullens, R.A. De Weger, and W. Den Otter. 1985. Macrophage T-lymphocyte interactions in the anti-tumor immune response: a mathematical model. J. Immunol. 134:2748.
15. De Boer, R.J. and P. Hogeweg. submitted. Macrophage T-lymphocyte interactions II: sneaking through intrinsic to helper T cell dynamics.
16. Berendt, M.J. and R.J. North. 1980. T cell-mediated suppression of anti-tumor immunity. An explanation for progressive growth of an immunogenic tumor. J. Exp. Med. 151:69.
17. Herberman, R.B. 1982. Cells suppressing cell-mediated immune responses of cancer patients. In: Human Suppressor Cell, Ed. B. Serrou. North Holland, Amsterdam P. 179.
18. Prehn, R.T. 1982. Antigenic heterogeneity: a possible basis for progression. In: Tumor Cell Heterogeneity: Origins and Implications. Eds. A.H. Owens, D.S. Coffey, and S.B. Baylin. Academic Press, New York and London P. 73.
19. Old, L.J., E. Stockert, E.A. Boyse, and J.H. Kim. 1968. Antigenic modulation. Loss of TL antigen from cells exposed to TL antibody. Study of the phenomenon in vitro. J. Exp. Med. 127:523.
20. Dullens, H.F.J., J. Hilgers, B.J. Spit, E. De Heer, R.A. De Weger, C.D.H. Van Basten, and W. Den Otter. 1982. Staging, growth properties and metastatic behaviour of a transplantable murine T cell lymphoma. Cancer Treat. Rep. 63:99.
21. Den Otter, W. 1981. The effect of activated macrophages on tumor growth in vitro and in vivo. Lymphokines 3:389.
22. De Boer, R.J. 1983. GRIND: Great Integrator Differential Equations. Bioinformatics Group, University of Utrecht, The Netherlands.
23. Gottwald, B.A. and G. Wanner. 1981. A reliable Rosenbrock integrator for stiff differential equations. Computing 26:355.
24. Lannin, D.R., S. Yu, and C.F. McKahn. 1982. Thymus-dependent response: too little and too late for immune surveillance. Transplantation 33:99.
25. Dullens, H.F.J., C. Venengoor, R.A. De Weger, F. Woutersen, R.A. Woutersen, and W. Den Otter. 1979. Comparison of various forms of therapy in two different mouse tumour systems. Cancer Treat. Rep. 63:99.
26. Miller, R.A. and O. Stutman. 1984. T cell repopulation from functionally restricted splenic progenitors: 10,000-fold expansion documented by using limiting dilution analysis. J. Immunol. 133:2925.
27. Ishii, Y., A. Matsuura, T. Takami, T. Uede, Y. Ibayashi, T. Uede, M. Imamura, K. Kikuchi, and Y. Kikuchi. 1984. Lymphoid cell subpopulations infiltrating into autologous rate tumors undergoing rejection. Cancer Res. 44:4053.
28. Ibayashi, Y., T. Uede, T. Uede, and K. Kikuchi. 1985. Functional analysis of mononuclear cells infiltrating into tumors: differential cytotoxicity of mononuclear cells from tumors of immune and nonimmune rats. J. Immunol. 134:648.
29. Jerne, N.K. 1984. Idiotypic networks and other preconceived ideas. Immunol. Rev. 79:5.
30. Prehn, R.T. 1976. Immunostimulation of the lymphodependent phase

of neoplastic growth. J. Natl. Cancer Inst. 59:1043.
31. Marchant, J. 1969. Sarcoma induction in mice by methylcholanthrene. Antigenicity tests of sarcomas induced in thymus grafted and control animals. Br. J. Cancer 23:383.
32. Mitchison, N.A. 1965. Induction of immunological paralysis in two zones of dosage. Proc. R. Soc. Lond. Ser. B 161:275.
33. Weigle, W.O. 1971. Recent observations and concepts in immunological unresponsiveness and autoimmunity. Clin. Exp. Immunol. 9:437.
34. Malkovský, M. and P.B. Medawar. 1984. Is immunological tolerance (non-responsiveness) a consequence of interleukin 2 deficit during the recognition of antigen?. Immunol. Today 5:340.
35. Malkovský, M., P. Medawar, R. Hunt, L. Palmer, and C. Doré. 1984. A diet rich in vitamin A acetate or in vivo administration of interleukin-2 can counteract a tolerogenic stimulus. Proc. R. Soc. Lond. B 220:439.
36. Bretscher, P. and M. Cohn. 1970. A theory of self-nonself discrimination. Paralysis and induction involve the recognition of one and two determinants on an antigen, respectively. Science 169:1042.
37. Teale, J.M., J.E. Layton, and G.J.V. Nossal. 1979. In vitro model for natural tolerance to self antigens. J. Exp. Med. 150:205.
38. Cleveland, R.P. and H.N. Claman. 1980. T cell signals: tolerance to DNFB is converted to sensitization by a separate nonspecific second signal. J. Immunol. 124:474.
39. Van Furth, R., M.M.C. Diesselhoff-Den Dulk, J.A. Raeburn, T.L. Van Zwet, R. Crofton, and A. Blussé Van Oud Alblas. 1980. Characteristics, origin and kinetics of human and murine mononuclear phagocytes. In: Mononuclear Phagocytes, Functional Aspects I, Ed. R. Van Furth. Martinus Nyhoff, The Hague P. 295.
40. Bell, G.I. 1978. Lymphocyte traffic patterns and cell-cell interactions. In: Theoretical Immunology, Eds. G.I. Bell, A.S Perelson, and G.H. Pimbley. Marcel Dekker, New York and Basel P. 341.
41. Schreier, M.H. and N.N. Iscove. 1980. Hematopoietic growth factors are released in cultures of H-2-restricted helper T cells accessory cells and specific antigen. Nature 287:228.
42. Trainer, D.L. and E.F. Wheelock. 1984. Phenotypic shifts in the L5178Y Lymphoma during progression of the tumor-dormant state in DBA/2 mice. Cancer Res. 44:1063.
43. Irvine, D.H., and M.A. Savageau. 1985. Network regulation of the immune response: alternative control points for suppressor modulation of effector lymphocytes. J. Immunol. 134:2100.
44. Irvine, D.H., and M.A. Savageau. 1985. Network regulation of the immune response: modulation of suppressor lymphocytes by alternative signals including contrasuppression. J. Immunol. 134:2117.
45. De Boer, R.J. and P. Hogeweg. submitted. Immunological tolerance arises due to the kinetics of IL2 production.
46. Strezl, S. 1966. Immunological tolerance as the result of terminal differentiation of immunologically competent cells. Nature 209:416.
47. Grossman, Z. 1982. Recognition of self, balance of growth and competition: horizontal networks regulate immune responsiveness. Eur. J. Immunol. 12:747.
48. Grossman, Z. 1984. Recognition of self and regulation of specificity at the level of cell populations. Immunol. Rev. 79:119.
49. Merrill, S.J. 1982. Foundations of the use of an enzyme-kinetic analogy in cell-mediated cytotoxicity. Math. Biosci. 62:219.

PART IV

EPIDEMIOLOGY AND THE IMMUNE SYSTEM

MODELS OF THE DYNAMICS OF ACQUIRED IMMUNITY TO HELMINTH INFECTION IN MAN

Roy M. Anderson
Department of Pure and Applied Biology,
Imperial College, London University,
London SW7 2BB
England

INTRODUCTION

Upon invading a host organism, parasitic species invariably trigger the defence mechanisms of the immune system. In vertebrate hosts, the system comprises of cells, antibodies, amplification factors and specialized organs. The immune system sometimes enables the host to regulate parasitic abundance and to build up a degree of acquired resistance to reinfection. However, in the case of most parasitic protozoa and helminths, the degree of acquired immunity illicited by infection is variable, and not so solid as that induced by many viruses or bacteria. In endemic areas of the world parasitic infections therefore tend to be persistent in character, where the human inhabitants are repeatedly exposed to reinfection and may harbour parasites for the majority of their lives. The major helminth infections of man (the intestinal nemotodes, the schistosome flukes and the filarial worms) are particularly remarkable in this sense, since man appears unable to develop fully protective immunity, despite repeated exposure to high levels of infection. In part, this is thought to be a consequence of the antigenic complexity of parasitic worms, and their often complex developmental cycles within the human host. Each developmental stage may express different surface or excretory antigens. As a consequence of this complexity, it is usually difficult to relate particular antigenic components of the parasite, to the generation of the immune response. Many problems surround the identification of antigens, which elicit protective responses and antigens with no apparent role in resistance (i.e between functional or non-functional antigens) (Wakelin, 1984).

Evidence of acquired immunity in man to helminth infection, is largely circumstantial in nature. The observation that average worm burdens tend to be lower in adults than children (age-intensity of infection profiles are often convex in forms) (Figs. 1, 2 and 3) is often quoted as evidence for immunity. The inference is that acquired resistance, built up from past exposure to infection in childhood, reduces parasite establishment, fecundity and survival in adults. However, similar patterns of change in the intensity of infection with age, could equally arise from age-related changes in contact with infection, given that adult parasite life expectancy is thought to be much less than human life expectancy (a few years as opposed to a few decades). Whether or not such patterns result from acquired immunity or age-related contact processes, is a matter of some controversy at present (Warren, 1978; Anderson and May, 1985). It is probable that both factors play important roles.

Laboratory studies of mammalian host-helminth parasite systems, clearly indicate that immunological responses can reduce parasite establishments, survival or fecundity in a manner dependent on the degree of antigenic stimulation (parasite load) (Wakelin, 1984).

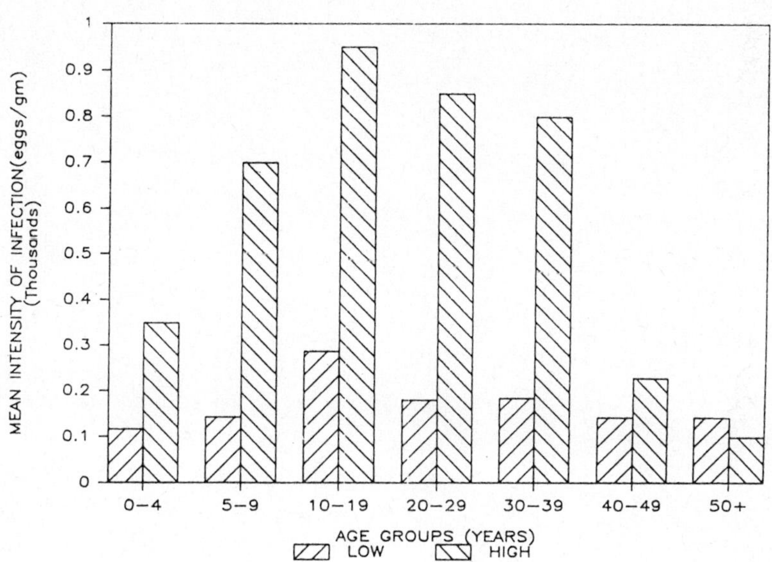

Figure 1. Age-intensity of infection (egg output/gram faeces) profiles for high and low transmission areas with endemic Schistosoma mansoni infection (data from Siongok et al., 1976; Abdel-Wahab et al., 1980). Convex patterns of change with age are more commonly associated with areas of high transmission.

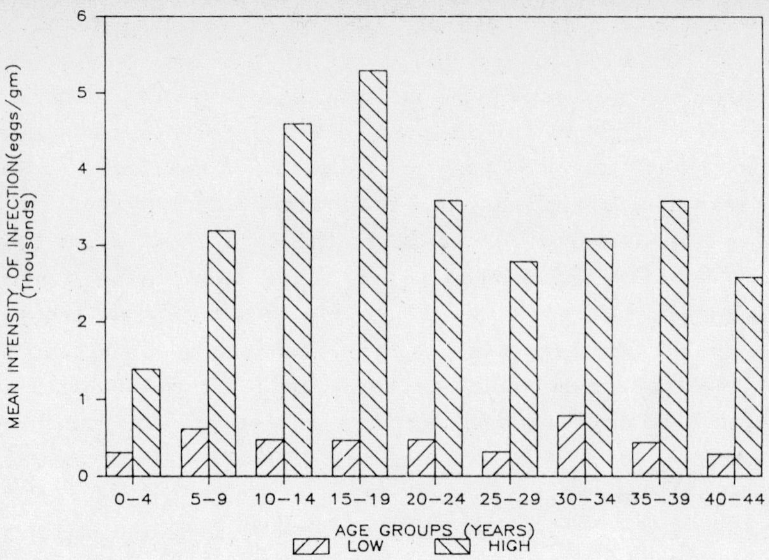

Figure 2. Similar to Figure 1 but recording changes in hookworm infection with age in areas of high and low transmission (data from Pesigan *et al*., 1958; Carr, 1926).

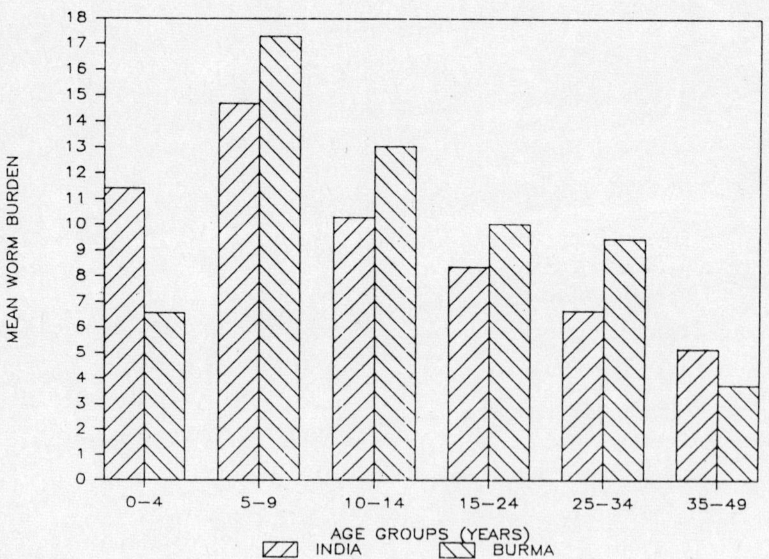

Figure 3. Similar to Figure 1 but recording the changes in *Ascaris lumbricoides* (roundworm) infection (mean worm burden) from a set of fishing villages in Southern India and some rural villages in Burma (data from Elkins, Haswell-Elkins and Anderson, 1985; Hlaing, 1985).

Despite the lack of firm evidence at present, it appears highly likely that similar responses play an important role in regulating helminth parasite abundance and transmission within human communities (Cohen and Warren, 1982).

This paper explores the role of acquired immunity, in regulating helminth parasite transmission and population growth, by means of the construction and analysis of simple mathematical models. Particular emphasis is placed on the influence of immunity on the patterns of change in mean worm load with the age of the host, variability in immunocompetence or exposure to infection within human communities and the impact of control measures on herd immunity. The paper is organised as follows. The first section, outlines the basic mathematical framework describing the parasite's dynamics and transmission in the absence of acquired resistance. The second, third and fourth sections, consider more complex models in which acquired immunity is dependent on the accumulated degree of exposure to infection. The fifth section examines the influence of age-related changes in contact with infection, and the sixth section explores the impact of heterogenity in exposure or immunological competance. After a brief discussion of age-related changes in parasite distributions with human communities, the final two sections examine the impact of control measures (chemotherapy and vaccination) on parasite transmission and herd immunity.

MATHEMATICAL MODELS

:) Deterministic Framework

Despite the volume of published work on the epidemiology of parasitic infections, relatively few attempts have been made to construct models of the transmission dynamics of helminth parasites. Early work includes the studies of Kositzin (1934), Hairston (1965), Macdonald (1965), Leyton (1968) and Tallis and Leyton (1969). More recently, a small but growing body of literature has focused on deterministic models for both directly and indirectly transmitted infections, and their use in the design of control programmes based on chemotherpeutic treatment (see Anderson, 1982; Anderson and May 1982, 1985).

A description of the temporal dynamics of parasite population growth, within human communities, can be given in terms of one variable, M(t,a); the mean adult worm burden in people of age a, at time t. The details of the parasites transmission via the segments of the life cycle (e.g. snail, insect vector or free-living infective stage) not involving man, may be 'collapsed' into a single non-linear partial differential equation for M(a,t). This simplifying assumption follows from the observation that the durations of stay of the parasite, in the free-living environment or in the snail or insect vector (ranging from a few days to a few weeks) are typically much shorter than adult parasite life expectancy in man (ranging from 1 to many years (see Anderson and May, 1982)). Mathematical models for helminth transmission, are usually based on a 'density' framework (the density of parasites within a host), as opposed to the 'prevalence' framework (the proportion of hosts infected) widely adopted for viral and bacterial infections. The mean, M(a,t), is simply a summary statistic of the full probability distribution of parasite numbers per person with a given community. These distributions are typically highly aggregated in form where the numerical value of the variance greatly exceeds that of the mean (the negative binomial probability distribution is a good model of observed patterns). The distribution of parasites is clearly important with respect to the net severity of density-dependent constraints acting to suppress parasite survival or fecundity within the host. In addition, the morbidity induced by infection is invariably proportional to worm load.

Within a deterministic framework, the distribution of parasite numbers per host can be mirrored by making a phenomological assumption, where the distribution is taken to be fixed and negative binomial in form, independent of the values of the rate parameters that control parasite and host population growth and the functional dependencies of the major variables (see Anderson and May, 1978; May and Anderson, 1978). Ideally, a full stochastic framework should be employed, but these models have proved difficult to investigate by analytical means, due to the non-linearities that arise from density-dependent constraints on parasite population growth within individual hosts. In the absence of acquired immunity a simple deterministic model of changes in M(a,t) with respect to host age a, and time t is as follows:

$$\partial M/\partial t + \partial M/\partial a = \Lambda(t) - \mu M \tag{1}$$

where

$$\Lambda(t) = (R_o \mu/L) \int_0^\infty l(a)\, M(t,a)\, f(M,k,z)da \tag{2}$$

Here $\Lambda(t)$ denotes the rate of host infection as a function of the basic reproductive rate of the parasite (the average number of offspring produced by a female parasite that attains reproductive maturity in the absence of density dependent constraints), R_o, the age specific survival rate of the host (= man), l(a), where life expectancy $L = \int_0^\infty l(a)\, da$, the death rate of the adult parasite, μ, (life expectancy $A = 1/\mu$) and the density dependent fecundity rate of the adult parasite denoted by the function f(M,k,z) (Anderson and May, 1982). With the assumptions that the distribution of worms per person is fixed and negative binomial in form with clumping parameter k (varies inversely with the degree of parasite contagion) and that the per capita parasite fecundity decays exporentially with increases in worm load, the function f is of the form;

$$f(M,k,z) = [1 + (1-z)\, M/k]^{-(k+1)} \tag{3}$$

Here z = exp (-b), where b denotes the severity of decrease in fecundity as worm burden rises. The model contains five major biological assumptions, namely; (1) the parasites are distributed in a negative binomial manner with clumping parameter k independent of host age; (2) parasite mortality is constant and independent of parasite or host age, or worm load; (3) regulation of parasite transmission results from density dependent constraints on fecundity; (4) the rate of infection ($\Lambda(t)$) is independent of host age and (5) the human host is unable to acquire immunity to infection.

At equilibrium (where $\partial M/\partial t = 0$) eqn. (1) reduces to a simple differential equation for M(a)

$$dM/da = \Lambda - \mu M(a) \tag{4}$$

with solution

$$M(a) = (\Lambda/\mu)(1-e^{-\mu a}) \tag{5}$$

where

$$\Lambda = (R_o \mu)/L \int_0^\infty l(a)\, M(a)\, f(M,k,z)\, da$$

If the life expectancy of the parasite is short in relation to that of its human host (A<<L), the mean worm burden rises rapidly as host age increases to reach a plateau (Λ/μ) such that the mean worm burden, M(a), in the majority of age classes, is essentially equal to the mean worm burden of the total population, M^*. As such a good estimate of Λ is given by:

$$\Lambda = R_o\, M^*\, f(M^*,k,z) \tag{6}$$

where

$$M^* = [R_o^{1/(k+1)} - 1][k/(1-z)] \tag{7}$$

Given that the worms are distributed in a negative binomial manner, the prevalence of infection (= proportion infected) P(a) is simply:

$$P(a) = 1 - [1+M(a)/k]^{-k} \tag{8}$$

The model defined by eqns. (5) and (8) has proved useful in studies of the epidemiology and transmission dynamics of certain directly transmitted intestinal nematode infections (such as Ascaris) where observed changes in worm load with age exhibit a rapid rise to a stable plateau as age increases (Anderson and May, 1982; Croll et al., 1981). More generally, however, observed profiles of changes in worm burden with human age, exhibit convex patterns where the average worm burden rises to a peak in the child to teenage classes, and declines in the older age groups (Figs. 1, 2 and 3). Such patterns are thought to arise as a consequence of two factors, namely; acquired immunity to infection in the older age classes, and age related changes in contact with infective stages (or infected vectors) (Anderson and May, 1985; Warren, 1978).

2) Acquired Immunity

Current understanding of immunity to helminth infection is largely based on experimental work involving laboratory host (rats or mice) - parasite systems. Laboratory studies reveal that rodent, canid and primate species, are able to mount immune responses to helminth invasion. In contrast to many viral, bacterial and protozoan infections, however, such responses provide only partial protection to reinfection following an initial exposure. The immune responses elicited by helminths tend to be complex and involve both antibody activity and cellular sensitization (Wakelin, 1984). With respect to the major parasites of man, current evidence suggests that people living in endemic areas are repeatedly exposed to infection such that a new born child will harbour worms for the majority of its life. Immunological responses to invasion are detectable, but they appear to be unable to provide fully protective immunity (= sterile immunity). They are thought to reduce parasite establishment, survival and fecundity in a manner related to the degree and duration of past exposure to infection (Wakelin, 1984). Laboratory studies involving the repeated exposure (= trickle infection) of rodent hosts to various helminth species (nematodes and digeneans) reveal that acquired resistance to infection builds up slowly over long periods of time (Crombie and Anderson, 1985; Anderson and Crombie, 1985).

Recent research has provided a starting point for the development of a mathematical framework to help explore the impact of acquired immunity on the transmission dynamics of helminth species (Anderson and May, 1985a, 1985b; Anderson 1985). The work is based on models which incorporate the assumption that the rates of parasite establishment or survival within the host are dependent on the accumulated past experience of infection. The general form of these models can be expressed as follows (where M(a,t) is as defined in eqn. (1));

$$\partial M/\partial t + \partial M/\partial a = F[\bar{M}(a,t)] - G[\bar{M}(a,t)]M \quad (9)$$

Here the functions F and G denote respectively, the per capita rates of parasite establishment (per host) and mortality (per parasite). The variable $\bar{M}$ records the accumulated sum of past experience of infection in a host of age a, at time t, where

$$\bar{M}(a,t) = \int_0^a M(a',t-(a-a'))da' \quad (10)$$

At equilibrium ($\partial M/\partial t=0$) eqn. (9) reduces to a differential equation for changes in mean worm burden with age;

$$dM/da = F[\bar{M}(a)] - G[\bar{M}(a)]M \quad (11)$$

where

$$\bar{M}(a) = \int_0^a M(a')da'$$

The principal features of current understanding of acquired immunity to helminths can be crudely captured by a model in which the rate of extablishment of new parasites and death of adult parasites are linear functions of the accumulated average experience of infection (Anderson and May, 1985). These assumptions can be represented as follows:

$$F[M(a)] = \Lambda[1- \Delta\int_0^a \Lambda e^{-\sigma_2(a-a')} da' - \epsilon\int_0^a M(a')e^{-\sigma_1(a-a')} da'] \quad (12)$$

$$G[M(a)] = \mu + \gamma\int_0^a M(a')e^{-\sigma_3(a-a')} da' \quad (13)$$

Here Λ denotes the per capita rate of infection. It is a function of the average fecundity of mature worms, infective stage life expectancy or infected vector life expectancy, host density and the probability of host contact with infective stages or infected vectors (Anderson and May, 1982). In eqn. (12) the parameters Δ and ϵ record the strengths of acquired immunity as it acts to decrease parasite establishement due either to exposure to infection (Δ) or to adult parasite burden (ϵ). The terms $1/\sigma_1$, and $1/\sigma_2$ reflect the average duration of the 'immunological memory' of past exposure and past worm loads respectively (if σ_i; = 0, memory is life-long; if $\sigma_i = \infty$ memory is absent). In eqn. (13) $1/\mu$ denotes adult parasite life expectancy in naive hosts, denotes the severity of rise in worm death rate as the accumulated experience of infection increases and $1/\sigma_3$ denotes the memory duration of past experience relevant to the immunologically mediated reduction in parasite survival within the host.

An understanding of the equilibrium properties of this complex model is facilitated by considering a special case in which acquired immunity is assumed to simply act to reduce parasite establishment in a manner dependent on past worm loads (i.e $\epsilon > 0$, $\Delta = \gamma = 0$). Under these conditions the mean worm burden at equilibrium in host of age a, M(a) is given by the solution of eqn. (11) as follows:

Case 1

For $(\mu - \sigma)^2 > 4\epsilon\Lambda$;

$$M(a) = A + (\Lambda/\lambda)\left[\frac{(p_1+\sigma)e^{p_1 a}}{p_1} - \frac{(p_2+\sigma)e^{p_2 a}}{p_2}\right] \quad (14)$$

where

$A = \Lambda\sigma/(\sigma\mu + \epsilon\Lambda)$, $\lambda = ([\mu-\sigma]^2 - 4\epsilon\Lambda)^{1/2}$, $p_1 = (\lambda - \mu - \sigma)/2$ and $p_2 = -(\lambda + \mu + \sigma)/2$.

The infection rate Λ may be defined as $\Lambda = C\hat{M}$ where C is a transmission coefficient and $\hat{M}$ is the mean worm burden in the whole population; $\hat{M} = \int_0^\infty M(a)\, e^{-a/L}\, da$ where L is human life expectancy (it is assumed that human survival decays exponentially with parameter 1/L). By integration of eqn. (14) we get

$$\hat{M} = \Lambda(1/L+\sigma)/[(1/L+\mu)(1/L+\sigma) + \epsilon\Lambda]$$

Thus

$$\Lambda = (\sigma+1/L)(\mu+1/L)(R_o-1)/\epsilon \quad (15)$$

where R_o is the basic reproductive rate of the parasite (see eqn. (2)).

The maximum worm load, M(a), is attained in age class a' where

$$a' = (1/\lambda)\ln([\mu-\sigma+\lambda]/[\mu-\sigma-\lambda]) \quad (16)$$

and

$$M(a') = \frac{\Lambda M(\infty)}{\lambda}\left[1 + \frac{(\mu-\sigma-\lambda)}{2}\left(\frac{\mu-\sigma+\lambda}{\mu-\sigma-\lambda}\right)^{(\lambda-\mu-\sigma)/2\lambda}\right]$$

given that $M(\infty) \to (\Lambda\sigma)/[\sigma\mu + \epsilon\Lambda]$

From eqn. (16) it can be seen that adult worm life expectancy $(1/\mu)$ is a major determinant of the age (a') at which the maximum worm load is attained (Fig. 4)

Case 2

For $(\mu - \sigma)^2 < 4\epsilon\Lambda$;

$$M(a) = A + e^{-(\mu+\sigma)a/2}\left\{\frac{2\Lambda}{\theta}\sin\left(\frac{a\theta}{2}\right)\left[1 - \frac{A(\mu+\sigma)}{2\Lambda}\right] - A\cos\left(\frac{a\theta}{2}\right)\right\} \quad (17)$$

where

$$\theta = [4\epsilon\Lambda - (\mu-\sigma)^2]^{1/2}$$

For life long immunological memory ($\sigma = 0$) eqn. (14) simplifies to:

$$M(a) = \frac{\Lambda e^{-\mu a/2}}{\lambda'}\left[e^{\lambda' a/2} - e^{-\lambda' a/2}\right] \quad (18)$$

where

$$\lambda' = [\mu^2 - 4\epsilon\Lambda]^{1/2}.$$

Alternatively if memory is non-existent ($\sigma \to \infty$) eqn. (14) reduces to

$$M(a) \simeq \frac{\Lambda}{\mu}[1 - e^{-\mu a}] \qquad (19)$$

The assumption of a linear dependency of $F(\bar{M})$ on the accumulated sum of past experiences is clearly a crude approximation. For instances if ϵ is large, the situation can arise in which the net rate of infection, $F(\bar{M})$, is negative in value. This can be interpreted as a very severe acquired response which reduces the rate of parasite establishment to zero and, in addition, increases the net death rate of adult worms (the negative value of $F(\bar{M})$ is added to the mortality rate μM). This problem, however, only arises in situations where $(\mu - \sigma)^2 < 4\epsilon\Lambda$ (i.e <u>case 2</u>). For <u>case 1</u> it can be shown that $F(\bar{M}) > 0$, for any value of M.

The equilibrium model (eqns (14) and (17) for the age-worm load distribution (= age-intensity profile of infection) is able to mimic a wide range of patterns in the way the average worm burden, M(a), varies with age, a. These patterns include monotonic increase in M(a) to a stable plateau; M(a) peaking within childhood, teenage or early adult

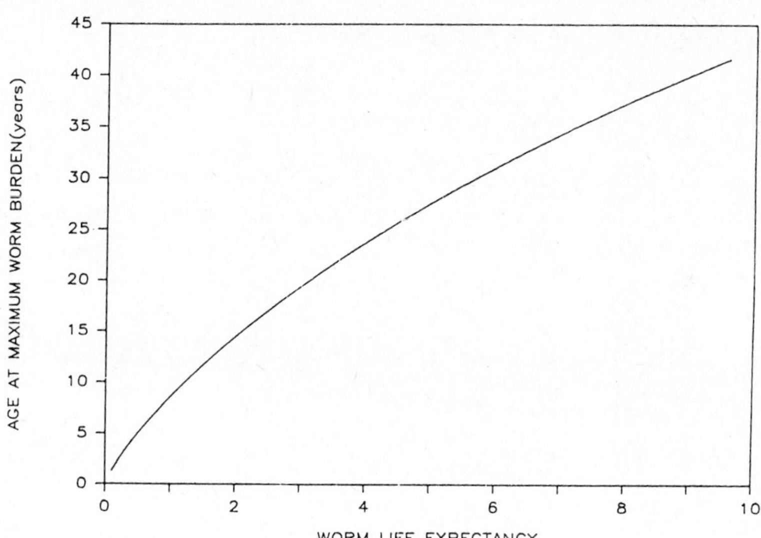

Figure 4. The relationship between the age at which the maximum average worm load is attained (M(a)) and the life expectancy of the parasite ($1/\mu$)(see equation (16) in the main text).

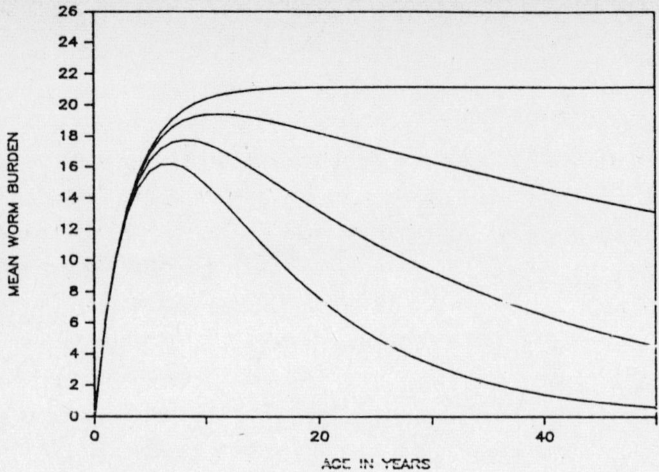

Figure 5 (a). Age-intensity of infection profiles generated by equation (14) (case 1) in the main text. Parameter values (all yr^{-1}); $\Lambda = 7$, $\mu = 0.33$, $\epsilon = 1.0 \times 10^{-6}$ (top line at a = 40), $\epsilon = 5.0 \times 10^{-4}$ (second from top line at a = 40), $\epsilon = 0.0015$ (second from bottom line at a = 40) and $\epsilon = 0.003$ (bottom line at a = 40).

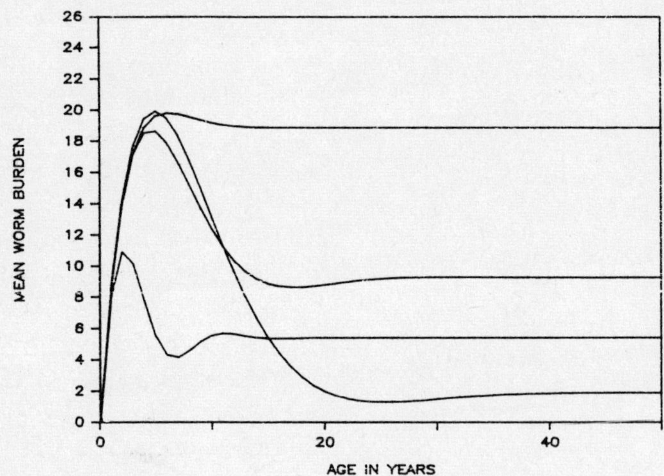

Figure 5 (b). Age-intensity of infection profiles generated by equation (7) (case 2) in the main text. Parameter values (yr), $\Lambda = 10$, $\mu = 0.33$; bottom line at a = 40, $\epsilon = 0.005$, $\sigma = 0.01$; top line at a = 40, $\epsilon = 0.01$, $\sigma = 0.5$; second from top line at a = 40, $\epsilon = 0.0075$, $\sigma = 0.1$; second from bottom line at a = 40, $\epsilon = 0.05$, $\sigma = 0.05$.

age groups, and then declining; and damped oscillations in intensity (for case 2) (Fig. 5). The shapes of these curves are very reminiscent of observed trends (Figs. 1, 2 and 3) for various plausible values of ϵ, σ, Λ and μ. They are determined by the interaction of the intensity of transmission (Λ), the acquired immunological response (ϵ), the duration of the memory of past experience ($1/\sigma$) and the life expectancy of the parasite ($1/\mu$). For a given severity of acquired response (ϵ constant) the worm burden curve tends to be convex-rising to a peak and then declining at older ages - if memory is long ($1/\sigma$ large), and/or transmission is intense (Λ large), and/or worm life expectancy is long. Monotonic growth to a stable plateau in older age classes arises if ϵ is very small (little acquired immunity) or σ large (short memory). These predictions are in qualitative agreement with observed trends: a decline in M(a) in older age groups is more apparent in areas of intense as opposed to light transmission (Fig. 1). Furthermore, the age of peak intensity of parasitic infection appears to be positively correlated with such crude estimates of parasite longevity that are available (short for the roundworm *Ascaris lumbricoides* and the whipworm *Trichuris trichuria* ($\simeq$ 1 year), medium for hookworms - *Necator americanus* and *Ancylostoma duodenale* (2-3 years) and schistosomes - *Schistosoma mansoni*, *S. haematobium* and *S. japonicium* (- 3-5 years) and long for the filarial nemotodes - *Onchocerca volvulus* (8-12 years) (Anderson and May, 1985).

3) Immunity Dependent on Past Exposure to Infection

A somewhat simpler model arises if it is assumed that acquired immunity is dependent on past exposure to infection, as opposed to past experience of worm burdens. This assumption is captured in the function F (M(a)) (see eqn (12)) with $\epsilon = 0$ and $\Delta > 0$. Given that ϵ in eqn (13) is set to zero, the model adopts the form (at equilibrium, where

$\partial M/\partial t=0$),

$$dM/da = \Lambda\,[1- \Delta\int_0^a \Lambda e^{-\sigma(a-a')}da'] - \mu M$$

with solution

$$M(a) = \frac{\Lambda}{\mu}\,[(1-e^{-\mu a})(1+\frac{\Delta\Lambda}{\mu-\sigma}) - \frac{\Delta\Lambda\mu}{\sigma(\mu-\sigma)}(1-e^{-\sigma a})]$$

As $a \to \infty$

$$M(\infty) \simeq [1- \frac{\Delta\Lambda}{\sigma}]$$

The maximum worm load occurs in age class a'

where

$$a' = \frac{1}{(\mu-\sigma)} \ln \left[1+ \frac{\mu-\sigma}{\Delta\Lambda}\right]$$

For the infection rate to remain positive at all ages the following constraint must be satisfied:

$$0 < \Delta\Lambda/\sigma < 1$$

The pristine infection rate, Λ, (realised in the absence of immunity) is a function of the basic reproductive rate of the parasite, R_o, where:

$$\Lambda = [(1/L+\sigma)/\Delta] \; [1-1/R_o]$$

The age intensity curve patterns generated by the model, are broadly similar to those created by the model in which acquired immunity was assumed to depend on worm burden as opposed to exposure. The only major difference, is that the linear dependence of infection rate on past exposure, is unable to generate oscillatory fluctuations in average worm load with changes in host age.

4) <u>More Complex Immunity Functions</u>

As mentioned is section 2, the assumption of a linear dependency of the rate of infection (F), on the accumulated past experience of infection ($\bar{M}$) or exposure to infection (Λ), is only a crude approximation. It has the merit of facilitating analytical studies of the equilibrium age distribution of M(a), but the disadvantage of creating negative infection rates if the value of ϵ is too large. This latter problem can be overcome by assuming that the function $F[\bar{M}(a)]$ adopts a slightly more complex form where, for example:

$$F[\bar{M}(a)] = \Lambda \,/ [1 + \bar{\gamma} \int_0^a e^{-\sigma(a-a')} M(a')\, a'] \tag{20}$$

Numerical studies of the equilibrium model ($\partial M/\partial t=0$) defined by eqn. (9) (with $F(\bar{M})$ as given in eqn. (20) and G(M) as specified in eqn (13) with $\gamma = 0$), reveal that the revised model yields patterns of change in M(a) with age, a, broad similar to those described for the simpler models (eqn (12)) in the previous sections (Fig. 6)

5) <u>Age Dependent Transmission</u>

Convex patterns of change in average worm load with host age may arise from age related changes in the force of infection (Λ). For schistosome infections of man, for example, transmission results from

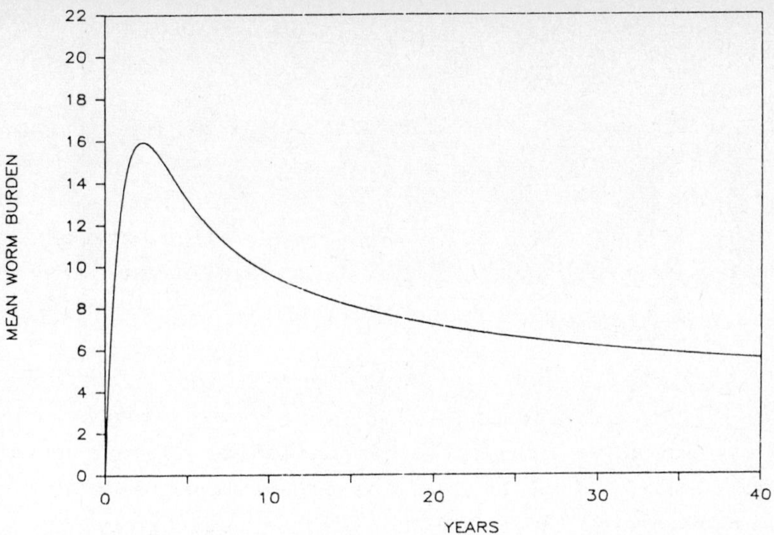

Figure 6. Age-intensity profile generated by equations (9) and (20) in the main text. Parameter values; $\Lambda = 20$, $\mu = 1$, $\bar{\gamma} = 0.01$, $\sigma = 0.1$ (yr^{-1}).

human contact with aquatic infective stages of the parasite (the cercaria) which are released from the snail intermediate host. It often appears that human contact with water in endemic areas, changes with age, such that young children and the older adult age groups have low water contact patterns (Dalton and Poole, 1978). It appears probable that many of the observed convex patterns of change in M(a) with age, arise from a combination of age-related contact with infection and acquired immunity.

The models described in the previous sections can be easily modified to encorporate age dependent rates of infection, by replacing the Λ term in equations (12) and (20) with a function $\Lambda(a)$. Under these circumstances, the equilibrium age distribution of infection may adopt a wide variety of patterns, depending on the functional form of $\Lambda(a)$ and the values of the parameter controlling the acquired immunological response to infection. A variety of patterns derived by numerical studies of the model (eqn (9), with $\partial M/\partial t = 0$, $F(\bar{M})$ as defined in eqn. (20) and $G(\bar{M}) = \mu$) are displayed in Figs. 7 and 8. As illustrated in Fig. 6, age dependent rates of infection can act to

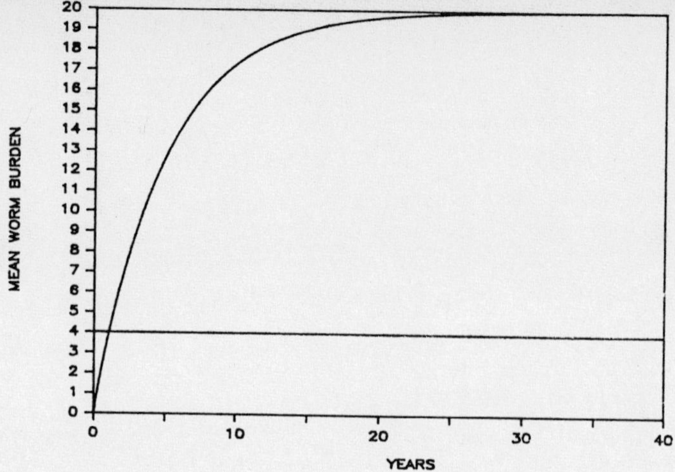

Figure 7. The interaction between acquired immunity and age-relate changes in contact with infection. (1) No immunity.
Graph (a) Predictions of equations (9) and (20) with parameter values $\Lambda = 4$, $\epsilon = 0$, $\mu = 0.2$ (yr^{-1}). The convex curve denotes changes i M(a) with age, and the straight line denotes the value of Λ .

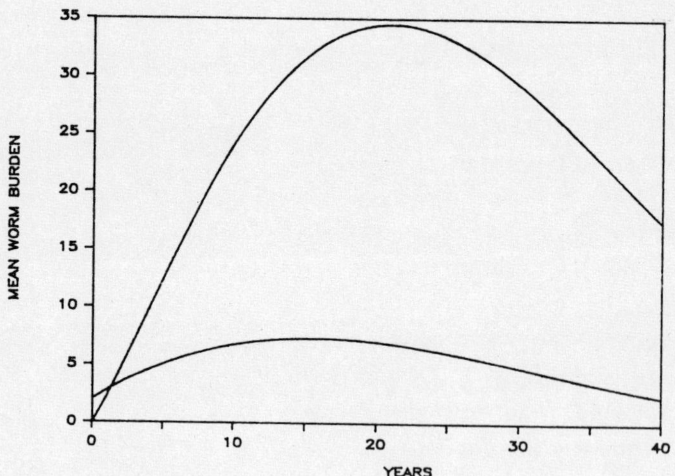

Graph (b) Similar to (a) but with an age-dependent infection rat (a). Parameter values; $\Lambda(a) = b_0 + b_1 + b_2 a^2 + b_3 a^3$ where $b_0 = 2$, b = 0.777, $b_2 = -0.33$, $b_3 = 0.00035$; $\epsilon = 0$, $\mu = 0.2$ (yr). The lowe convex curve denotes Λ(a) while the upper curve records M(a).

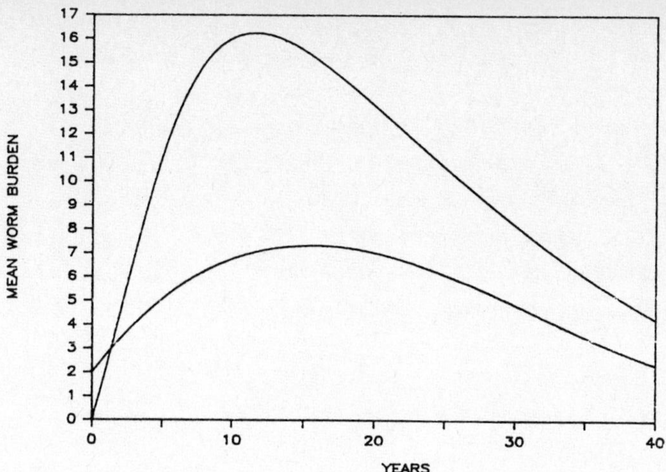

Figure 8. The interaction between acquired immunity and age-related changes in contact with infection (2) with immunity.
Graph (a) Prediction of equations (9) and (20) with parameter values; $\Lambda(a)$ as defined in Figure 7(b), ϵ = 0.001, σ = 0.01, μ = 0.2 (yr^{-1}). The bottom curve denotes $\Lambda(a)$ and the top curve M(a).

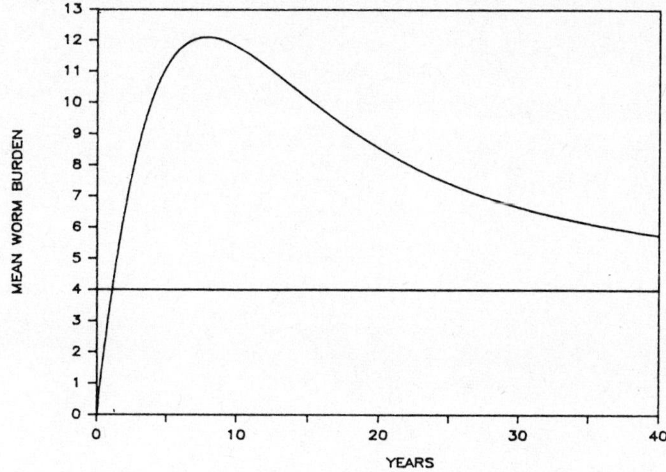

Graph (b) Similar to (a) but with parameter values Λ = 4, ϵ = 0.01, σ = 0.01, μ = 0.2. The curve denotes M(a) and the straight line Λ.

shift the maximum mean load to an older, or younger age class, than would be the case for constant Λ (given that $\Lambda(a)$ adopts a maximum value in a different age class that that in which M(a) is maximum in the absence of age dependency in the force of infection). At present, little is known about the manner in which Λ changes with age for the major helminth infections of man. For a given infection, it appears probable, however, that the pattern of change in Λ with age will vary in different human communities, depending on the prevailing social, behavioural and environmental conditions.

6) Genetic Variability in Immunological Responsiveness

Observed distributions of parasites are highly aggregated with most people harbouring few worms, and a few people harbouring the majority of parasites. Often greater that 70% of the worms are harboured by less than 15% of a community. Recent research suggests that, for certain helminth infections, these 'wormy people' are predisposed to this state by as yet undetermined genetic, behavioural or social factors (Schad and Anderson, 1985). Laboratory studies of animal models suggest that host genetics is an important determinant of immunological responsiveness to helminth invasion (Wakelin, 1984). There is little reason to suppose that human populations are different.

The model of acquired immunity can be extended, to encompass variability in the way different groups of individuals within a community, either respond to parasitic invasion (genetically based where ϵ and σ vary) or are exposed to infection (behavioural differences where Λ varies). For example, if their are n different groups of people, (with parameter values Λ_i, ϵ_i, σ_i, and μ_i in group i), under the linear assumption for the function $F(\bar{M})$ (with Δ and γ set to zero) the equilibrium age distribution of mean worm burdens, $M_i(a)$, in group i is given by:

$$dM_i(a)/da = \Lambda_i[1-\epsilon_i \int_0^a M_i(a')e^{-\sigma_i(a-a')}da'] - \mu_i M_i(a) \qquad (21)$$

The range of patterns of change with age, in the overall mean worm burden in age class a, within the total population, M(a), (where $M(a) = \sum_{i=1}^{n} M_i(a) f_i$ and f_i denotes the fraction of the age class in group i) that can be generated by such 'heterogeneous models' is bewilderingly large. A few special cases are considered below.

a) No Immunity

Consider the simplest case in which the population is homogeneous with respect to contact with infection and immunological responsiveness, and where acquired immunity is absent. The equilibrium age distribtion of worm loads, M(a), in age class a is given by the solution of a simple immigration - death process where

$$M(a) = (\Lambda/\mu)\,[1-e^{-\mu a}] \tag{22}$$

A stochastic model of this process reveals that the probability of observing j worms in a person of age a, $P_j(a)$, is distributed as a Poisson variate with probability generating function (p,g,f.), $\Pi(z,a)$, given by:

$$\Pi(z,a) = \exp[(z-1)M(a)] \tag{23}$$

The expectation (E{j,a}) and variance of j(V{j,a}) in age class a are simply:

$$E\{j,a\} = V\{j,a\} = M(a) \tag{24}$$

The distribution of parasites in the total population, (irrespective of host age) is a mixture of Poisson distributions with p.g.f. H(z) where:

$$H(z) = \int_0^{\infty} [\Pi(z,a)e^{-a/L}/L]\,da \tag{25}$$

and L denotes human life expectancy. Equation (25) is based upon the assumption that human survival decays exponentially with age at a constant rate 1/L (Type II survivorship). The mean and variance of this distribution are given by:

$$E\{j\} = \Lambda/(\mu + 1/L)$$

and

$$V\{j\} = E\{j\}\left[\frac{E\{j\}}{(2\mu L+1)} + 1\right] \tag{26}$$

The distribution is aggregated or contagious in form, since V{j} > E{j} . The variance to mean ratio (V{j}/E{j}) rises linearly with the mean, with slope $1/(2\mu L+1)$ and an intercept of unity. Since parasite life expectancy ($1/\mu$) is always much less than that of its host (L) the slope is much smaller that unity in value. In other words, the parasites are not highly aggregated in their distribution within the total host population. Within each age class the parasites are of course randomly distributed.

For a non-homogeneous host population, the situation is somewhat different. Consider a simple case in which the host population consists of two groups (1 and 2), who constitute fractions f_1 and f_2 of the total population (where $f_1 + f_2 = 1$). It is assumed that the infection rates and parasite death rates differ in the two groups with values Λ_1, Λ_2 and μ_1, μ_2. The p.g.f. for the probability of observing j parasites in a host of age a, $\Pi(z,a)$ is now:

$$\Pi(z,a) = f_1 e^{M_1(a)(z-1)} + f_2 e^{M_2(a)(z-1)}, \text{ where} \tag{27}$$

$M_i(a) = [\Lambda_i/\mu_i][1-e^{-\mu_i a}]$. (28).The mean and variance of the distribution of parasites are:

$$E\{j\} = M_1f_1 + M_2f_2 \quad (29)$$

$$V\{j\} = f_1M_1 + f_2M_2 + f_1f_2[M_1-M_2]^2 \quad (30)$$

The distribution within an age class is aggregated in form with a variance to mean ratio greater than unity in value.

The p.g.f. of the probability of observing j parasites irrespective of the age of the host, H(z) is as defined by eqn. (25) where $\pi(z,a)$ is given by eqn. (27). The mean and variance of this distribution are:

$$E\{j\} = \frac{f_1\Lambda_1}{(\mu_1+1/L)} + \frac{f_2\Lambda_2}{(\mu_2+1/L)} \quad (31)$$

and

$$V\{j\} = \frac{f_1\Lambda_1}{(\mu_1+1/L)}\left[\frac{2\Lambda_1}{(2\mu_1+1/L)} + 1\right] + \frac{f_2\Lambda_2}{(\mu_2+1/L)}\left[\frac{2\Lambda_2}{(2\mu_2+1/L)} + 1\right] - [E\{i\}]^2 \quad (32)$$

If $\mu >> 1/L$ (as is normally the case for helminth parasites) eqn (32) simplifies to:

$$V\{j\} = f_1f_2\left[\frac{\Lambda_1}{\mu_1} - \frac{\Lambda_2}{\mu_2}\right]^2 \quad (33)$$

from which it is clear that for appropriate combinations of parameter values, $V\{j\} >> E\{j\}$. In other words the distribution can be highly overdispersed in character. The overall conclusion to be drawn is that hetrogeneity in infection rates, (Λ_i) and parasite death rates, (μ_i) can result in overdispersed distribution of parasite numbers per host, not only within the total population, but also within each age class. In certain instances, these distributions can be highly aggregated in character (as often observed in natural situations).

b) With Acquired Immunity

Taking the homogeneous case first, consider a model in which the infection rate, $F(\bar{M})$, declines linearly as the sum of past experiences of infection increases $(\bar{M})$, where the memory component of the immunity is life-long ($\sigma = 0$) and given that $\mu^2 > 4\epsilon\Lambda$.

The mean worm burden at age a, M(a) is as defined in eqn(18). Assuming that the parasites are randomly distributed in any one age class, then the p.g.f. of the probability distribution of observing j parasites in a host, irrespective of age, H(z) is again as defined in eqn (25). The mean and variance of this distribution can be derived in the usual way from eqn (25) where, for example,

$$E\{j\} = \Lambda / [L(\frac{\mu}{2} - \frac{\lambda'}{2} + \frac{1}{L})(\frac{\mu}{2} + \frac{\lambda'}{2} + \frac{1}{L})] \qquad (34)$$

given that $\lambda' = [\mu^2 - 4\epsilon\Lambda]$

The general conclusion to emerge is that for the homogeneous case, acquired immunity can act to enhance the degree of overdispersion of the parasites, within the total host population, when compared with the patterns generated by models with no immunity (see eqn 26). Note, however, that within each age class, with or without immunity, the distribution is taken to be Poisson in form. The reason why immunity can generate more pronounced overdispersion, is simply related to its ability to create greater variability in the average worm loads in different age classes (i.e convex age intensity curves) when compared with the montonic growth patterns arising from the simple immigration-death process (no immunity).

For the heterogeneous case, we again arrive at a mixture of Poisson variates, for the probability distribution of parasite numbers per host within each age class. If their are n types of people (each with differing infection rates and immunological competences), then the p.g.f, $\pi(z,a)$ for the distribution within an age class is:

$$\pi(z,a) = \sum_{i=1}^{n} f_i e^{M_i(a)(Z-1)} \qquad (35)$$

from which the mean and variance can be derived. For two groups E{j} and V{j} are as defined in eqns (29) and (30).

The infection rates for each group (Λ_1 and Λ_2) (see eqn (21)) are given by the relationship:

$$\Lambda_i = R_{oi}(\mu_i + 1/L)\bar{M}, \qquad (36)$$

where R_{oi} is the basic reproductive rate of the parasite in host group i and $\bar{M}$ is the overall mean worm burden (over all age classes and types of people). More precisely

$$\bar{M} = \sum_{i=1}^{2} (f_1/L) \int_0^\infty M_i(a)\, e^{-a/L}\, da \qquad (37)$$

The solution of eqn (21) for the two group case (n = 2) can easily be derived to yield expressions for $M_1(a)$ and $M_2(a)$. However, insights into the impact of heterogeneity on the dynamics of the parasite population, are not easily obtained by inspection of these results. A few simple numerical examples help to clarify some of the main properties of the model. First note that in the absence of heterogeneity, the simple acquired immunity model, predicts a distribution of parasites per host in each age class of the population which is random (= Poisson) in form.

Over all age classes, the distribution will be overdispersed or aggregated as a consequence of sampling from a mixture of Poisson distributions (see eqns 25). In section 1 it was assumed that this distribution was negative binomial in nature (see eqns (1) - (3). The heterogeneous model, however, allows us to determine this distribution as a function of the different population parameters of the parasite within the various groups of people in the community (either within an age class or throughout the total population).

Consider first, heterogeneity in exposure to infection between the two groups. We assume that all the parameter values (i.e μ_i, ϵ_i and σ_i) are the same excepting the basic reproductive rates of the parasite (R_{oi}) in the two groups. Different R_{oi} values lead to different infection rates (the Λ_i's, see eqn (36)). An example of patterns of change in mean worm burden with age in group 1 ($M_1(a)$), group 2 ($M_2(a)$) and the overall mean worm burden M(a) is displayed in Fig 9 for given values of f_1 and f_2 (the fractions of the population in groups 1 and 2). Note how the overall mean, M(a), can mask trends in a small fraction of wormy people (high Λ) if the majority of the population have a low exposure rate (low Λ), and vice versa (Fig 9). By making the infection rates different in each group, but constant within a group we have assumed that one group (with a high Λ) is predisposed to heavy infection (in this case as a result of behavioural, social or spatial factors influencing contact with infective stages). Similar patterns arise if we hold Λ constant for both groups, but vary the immunological responsiveness between groups (either via ϵ, σ or μ). For example, a high ϵ value would denote 'good responders' and a low ϵ value 'poor responders' (Fig. 9). Predisposition in this case, arises from genetic heterogeneity in immunological (or non specific) responsiveness. This type of analysis can easily be extended to n different groups of people, who vary in either their exposure to infection or their abilities to acquire immunity.

7) Age Related Changes in Parasite Aggregation

A measure of the degree of parasite overdispersion within an age class is provided by the negative binomial parameter, k(a). The value of k(a) varies inversely with the degree of parasite contagion and, for the two group case, is defined as:

$$k(a) = \frac{M_1(a)f_1 + M_2(a)f_2}{f_1 f_2[M_1(a)-M_2(a)]^2} \tag{38}$$

where f_1 and f_2 denote the fractions in group 1 and 2, and $M_1(a)$ and

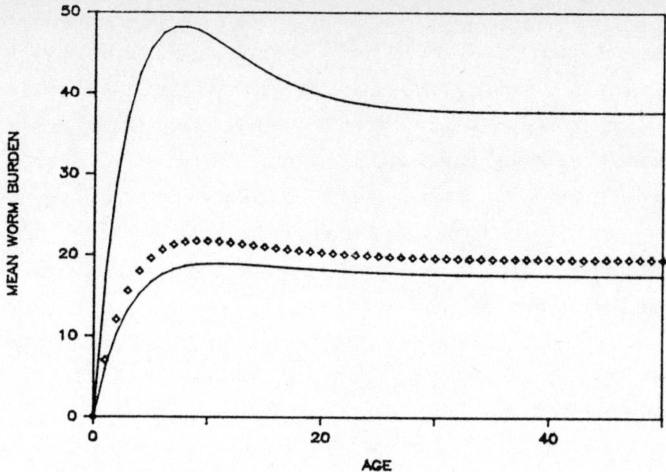

Figure 9. Heterogeneity in exposure to infection and immunological competence. Graph (a) Heterogeneity in exposure. The graph records changes in worm loads with age as predicted by equation (21) in the main text within two groups of people. Group 1 constitutes 90% of the population (f_1 = 0.9) and have a low exposure rate (Λ = 7). Group II constitute 10% of the population (f_2 = 0.1) and have a high exposure rate (Λ = 20) (other parameter values are identical for each group, where ϵ = 0.001, μ = 0.33, σ = 0.1 (yr^{-1}). The top solid line denotes changes in M(a) in the high exposure segment of the population and the bottom solid line changes in the low exposure group. The symbolled line denotes the overall population mean.

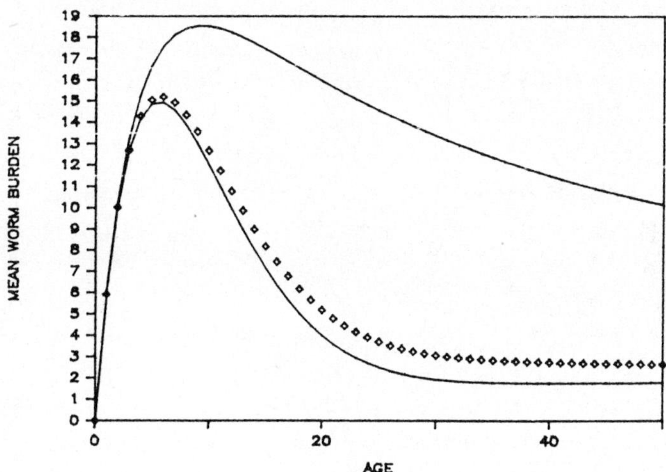

Graph (b) Heterogeneity in immunocompetence. Similar to graph (a) but with constant and variable between the two groups (μ = 0.33, Λ = 7, σ= 0.01). In the 'high responders' (group 1, f_1 = 0.9) ϵ = 0.005 while in the low responders (the worm fraction, group II, f_2 = 0.1) ϵ = 0.001). The symbolled line is the overall population mean worm load.

$M_2(a)$ are the mean worm burdens at age a. More generally k(a) is defined as:

$$k(a) = M(a)^2/[V(a)-M(a)]$$

where M(a) is the overall mean worm burden at age a (over all groups) and V(a) is the overall variance.

Heterogeneity in contact with infection or immunological responsiveness, can generate age-related changes in the degree of parasite contagion within the population, even though the parameters Λ_i, ϵ_i, σ_i and μ_i are independent of age.

Observed changes in k with age, tend to be convex in form with high degrees of clumping in young and old age groups (small k values) and lower levels in the teenage and young adult groups (Elkins, Elkins and Anderson, 1985). Patterns of this type can be generated by the heterogeneous acquired immunity model, although other factors such as age-related changes in contact with infection may also create similar trends.

8) Parasite Control by Mass Chemotherapy

Helminth control in developing countries may be achieved by a variety of methods which include mass chemotherapy, improved education, santitation and hygiene or, in the case of indirectly transmitted infections, by vector control. The availability of cheap, safe and effective drugs for the majority of the major helminth parasites of man, has resulted in the widescale adopted of mass chemotherapy in many areas of the world.

Chemotherapy acts to increase the death rate, μ, of the adult parasites in a manner related to the frequency, intensity and efficacy of drug treatment. For example, if a proportion p of the population are treated by a drug with efficacy h (defined as the proportion of the worm population within an individual that is killed by a single treatment) then the extra death rate imposed by the treatment g, over a time interval Δt is defined as $g = -\ln(1-ph)/\Delta t$ (Anderson, 1981). The per capita death rate of the parasite, $\hat{\mu}$, under mass chemotherapy where treatment is administered randomly within the population (each individual has an equal probability of treatment in any given time interval) is given by $\hat{\mu} = \mu + g$ where μ is the natural mortality rate of the parasite. To eradicate the parasite, it is necessary to reduce the basic reproductive rate of the parasite to less than unity in value ($R_0 < 1$). For the simple acquired immunity model (eqns (14) and (17)), this can be achieved provided the rise in the death rate of the parasite is sufficient to reduce the basic reproductive rate of the parasite (R_o) below unity in value (Anderson, 1981). More precisely, if μ is the parasite death rate in the absence of treatment, and μ' the death rate in the treated community, to eradicate the infection $\mu'/\mu > R_o$ (given that $1/L >> 1/\mu$).

Most commonly eradication is not the aim. Community chemotherapy is usually employed to simply reduce the incidence of disease morbidity arising from infection. As such, the frequency and intensity of anthelmintic application is invariable less than that required to reduce R_o to less than unity in value. One worry under these circumstances, concerns the impact of low to moderate levels of mass chemotherpay on the degree of herd immunity to helminth infection, prevailing within the treated community. Under certain circumstances, it seems likely that mass drug treatment can effectively act to reduce the degree of herd immunity below the level pertaining prior to the introduction of control measures.

This point is illustrated in <u>Fig 10</u> where the consequences of gradually increasing the parasite death rate (by chemotherapy), are displayed in the context of changes in the equilibrium age-mean worm burden profiles (generated by eqn. (14)). Note that moderate to high levels of treatment, can raise the mean worm burdens in adult age classes above the levels pertaining prior to control. Fortunately, however, helminth parasites are more commonly a cause of morbidity in young children as opposed to adults, and thus the problem illustrated in Fig 10 may be of limited relevance in practice.

9) Parasite control by Vaccination

Helminth parasite vaccines are unavailable at present, although much current research is focused towards their development. Given that naturally acquired infections do not generate fully protective or sterile immunity in man, it appears probable that helminth vaccines (when developed), will only provide partial and perhaps short lived protection against parasitic invasion.

A crude model of the impact of vaccination can be formulated as follows. Suppose individuals of age a are inoculated with parasite antigen (perhaps produced by genetic engineering techniques) which triggers immunity in a manner linearly related to the accumulated sum of inoculated antigen. Let the quantity of antigen inoculated at age

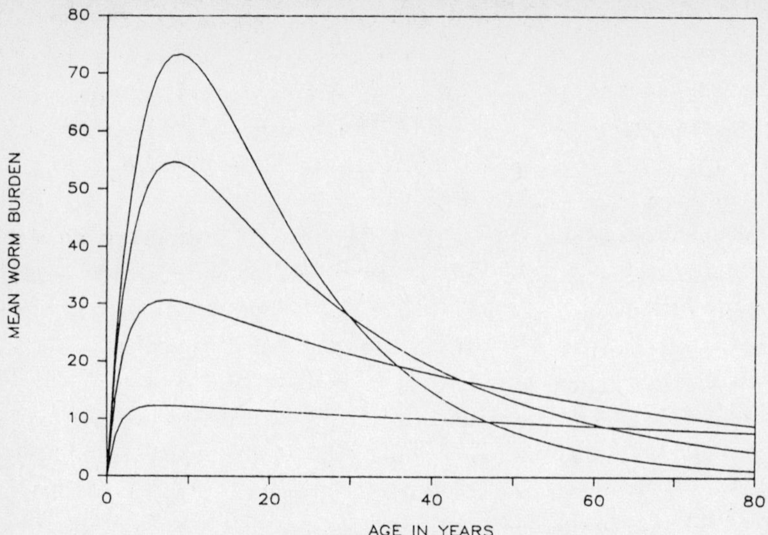

Figure 10. The impact of mass chemotherapy on the equilibrium age-intensity profile of infection. The predictions are generated by equation (14) in the main text. Mass chemotherapy is assumed to act to increase the death rate, μ, of the adult parasites. Parameter values, $\sigma = 0$, $\epsilon = 0.005$, μ = variable. In the bottom line at a = 80, μ = 0.25 (no control); in the second from bottom line at a = 80, μ = 0.33 (light control); in the second from top line at a = 80, μ = 0.5 (moderate control) and in the top line at a = 80, μ = 0.75 (intense control).

a, be V(a), where the units of V are defined as units of whole parasites in the context of their ability to trigger acquired immunity. A simple extension of the model defined in eqn (14)d gives (at equilibrium),

$$dM/da = \bar{\Lambda}\,[1 - \epsilon \int_0^a [V(a') + M(a')]\, e^{-\sigma(a-a')}\,da'] - \mu M \qquad (39)$$

This equation contains the assumption that the vaccine acts to reduce parasite establishment in a manner linearly dependent on the sum of past inoculations of antigen, where the strength of the acquired response triggered by antigen quantity V, is identical to that generated by M adult worms. Furthermore, the duration of 'immunological memory', $1/\sigma$ triggered by either M worms, or a quantity V of inoculated antigen is assumed to be identical.

Under type II human survivorship (exponential decay with parameter 1/L, where L is human life expectancy) the net infection rate in eqn (39), is given by

$$\bar{\Lambda} = \frac{(1/L + \sigma)(1/L + \mu)}{\epsilon} \left\{ R_0 [1 - \frac{\epsilon}{(1+\sigma L)} \sum V_i e^{-a_i/L}] - 1 \right\} \qquad (40)$$

where V_i is the per capita quantity of antigen administered to individuals in age class a_i. To eradicate the infection, it is necessary to reduce the value of to zero in value. To achieve this, the following condition must be satisfied.

$$R_o[1 - \frac{\epsilon}{(1+\sigma L)} \sum_i V_i^{-a/L}]<1 \qquad (41)$$

If individuals are vaccinated at random, (irrespective of age) at a rate τ with a constant quantity of antigen then the eradication criteria is defined as (assuming that $\sigma, \mu >> 1/L$)

$$\frac{\epsilon V}{\sigma} > (1-1/R_o)/\tau \qquad (42)$$

Here the quantity $\epsilon V/\sigma$ denotes the 'strength' of the vaccine with respect to the quantity of antigen inoculated (V), the effectiveness of the antigen in stimulating a protective immunological response (ϵ) and the average duration of the immunological memory ($1/\sigma$). If the vaccine 'strength' is low, the rate of vaccination (τ) must be high to achieve eradication.

CONCLUSIONS

The models described in this paper, are clearly very crude mimics of the known complexity of immunological responses to helminth parasitic infections. Although they generate a variety of epidemiological patterns that are similar to those actually observed, predictions must remain tentative at present, until improved understanding of acquired immunity in man can result in model refinement and extension. The main purpose of this theoretical study, is to highlight some of the possible population-level implication of immunity to helminth invasion.

Of particular interest in this respect, is the analysis of heterogeneity in immunological competance or exposure to infection. The recent demonstration of predisposition to light or heavy helminth infection in human communities (caused by as yet, unidentified genetic, social or behavioural mechanisms) suggests that real populations are indeed heterogeneous with respect to contact with infective stages, or in their ability to mount effective immunological responses against parasite invasion. (Schad and Anderson, 1985; Anderson and Medley, 1985). It therefore seems highly probable that observed change in mean worm load with age mask interests trends in individuals or groups of people. Much information is lost by immediate recourse to average trends in intensity of infection. The models suggest that very complex patterns of change in worm load with age can arise, perhaps involving oscillatory fluctuations. Longitudinal studies of individual patients (both 'wormy' and 'non-wormy' people) could therefore be of great value in assessing the nature and importance of acquired immunity.

Theoretical study also provides some useful guidelines concerning the impact of control measures on parasite transmission. Most importantly, the analyses suggest that mass chemotherpay, at a level less than that required for eradication, may raise worm burdens in older age classes over the levels pertaining prior to control if acquired immunity is an important constraint on parasite population growth. More generally, the models enable criteria to be established, which define the frequency and intensity of control (whether chemotherapy or vaccination) required to eliminate parasite transmission within a given community.

ACKNOWLEDGEMENTS

I am indebted to Robert May for much help and invaluable advice on the research presented in this paper. Financial support was kindly provided by the Rockefeller Foundation.

REFERENCES

Abdel-Wahab, M.F., Strickland, G.T., El-Sahly, A., Ahmed, L., Zakaria, S., El Kady, N. and Mahmoud, S. (1980) Schistosomiasis mansoni in an Egyptian village in the Nile Delta. American Journal of Tropical Medicine and Hygiene 29, 868-874.

Anderson, R.M. (1980) The dynamics and control of direct life cycle helminth parasites. Lecture Notes in Biomathematics 39, 278-332.

Anderson, R.M (ed) (1982) Population dynamics of infectious diseases: theory and applications. Chapman and Hall, London.

Anderson, R.M. (1985) Mathematical models for the study of the epidemiology and control of ascariasis in man. In Ascariasis and its public health significance (ed. D. W. Crompton) pp. 39-67. Taylor and Francis, London.

Anderson, R.M and Crombie, J.A. (1985) Experimental studies of age-intensity and age-prevalence profiles of infection: Schistosoma mansoni in snails and mice. In Host-Parasite Populations: Ecology and Genetics (eds. D.A. Rollinson and R.M. Anderson) John Wiley, New York.

Anderson, R.M. and May, R.M. (1978) Regulation and stability of host-parasite population interactions: I. Regulatory processes. Journal of Animal Ecology 47, 219-247.

Anderson, R.M. and May, R.M. (1982) Population dynamics of human helminth infections: control by chemotherapy. Nature 297, 557-563.

Anderson, R.M. and May, R.M. (1985a) Herd immunity to helminth infection: implications for parasite control. Nature 315, 493-496.

Anderson, R.M. and May, R.M. (1985b) Acquired immunity to parasitic infection: mathematical models of transmission dynamics. Parasitology (submitted).

Anderson, R.M. and Medley, G.F. (1985) Community control of helminth infections of man by mass and selective chemotherapy. Parasitology 90, 629-660.

Carr, H.P., (1926) Observations upon hookworm disese in Mexico. American Journal of Hygiene 6, 42-61.

Cohen, S. and Warren, K.S. (1982) Immunology of Parasitic Infections. Blackwell Scientific Publications, Oxford.

Crombie, J.A. and Anderson, R.M. (1985) Population dynamics of Schistosoma mansoni in mice repeatedly exposed to infection. Nature 315, 491-193.

Dalton, P.R. and Poole, D. (1978) Water contact patterns in relation to Schistosoma haematobium infection. Bulletin of the World Health Organization, 56, 417-426.

Elkins, D.B., Haswell-Elkins, M. and Anderson, R.M (1985) The epidemiology and control of intestinal helminths in Southern India. I. Study design, pretreatment observations and results of treatment. Transactions of the Royal Society of Tropical Medicine and Hygiene (in press).

Hairston, N.G. (1965) On the mathematical analysis of schistosome populations. Bulletin of the World Health Organisation 33, 45-62.

Hlaing, T. (1985) Epidemiology of ascariasis in Burma. In. Ascariasis and its public health significance (ed by D.W.T. Crompton) Taylor and Francis, London (in press).

Kostitzin, V.A. (1934) Symbiose, parasitisme et evolution. Hermann, Paris.

Leyton, M.K. (1968) Stochastic models in populations of helminthic parasites in the definitive host. II. Sexual mating functions. Mathematical Biosciences 3, 413-419.

Macdonald, G. (1985) The dynamics of helminth infections with special reference to schistosomes. Transactions of the Royal Society of Tropical Medicine and Hygiene 59, 489-506.

May, R.M. and Anderson, R.M. (1978) Regulation and stability of host-parasite population interactions. II. Destabilizing processes. Journal of Animal Ecology 47, 249-267.

Pesigan, T.P., Farooq, M., Hairston, N.G., Jaurequi, J.J., Garcia, E.G., Santos, A.T., Santos, B.C. and Bessa, H.A. (1958) Studies on _Schistosoma japonicum_ infection in the Phillipines. I. General consideration and epidemiology. _Bulletin of the World Health Organisation_ _18_, 345-455.

Schad, G.A. and Anderson, R.M. (1985) Predisposition to hookworm infection in man. _Science_ _228_, 1537-1540.

Siongok, T.K.A., Mahmoud, A.A.F., Ouma, J.H., Warren, K.S., Muller, A.S., Handa, A.K. and Houser, H.B. (1976). Morbidity in _Schistosomiasis mansoni_ in relation to intensity of infection. Study of a community in Machakos, Kenya. _American Journal of Tropical Medicine and Hygiene_ _25_, 273-284.

Tallis, G.M. and Leyton, M.K. (1969) Stochastic models of populations of helminthic parasites in the definitive host. I. _Mathematical Biosciences_ _4_, 39-48

Wakelin, D. (1984) _Immunity to Parasites_. Edward Arnold, London.

Warren, K. (1978) Regulation of the prevalence and intensity of schistosomiasis in man. Immunology or ecology. _Journal of Infectious Diseases_ _127_, 595-601.

Dynamics of Childhood Infections in High Birthrate Countries

Angela McLean
Department of Pure and Applied Biology
Imperial College, London University,
Prince Consort Road,
London SW7 2BB
England

Abstract

The majority of the mathematical literature concerned with disease ynamics is concerned with transmission in populations of fixed size here net births balance net deaths. The current generation of models o not take account of case fatalities nor of positive population rowth rates and are therefore of limited use to aid in data nterpretation or for the design of optimal control policies in eveloping areas. A deterministic model for the epidemiology of an nfectious disease which induces lifelong immunity is described. The odel allows for age dependent case fatality rates and for population rowth. Both equilibrium and dynamical results are discussed; the ormer in connection with the estimation of disease parameters from ublished data, and the latter with reference to the investigation of he possible effects of different vaccination strategies. Measles is sed as an example throughout, and reference is made to the available ata on the epidemiology of measles in tropical regions.

Introduction

Vaccine preventable, infectious diseases were responsible for the eath of more than five million children in 1983 (Henderson, 1984). ost of these deaths occurred in countries whose demography is haracterised by comparatively rapid growth of the population. These ortality figures have triggered extensive immunization initiatives by nternational agencies such as the World Health Organisation. To acilitate the design and to investigate the effect of different accination strategies, a mathematical model has been developed to irror events in such countries. The two properties which distinguish the model from previously published studies are a positive populatio growth rate, and an increased death rate associated with infection properties which are specifically excluded from most pre-existin mathematical models for the dynamics of directly transmitted diseases.

The five million deaths mentioned above were caused by si diseases, namely; measles, pertussis, polio, tetanus, tuberculosis an diptheria. Throughout this body of work measles has been used as a example of a vaccine preventable, directly transmitted disease. Th great severity of measles (one half of the above mentioned deaths wer as a result of measles (Henderson, 1984)) means that its epidemiolog is reasonably well documented at least in more developed areas. This i partly as a result of vaccination campaigns which often generat complimentary epidemiological study programmes. More rarely, som surveys were conducted before vaccination was introduced. Th availability of empirical data is, however, less than satisfactory i the majority of tropical regions. Although there are studies tha compare well with the serological surveys collected by Black (Black 1959), there are none to compare with the long term case notificatio records for measles in the U.K. and the U.S.A. (Anderson, Grenfell May 1984).

Interpretation of Serological Profiles

As stated above the current generation of models are not ideall suited to the interpretation and analysis of data collected i developing areas (that is in situations where there are appreciabl case fatalities and the total population is not constant). One exampl of their inapplicability is in the interpretation of serologica profiles. If there are no case fatalities, the serological profile is true record of the proportions at each age that have experienced th disease. As such it can be used to gain information on transmissic rates and on the basic reproductive rate (the average number o secondary cases generated by one primary case in a susceptibl population (Anderson & May, 1982)). If however, the transition frc susceptible to immune status incurs an increased risk of death, tł serological profile becomes only a record of those who have <u>survive</u> the disease. The heightened death rate concommitant with experiencir the disease must therefore be taken into account when using serologica profiles as sources of information on the force of transmission withi a defined population.

Serological Profiles from Various Countries

Insights into the different epidemiological patterns of measles in the U.S. and in various countries of the southern hemisphere may be gained by examination of serological profiles (the proportion seropositive in different age classes). The five serological profiles illustrated in figure 1 are all taken from unvaccinated communities.

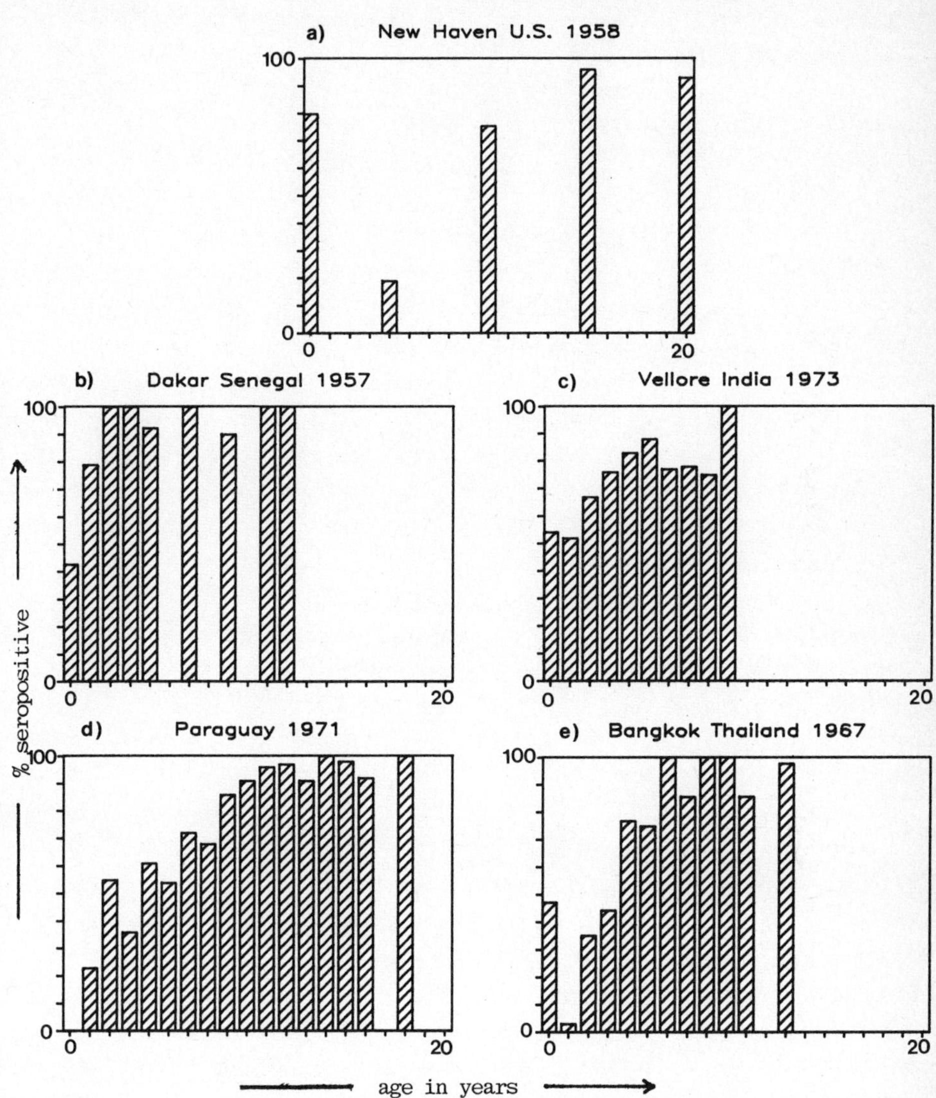

igure 1. Serological profiles from different countries. Data are from a) Black, 1959; (b) Boue, 1964; (c) John & Jesudos, 1973; (d) olubjatnikov, 1971; (e) Ueda et al, 1967.

The most obvious difference is the younger average age at infection in tropical countries when compared with developed areas. Most striking is the profile from Dakar with 100% of the population seropositive by age two years. There is also a general trend for lower average ages at infection in urban than in rural communities. Since case fatalities will act to reduce the observed rate of increase of seropositives with age (i.e. the steepness of the slope of the serological profile), differences in ages at attack between developing and developed areas are even greater than suggested in figure 1.

Severe Measles

It is not only the epidemiological patterns that differ between developed and less developed countries. In many children, the clinical manifestations are substantially different from those seen in children in the more developed countries. The symptoms, which have been given the name severe measles, were first documented by Morley (Morley, 1962; Morley, 1974). After development of the normal red rash, there is a subsequent darkening to a deeper red or even violet colour. This is followed by desquamation much more extensive than that seen in European and North American children. At the same time, similiar reactions on other epithelial surfaces produce; conjunctivitis, sore mouth, laryngitis, bronchopneumonia, and diarrhoea. It is the diarrhoea that is most dangerous for children whose nutrition may already be poor, and who cannot easily survive weight loss of the order of 10% typically associated with infection.

Synopsis of Subsequent Sections

The paper is arranged as follows. First, the mathematical model and its parameters are described. The remaining subject matter is split into two broad categories of statics and dynamics. In the statics section the first question examined is the interpretation of serological profiles in the presence of a disease related death rate. After a brief note on the connection between disease related death rates and case fatality rates, the framework constructed in the first sub-section is used to derive equilibrium results for the basic reproductive rate R_0, the average age at infection A, and the critical vaccination level for eradication pc. The final section considers the temporal behaviour of the model and examines the results of numerical simulations of changes in disease prevalence under different vaccination strategies.

Description of the Model

The model used is identical to that described in Anderson and May (1985) except in three respects. The human population is allowed to grow rather than remaining fixed in size; there is a death rate applying only to those in the infectious state; and the per capita rate of acquisition of infection by susceptibles [$\lambda(a,t)$] is assumed to depend on the <u>proportion</u> of infectives in the community as opposed to their <u>number</u>. It is therefore an age structured compartmental model of the general form as illustrated in figure 2, and described by the following system of partial differential equations:

$$\frac{\partial M}{\partial a} + \frac{\partial M}{\partial t} = -(\delta + \mu(a))M(a,t) \qquad (1)$$

$$\frac{\partial X}{\partial a} + \frac{\partial X}{\partial t} = \delta M(a,t) - (\lambda(a,t) + \mu(a))X(a,t) \qquad (2)$$

$$\frac{\partial H}{\partial a} + \frac{\partial H}{\partial t} = \lambda(a,t)X(a,t) - (\sigma + \mu(a))H(a,t) \qquad (3)$$

$$\frac{\partial Y}{\partial a} + \frac{\partial Y}{\partial t} = \sigma H(a,t) - (\gamma + \alpha(a) + \mu(a))Y(a,t) \qquad (4)$$

$$\frac{\partial Z}{\partial a} + \frac{\partial Z}{\partial t} = \gamma Y(a,t) - \mu(a)Z(a,t) \qquad (5)$$

The definitions of the compartments or states M-X-H-Y-Z are as follows:

- infants protected from infection by the presence of maternal antibodies
- indiviuals susceptible to infection
- infected, but not yet infectious individuals
- infectious individuals
- immunes - it has been assumed that immunity is lifelong.

A further definition N(a,t) - the total population of age a at time t, can be made and since;

N(a,t)=M(a,t)+X(a,t)+H(a,t)+Y(a,t)+Z(a,t)

the dynamics of the total population are described by:

$$\frac{\partial N}{\partial a} + \frac{\partial N}{\partial t} = -\mu(a)N(a,t) - \alpha(a)Y(a,t) \tag{6}$$

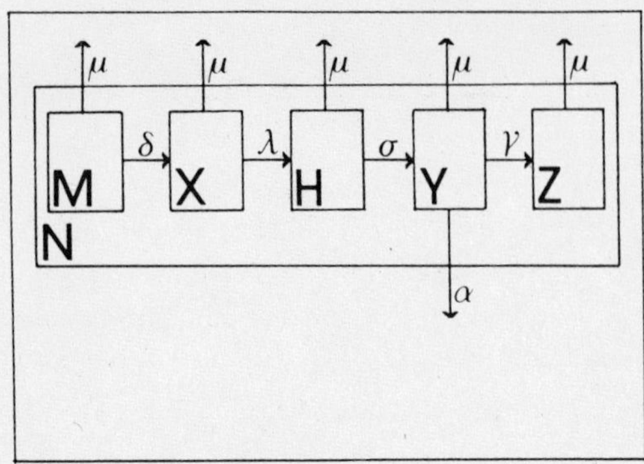

Figure 2. Scheme of flows between compartments in the model. Note in particular that the total population N loses individuals at a higher rate from the Y compartment than from the others.

The definition of the per capita force of infection $\lambda(a,t)$ is:

$$\lambda(a,t) = \frac{\int_0^\infty \beta(a,a')Y(a',t)da'}{\int_0^\infty N(a',t)da'} \tag{7}$$

The model structure is completed by giving boundary conditions along the lines $a=0, t>t_o$ and $t=t_o, a>0$

$$M(0,t) = \int_0^\infty m(a)N(a,t)da$$

$$X(0,t) = H(0,t) = Y(0,t) = Z(0,t) = 0$$

ie all infants are born with maternal antibodies,

and the quantities

$$M(a,t_o)\ ,\ X(a,t_o)\ ,\ H(a,t_o)\ ,\ Y(a,t_o) \text{ and } Z(a,t_o)$$

are all fixed, that is the system is completely described at time t_o The model parameters are summarised in table 1

The Parameter $\beta(a,a')$

In classical non-age structured deterministic models, (Bailey 1975), individuals move from the susceptible to the infected state a rate βXY. That is at a rate proportional to the product of the numbe of susceptible and the number of infectious individuals (the so calle 'mass action' assumption). The constant of proportionalit

Table 1
Summary of Models Parameters

parameter	biological interpretation	age dependent /independent	type of data measured from	range of values
δ	rate of loss of maternal antibodies	independent	serological surveys of young age classes which exclude known cases	2 - 5
$\mu(a)$	background death rate	dependent	demographic tables	0 - .15
$\lambda(a,t)$	per capita rate of acquisition of infection	dependent	serological surveys and age specific case notifications	0 - 1.8
σ	$1/\sigma$ is the mean incub- ation period	independent	clinical observations	73 - 45 ie $1/\sigma$ is 5 - 8 days
γ	$1/\gamma$ is the mean duration of infectious- ness	independent	clinical observations	91 - 60 ie $1/\gamma$ is 4 - 6 days
$\alpha(a)$	disease related death rate	dependent	case fatality rates	0 - 25

β represents the combination of two biological quantities; firstly the degree of contact between infectious and susceptible individuals, and secondly the probability that contact between an infectious and a susceptible individual will result in infection. The function $\beta(a,a')$ is exactly analogous to the constant β, with the extension that the two components mentioned above are deemed dependent on the ages of the infectious and susceptible individuals. So $\beta(a,a')$ combines the following two quantities; the degree of close contact between susceptible people of age a and infectious people of age a', and the propensity for a susceptible person aged a to develop the infection after exposure to an infectious person aged a'. This study follows previous work on age structured epidemic models (Schenzle, 1984; Anderson & May, 1985) in dividing a lifetime into n discrete age classes and assuming that, for susceptible individuals in the ith age class and infectious individuals in the jth age class, $\beta(a,a')$ is a constant with value β_{ij}. Thus $\beta(a,a')$ is a step function which can be represented by an n by n matrix of constants. The two components of (a,a') are far too complex to measure directly, but using the definition of the force of $\lambda(a,t)$ it is possible to find values for the β_{ij} by an indirect method.

Let $\lambda_i(t)$ be defined

$$\lambda_i(t) = \lambda(a,t)\Big|_{(ai-1,ai]}$$

then by definition

$$\lambda_i(t) = \frac{\sum_{j=1}^{n} \beta_{ij}\bar{Y}_j(t)}{\int_0^\infty N(a,t)da}$$

where $\bar{Y}_j(t) = \int_{a_{j-1}}^{a_j} Y(a',t)da'$. As already mentioned above under the assumption that each $\lambda_i(t)$ is equal to a constant λ_i, it is possible to estimate the λ_i from age prevalance data. Having measured the λ_i from the data, a set of $\bar{Y}_j$ are calculated from the equilibrium age distribution for Y(a) derived from the assumption that $\partial\lambda/\partial t = 0$. If the β_{ij} matrix is then restricted to having only n elements, these $\beta_1, \ldots, \beta_n$ are trivially derived by algebraic methods from the $\lambda_1, \ldots, \lambda_n$ and the $\bar{Y}_1, \ldots, \bar{Y}_n$. The distillation of $\lambda(a,t)$ into n discrete functions $\lambda_i(t)$ can be extended to the disease related death rate $\alpha(a)$ as follows.

$$\alpha(a) = \begin{cases} \alpha_1 & \text{for } 0 < a < a_1 \\ \vdots & \\ \alpha_j & \text{for } a_{j-1} < a < a_j \\ \vdots & \\ \alpha_n & \text{for } a_{n-1} < a < \infty \end{cases}$$

Where the age classes are the same as those over which $\beta(a,a')$ is constant.

The Model at Equilibrium : Statics

The work in this section is based upon the assumption that over a long time span the force of infection $\lambda(a,t)$ will remain approximately constant at any given age. This is equivalent to assuming that the age distribution of the infective individuals is stable. Although not analytically proven as yet, this assumption is supported by numerical results discussed in the dynamics section. On the basis of this assumption, all time derivatives can be set to zero resulting in a system of ordinary differential equations describing the equilibrium age distribution of the system. Subsequently it is possible to derive a method for estimating the force of infection from age-prevelance data. In addition such epidemiological measures as the average age at infection A, the critical vaccination proportion p_c and the basic reproductive rate R_o can be expressed in terms of the model's parameters.

The Extended Model

The first aim was to be able to measure the force of infection from available age prevelance data. Such data take two forms: the first being serological profiles (proportion seropositive by age); and the second being cumulative percentages of cases by age. Both of these are measures, not of the numbers in each state at a given age, but of the proportions of the total population in each state at a given age. These proportions are named $\hat{M}$, $\hat{X}$, $\hat{H}$, $\hat{Y}$ and $\hat{Z}$. That is

$$\hat{M}(a,t) = \frac{M(a,t)}{N(a,t)} \qquad \text{etc.}$$

As the rate of change of the total population N(a,t) is governed not only by population size, but also by the number of individuals in the infectious state (equn 6), straightforward division of equations 1 through 5 will give a set of equations for $\hat{M}$ to $\hat{Z}$ whose right hand sides all contain terms involving products of $\hat{Y}(a,t)$ and whichever variable is under consideration. This seems to make the problem much more difficult. However, the introduction of a 6th state, 'excess deaths', allows the definition of a different but related set of proportions which serve to clarify the problem. Conceptually this sixth class represents those individuals who have died as a result of contracting the disease and who would not have died from some other cause. The numbers in this class at age a and time t, E(a,t), are therefore described by the equation

$$\frac{\partial E}{\partial a} + \frac{\partial E}{\partial t} = \alpha(a)Y(a,t) - \mu(a)E(a,t) \qquad (8)$$

It is now possible to define a new 'would-be' total population

$$W(a,t) = N(a,t) + E(a,t)$$

That is, the total living population plus those who are dead as a result of the infection. This total population W(a,t) obeys the following partial differential equation.

$$\frac{\partial W}{\partial a} + \frac{\partial W}{\partial t} = -\mu(a)W(a,t) \qquad (9)$$

The new extended system is summarised in figure 3.

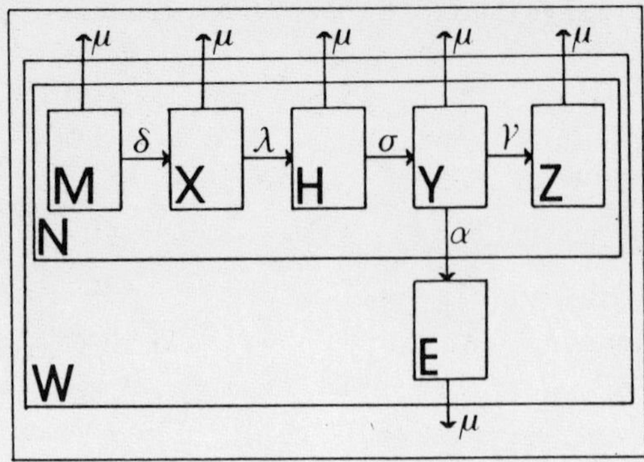

Figure 3. Scheme of flows between compartments in the extended model. By defining a new compartment E, and an alternative total population W, a situation is achieved where losses from the 'total' population W are at a uniform rate from each compartment.

Definition of the 'd Variables

We now define a complete new set of variables

$$M'(a,t) = \frac{M(a,t)}{W(a,t)} \quad X'(a,t) = \frac{X(a,t)}{W(a,t)} \quad H'(a,t) = \frac{H(a,t)}{W(a,t)}$$

$$Y'(a,t) = \frac{Y(a,t)}{W(a,t)} \quad Z'(a,t) = \frac{Z(a,t)}{W(a,t)} \quad E'(a,t) = \frac{E(a,t)}{W(a,t)}$$

and note the partial differential equations governing their dynamics.

$$\frac{\partial M'}{\partial a} + \frac{\partial M'}{\partial t} = -\delta M'(a,t) \tag{10}$$

$$\frac{\partial X'}{\partial a} + \frac{\partial X'}{\partial t} = \delta M'(a,t) - \lambda(a,t)X'(a,t) \tag{11}$$

$$\frac{\partial H'}{\partial a} + \frac{\partial H'}{\partial t} = \lambda(a,t)X'(a,t) - \sigma H'(a,t) \tag{12}$$

$$\frac{\partial Y'}{\partial a} + \frac{\partial Y'}{\partial t} = \sigma H'(a,t) - (\gamma + \alpha(a))Y'(a,t) \tag{13}$$

$$\frac{\partial Z'}{\partial a} + \frac{\partial Z'}{\partial t} = \gamma Y'(a,t) \tag{14}$$

$$\frac{\partial E'}{\partial a} + \frac{\partial E'}{\partial t} = \alpha(a)Y'(a,t) \tag{15}$$

The boundary conditions are as follows;

$$M'(0,t) = 1$$

$$X'(0,t) = H'(0,t) = Y'(0,t) = Z'(0,t) = E'(0,t) = 0$$

and the initial condition may be trivially derived from the initial condition specified for equations 1 to 5 with the additional specification of $E(a,t_o)$.

Under the assumption that $\lambda(a,t)$ and $\alpha(a)$ are constant over given age ranges and that $\partial\lambda(a,t)/\partial t = 0$, the equilibrium values of this set of equations are easily found by solving the related piecewise-linear ordinary differential equations which are obtained when the time derivatives in equations 10-15 are set to zero. This then gives expressions for the age distributions of each of the states at equilibrium in terms of the model's parameters.

Relationship between the 'd and the ^d Variables

It then remains only to clarify the relationship between these 'd variables and the quantities which are of epidemiological interest, the ^d variables.

Since

$$N(a,t) = W(a,t) - E(a,t)$$

and

$$E(a,t) = W(a,t)\ E'(a)$$

$$\hat{M}(a,t) = \frac{M(a,t)}{N(a,t)} = \frac{M(a,t)}{W(a,t)-E(a,t)} = \frac{M(a,t)}{W(a,t)(1-E'(a))} = \frac{M'(a)}{(1-E'(a))}$$

and similiarly for X, H, Y and Z.

From serological profiles, the proportion susceptible at each age, $\hat{X}(a)$, is known. Having derived an algebraic expression for $\hat{X}(a)$ in terms of the model parameters, if all the parameters other than the force of infection are known, it takes only an application of a root-finding algorithm to the function

$$F(\lambda) = \hat{X}(a)(1-E'(a)) - X'(a)$$

to obtain the age-specific values for the force of infection, the λ_i.

The Calculation of the α_j

Clearly the magnitude of E'(a) governs the extent by which this estimated value of the force of infection differs from the value that would be obtained using a method that does not take account of case fatalities. Since

$$E'(a) = \int_0^a \alpha(a')Y'(a')da'$$

this in turn depends upon the magnitude of $\alpha(a)$, which is determined by the case fatality rate. Given a set of age specific case fatalities $p_1, p_2, \ldots, p_n$ for age classes $0 - a_1, a_1 - a_2, \ldots, a_{n-1} - \infty$ a set of disease-related death rates for these same age classes are derived in the following way. The parameter p_j represents the proportion of those people aged between a_{j-1} and a_j leaving the infectious state, who go into the excess death state.

That is,

$$p_j = \frac{\int_{a_{j-1}}^{a_j} \alpha_j Y(a)da}{\int_{a_{j-1}}^{a_j} (\gamma + \alpha_j)Y(a)da} = \frac{\alpha_j}{(\gamma + \alpha_j)}$$

so

$$\alpha_j = \frac{\gamma p_j}{(1-p_j)}$$

For the younger age classes where the case fatality rate can be as high as 26% (Aaby, 1983) taking account of death from disease can alter the estimated force of infection by as much as 17% when compared with estimates derived from methods which ignore disease related deaths. Since so much of interest in the study of the dynamics of measles in less developed countries occurs in the first few years of life, such an underestimation of the force of infection at these young ages is of considerable practical relevance.

Demography, Definitions and an Approximation

In the following analysis a reduced system is considered for the sake of clarity. The maternal-antibody protected class is dropped and the boundary condition altered to

$$X(0,t) = \int_0^\infty m(a)N(a,t)da$$

to accomodate this change. Consideration is restricted to the case where there is only one age class and the mortality functions $\mu(a)$ and $\alpha(a)$ are constants. Before deriving expressions for other epidemiological parameters, various definitions help clarify the following analyses. The total number of susceptibles and infectives are denoted by $\bar{X}(t)$ and $\bar{Y}(t)$ respectively, and the total population is denoted $\bar{N}(t)$. Following May and Anderson (1985) a further definition is made thus:

$$B = \frac{\bar{N}(t)}{N(0,t)}$$

That is B is the reciprocal of the average birth rate.

In order to investigate epidemiological parameters such as the average age at infection, it will be necessary to note a few pertinent results from the theory of mathematical demography (Pollard, 1973). The 'would be' population W(a,t) which obeys equation number 9 can be thought of as undergoing an age structured birth-death process if we make the following alteration to the fertility function.

$$N(0,t) = \int_0^\infty m(a)N(a,t)da = \int_0^\infty m(a)(1-E'(a))W(a,t)da$$

if we define

$$\tilde{m}(a) = m(a)(1-E'(a))$$

we have

$$N(0,t) = \int_0^\infty \tilde{m}(a)W(a,t)da.$$

But since

$$W(0,t) = N(0,t)$$

we have

$$W(0,t) = \int_0^\infty \tilde{m}(a)W(a,t)da \tag{16}$$

It is well known (Pollard, 1973) that under the conditions defined by equations 9 and 16 the 'would be' population settles to a stable age distribution with overall growth at rate $\tilde{r}$, where $\tilde{r}$ satisfies the Euler relation

$$\int_0^\infty \tilde{m}(a)e^{-(\tilde{r}+\mu)a}da = 1$$

and the stable age distribution is given by

$$W(a,t) = W(0,t)e^{-(\tilde{r}+\mu)a}$$

The total population $\bar{N}(t)$ also grows at rate $\tilde{r}$.

Since

$$N(a,t) = W(a,t) - E(a,t) = W(a,t)(1 - E'(a))$$

$$\frac{d\bar{N}(t)}{dt} = \int_0^\infty \frac{\partial N(a,t)}{\partial t} da = \tilde{r}\bar{N}(t)$$

Hence

$$\bar{N}(t) = \bar{N}(0)e^{\tilde{r}t} \tag{17}$$

Next the equilibrium value of $\bar{X}(t)$ is found and then an approximation to the equilibrium value of $\bar{Y}(t)$ is derived.

$$\bar{X}(t) = \int_0^\infty X(a,t)da = \frac{W(0,t)}{(\tilde{r}+\mu+\lambda)} \tag{18}$$

An approximation to the equilibrium value of Y'(a) is now derived. The equilibrium value of Y'(a) in terms of the model parameters is as follows:

$$Y'(a) = \frac{\sigma\lambda}{(\sigma-\lambda)}\left\{\frac{e^{-\lambda a} - e^{-(\gamma+\alpha)a}}{(\gamma+\alpha-\lambda)} - \frac{e^{-\sigma a} - e^{-(\gamma+\alpha)a}}{(\gamma+\alpha-\sigma)}\right\}$$

If terms of order of magnitude $e^{-\sigma a}$ and $e^{-\gamma a}$ are dropped this expression simplifies to:

$$Y'(a) \simeq \frac{\lambda X'(a)}{(\gamma+\alpha)}$$

and therefore

$$\bar{Y}(t) \simeq \frac{\lambda \bar{X}(t)}{(\gamma+\alpha)} \tag{19}$$

The necessary tools are now available to derive expressions for the equilibrium values of three important epidemiological quantities, namely, the average age at infection A, the basic reproductive rate R_o, and the critical proportion to be vaccinated for eradication, p_c.

The Average Age at Infection

The average age at infection is defined as follows:

$$A = \frac{\int_0^\infty a\,\lambda(a)X(a,t)da}{\int_0^\infty \lambda(a)X(a,t)da}$$

$$X(a,t) = W(a,t)X'(a) = W(0,t)e^{-(\tilde{r}+\mu+\lambda)a}$$

thus

$$A = \frac{\lambda W(0,t)\int_0^\infty ae^{-(\tilde{r}+\mu+\lambda)a}da}{\lambda W(0,t)\int_0^\infty e^{-(\tilde{r}+\mu+\lambda)a}da} = \frac{1}{(\tilde{r}+\mu+\lambda)}$$

Consideration of the relative sizes of $\tilde{r}$, μ and λ leads to the relation

$$A \simeq \frac{1}{\lambda}$$

This relationship (noted in previous works on age structured epidemic models (Anderson & May, 1985)) is of interest because of its implications for the effect of vaccination programmes. When the force of infection is lowered as a result of vaccination, the average age at infection will rise. In a situation where the risk of serious disease resulting from infection is at its highest in the young age groups, this effect of immunisation is obviously beneficial.

The Basic Reproductive Rate

The basic reproductive rate R_o represents the number of new cases that will arise if a single infectious individual is introduced into a totally susceptible population. The effective reproductive rate R is the number of new cases that will arise as a result of the introduction of one more infectious individual into a population containing susceptible and immune individuals. The quantities are related in the following manner (see Anderson & May 1983)

$$R = R_o \frac{\bar{X}}{\bar{N}}$$

In a situation where the total human population is static, at equilibrium the reproductive rate R is equal to 1. In this model, however, where the force of infection $\lambda(a,t)$ is a function of the proportion of the population that are infectious and the total population is growing, in order for the disease to remain at equilibrium the number of infectious individuals must increase at the same rate as the total population. An individual is on average infectious for time $1/(\gamma+\alpha)$. So at the start of his infectious period the total population is (equn 17)

$$\bar{N}(0)e^{\tilde{r}t}$$

and at the end it is

$$\bar{N}(0)e^{\tilde{r}(t+1/(\gamma+\alpha))}$$

i.e. the total population increases by a factor $e^{\tilde{r}/(\gamma+\alpha)}$. Hence for the disease to remain at equilibrium

$$R = e^{\tilde{r}/(\gamma+\alpha)}$$

so at equilibrium

$$R_o = \frac{\bar{N}(t)e^{\tilde{r}/(\gamma+\alpha)}}{X(t)}$$

$$= [\bar{N}(t)e^{\tilde{r}/(\gamma+\alpha)}(\tilde{r}+\mu+\lambda)]/W(0,t)$$

but

$$W(0,t) = N(0,t)$$

and

$$\frac{\bar{N}(t)}{N(0,t)} = B$$

where B is the reciprocal of the average birth rate.

Hence,

$$R_o = \frac{B}{A} e^{\tilde{r}/(\gamma+\alpha)}$$

The interest in this result lies in comparing values of R_o for industrialized and developing countries. In developing countries the average age at infection is low, but the high birth rate and consequent low value of B balances this, yielding the surprising result that R_o is no greater in developing countries than in developed regions. Some numerical values for Ro are shown in table 2 to illustrate this point.

In calculating these values the term $e^{\tilde{r}/(\gamma+\alpha)}$ has been ignored (since $e^{\tilde{r}/(\gamma+\alpha)} \simeq 1$)

Table 2
Examples of Values for R_o

Country	Year	A	B	R_o	Reference for value of A
Chile	1962	3.4	42.5	12.5	Ristori et al, 1962
US	1965	5	68.3	13.7	Collins, 1929
Ghana	1960-68	2.5	30.6	12.2	Morley, 1969
Kenya	1974	3.5	26.1	7.5	W.H.O., 1979
India	1976	3	35.3	11.8	Bhau et al, 1976
Senegal	1964	1.8	31.1	17.3	Boue 1964

N.B. all values for B are calculated from; U.S. Agency for International Development, 1977

The Critical Vaccination Proportion

To conclude the the statics section, the proportion of the population that need be vaccinated in order to achieve eradication of an infection is derived, first from the definition of the force of infection, and then with a heuristic argument.

When there is only one age class, the definition of the force of infection is

$$\lambda = \beta \frac{\bar{Y}(t)}{\bar{N}(t)}$$

Where β is a constant determined by factors that will not be affected by vaccination

$$\beta = \frac{\lambda \bar{N}(t)}{\bar{Y}(t)} \quad \text{substituting equn 19 for Y(t)}$$

$$= \frac{B(\gamma+\alpha)}{A_o}$$

where A_o represents the average age at infection <u>before</u> vaccination is introduced. Now suppose a fraction p of each cohort is successfully immunized at birth. The force of infection under these circumstances is still defined as:

$$\lambda = \beta \frac{\bar{Y}(t)}{\bar{N}(t)}$$

that is

$$\lambda = \frac{\beta\lambda W(0,t)\left[\int_0^\infty e^{-(\tilde{r}+\mu+\lambda)a}da\right]X'(0)}{\bar{N}(t)(\gamma+\alpha)}$$

but the initial condition has changed from X'(0)=1 to X'(0)=(1-p)

$$\lambda = \frac{\beta\lambda W(0,t)\left[\int_0^\infty e^{-(\tilde{r}+\mu+\lambda)a}da\right](1-p)}{\bar{N}(t)(\gamma+\alpha)}$$

so

$$(1-p) = \frac{\bar{N}(t)(\gamma+\alpha)}{W(0,t)\left[\int_0^\infty e^{-(\tilde{r}+\mu+\lambda)a}da\right]\beta}$$

now at eradication

$$p = p_c,\ \lambda = 0$$

and

$$\bar{N}(t) = \bar{W}(t) = W(0,t)\left[\int_0^\infty e^{-(\tilde{r}+\mu)a}da\right]$$

so

$$(1-p_c) = \frac{(\gamma+\alpha)}{\beta}$$

$$= \frac{A_o}{B}$$

The critical vaccination proportion for eradication is therefore

$$p_c = 1 - \frac{A_o}{B}$$

This same result is achieved by the following heuristic argument. In order to eradicate the disease the effective reproductive rate R must be reduced so that $R < e^{\tilde{r}/(\gamma+\alpha)}$. That is

$$R_o \frac{\bar{X}(t)}{\bar{N}(t)} < e^{\tilde{r}/(\gamma+\alpha)}$$

but $\bar{X}(t)/\bar{N}(t)$ cannot be greater than (1-p), that is the proportion of the population that are susceptible is at most all those who are not vaccinated. So the eradication criterion becomes

$$R_o(1-p) < e^{\tilde{r}/(\gamma+\alpha)}$$

$$p > 1 - \frac{e^{\tilde{r}/(\gamma+\alpha)}}{R_o}$$

$$p > 1 - \frac{A_o}{B}$$

$$p_c = 1 - \frac{A_o}{B} \simeq 1 - \frac{1}{R_o}$$

As discussed above B/A_o is approximately constant. This has the very important implication that the proportion of each cohort that needs to be immunized to eradicate measles in developing countries is the same as that neccessary for eradication in developed countries (see Dietz, 1975 and Anderson & May 1982, 1983).

Temporal Behaviour of the Model : Dynamics

Whilst results based on conditions at equilibrium are useful for investigating such questions as critical vaccination levels required for eradication, a true picture of the temporal behaviour of the model can only be achieved by numerical solution of the system of partial differential equations. Results from such numerical work are presented here, using as an example data which reflect the situation in West Africa. All model parameters were derived from published data (Abdurrahman et al, 1982; Aaby et al, 1983; Boue, 1964; Billewicz & McGregor, 1981).

Using a step length of three days, Euler's method was used to solve the equations (1-5) along the characteristic lines $t = a + \text{constant}$. The initial conditions were set by

(i) solving the ordinary differential equations obtained by dropping time derivatives,

(ii) transforming these solutions so that they conformed to the stable age distribution determined by the age specific vital rates, and then

(iii) perturbing the whole system by a shift of 40% of the susceptible class into the immune class. The perturbation allows the investigation of the dynamics of the system as it returns to equilibrium, in particular the investigation of the effect of different levels of vaccination.

Observed Patterns

In the early 1960's before measles vaccines were used, Morley recorded annual cycles in admissions to the general hospital in Ilesha, West Nigeria (Morley, 1962). Similiar patterns have been recorded in The Cameroun for the early 1970's after initiation of a control programme (Guyer & McBean, 1981)(figure 4). Studies of the effects of measles immunization programs (Guyer & McBean, 1981; Helmholz & Seck, 1975) show the expected fall in incidence levels and also an upward shift in the age distribution of cases. As the highest case fatality rates occur in the very young age classes, this is very encouraging from the point of view of reducing child mortality.

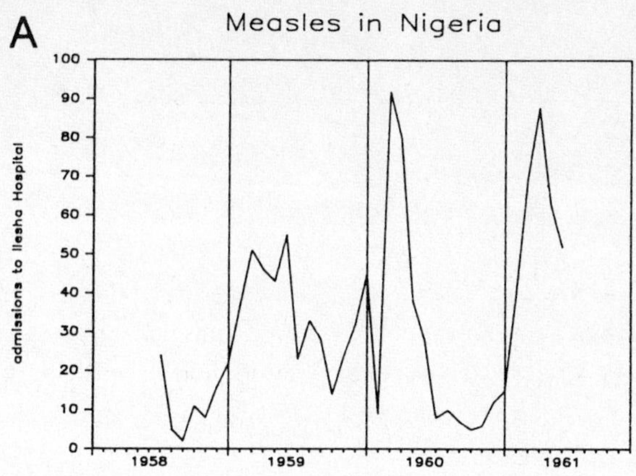

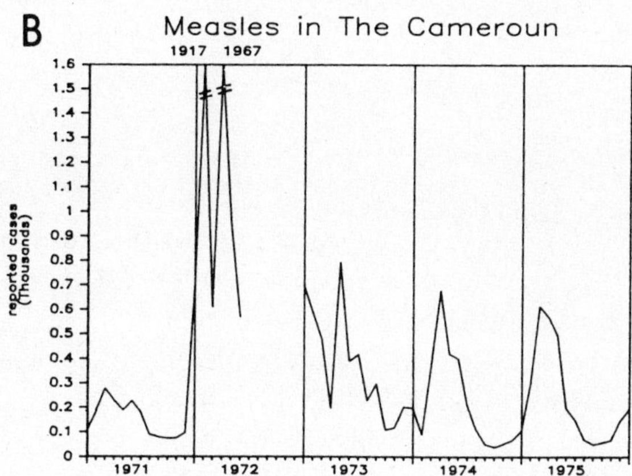

'igure 4. Annual measles epidemics in West Africa. (a) Admissions to :lesha general hospital 1958-1961. Morley, 1962. (b) Reported cases in :ameroun 1971-1975. Guyer & McBean, 1981.

'he Age Distribution of Cases

The first result to be extracted from the investigation of the lynamical behaviour of the system was a check on the assumption that .he age distribution of infectious individuals is indeed stable. A simulation run of 25 years without vaccination was performed, and the age distributions of the infectives at time 0, 10 and 25 years were compared. As can be seen in figure 5 they are practically identical. This result backs up the equilibrium assumption which underpinned the work in the statics section.

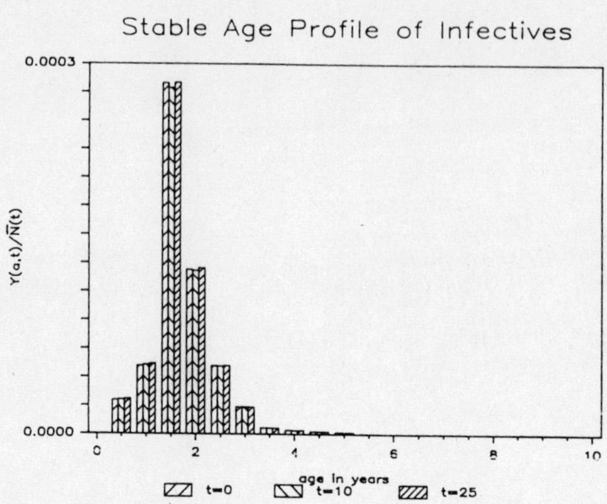

Figure 5. Age distribution of cases at three different points in time. Results from a simulation run with no vaccination. This result backs up the assumption that $\partial\lambda(a,t)/\partial t = 0$ which is essential for the work in the statics section.

Comparison of Four Different Levels of Vaccination

In this section the results of four different levels of vaccination are compared. The simulation was run for two years before introducing vaccination of each cohort at age exactly nine months. The levels of vaccination compared are 0% 50% 70% and 95% of susceptibles. Figure 6 illustrates the temporal behaviour of the model when no vaccination is applied. The number of cases oscillates with period just under 1 year, and quickly returns to equilibrium. Comparison of the profile at the start and at time 15 years gives further evidence of the stability of the age profile of infectives when there is no vaccination.

A good way to consider the effect of vaccination is to look at the shape of the serological profile as it changes through time. In figure 7 the shape of the serological profile with no vaccination and with 95% vaccination can be compared. Before continuing it should be stressed that an individual may appear as immune in the serological profile for

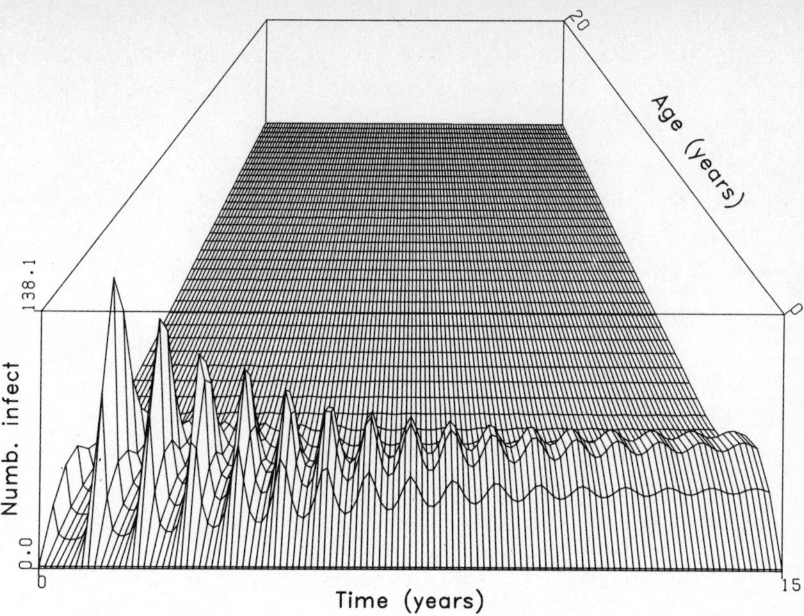

Figure 6. Oscilatory behaviour of the model without vaccination.

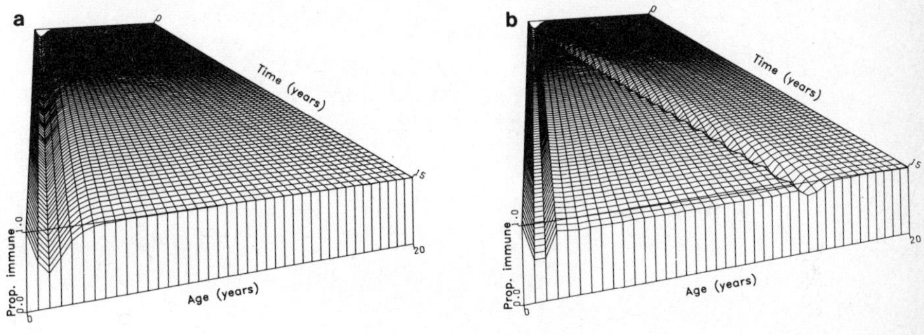

Figure 7. Serological profiles with (a) no vaccination and (b) 95% vaccination.

any one of three reasons; namely, protection by maternal antibodies, natural immunity after surviving the disease or vaccine-induced immunity. The trough running diagonally across figure 7(b) presents a nice illustration of the effect of herd immunity. The cohort with a low proportion immune who cause this trough are aged 14 and 15 at time 15 years. They were therefore aged 1 and 2 when vaccination was started . That is they were the last two cohorts not to be vaccinated. However even though they were not vaccinated themselves, they have received protection as a result of the drop in the force of infection which follows the introduction of mass immunization. Therefore they, as a cohort, have less natural immunity than their older peers, and less vaccine induced-immunity than the younger individuals. A second point to note from figure 7(b) is that the level of immunity in the vaccinated cohorts is not as high as 95%. This is because with the rate of loss of maternal antibodies used in these simulations, at age 9 months 12% of each cohort are still protected by maternal antibodies. Vaccination of a child that still has maternal antibodies does not induce a protective response. Hence vaccination of 95% of each cohort is equivalent to effective vaccination of only 84%. This illustrates a major dilemma - the earlier you vaccinate the more vaccine you waste on individuals who are still protected by maternal antibodies, but the later you vaccinate the less effect vaccination has.

In figure 8 the distribution of cases after 15 years at each of the vaccination levels, is illustrated. It shows a definite trend of increasing age at infection with increasing vaccination levels, as predicted by the equilibrium investigations, and recorded in the field. The most important effect of this will be reduced disease related mortality.

Turning finally to the consideration of case fatalities, figures 9(a), (b), (c) and (d) illustrate the numbers in the excess deaths class, through time at vaccination coverage levels of 0%, 50%, 70% & 95% respectively. It should be recalled that this class measures those who have died as a result of the disease who would not have died from some other cause. So individuals enter the class at a rate determined by the number of cases and the age-specific case fatality rates, and leave it at an age-specific rate equal to the death rate as applied to living members of the community. So in figure 9(a) there is a sharp rise up to age 2.5 years as a result of the large numbers of cases and high case fatality rates in the young age classes. The graph then falls off, as the child mortality rate from other causes comes into play.

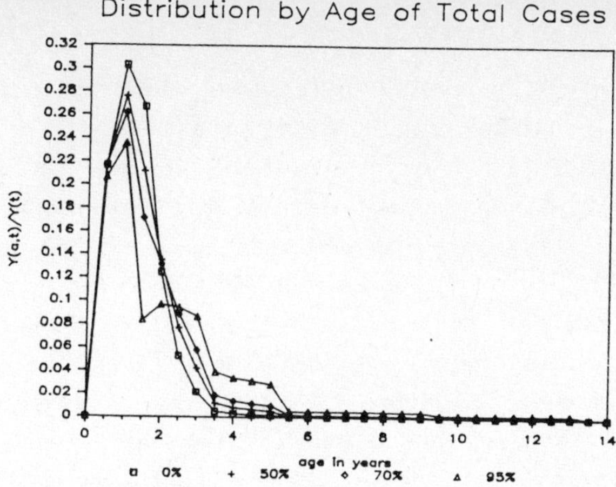

Figure 8. Comparison of the distribution by age of the total number of cases at different vaccination levels. The rise at two years old in the 95% vaccination curve occurs as a result of an increase in the number of susceptibles. This is due to the waning of maternal antibodies in individuals who were still protected by maternal antibodies at age 9 months and were therefore not successfully vaccinated.

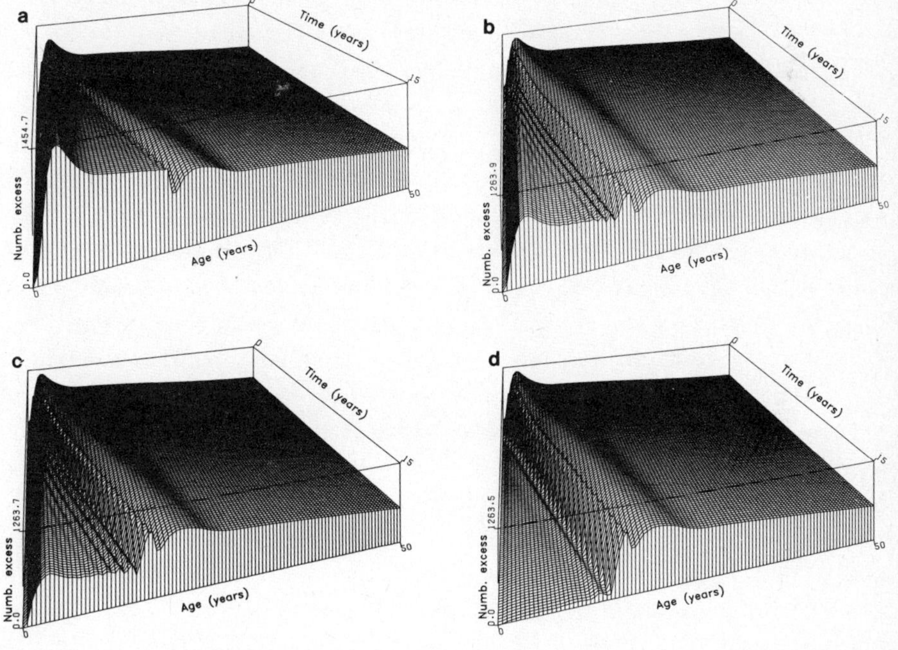

Figure 9. Excess deaths under different vaccination regimes. (a) no vaccination (b) vaccination of 50% of 9 month olds (c) vaccination of 70% of 9 month olds (d) vaccination of 95% of 9 month olds.

Discussion and Conclusions

In considering the limitations of this model one particular problem is of special relevance. The removal of case fatalities from the infectious state results in a shortening of the average infectious period from $1/\gamma$ to $1/(\gamma+\alpha)$. Since deaths which are counted in the calculation of case fatality rates occur anything up to one month after the onset of measles symptoms, the reduction in average duration of infectiousness which occurs in the current model is probably a poor reflection of what actually happens. This problem could be approached by introducing yet another compartment, namely an intermediate state between leaving the infectious state and joining the immune or excess death states. This compartment would represent those no longer infectious, but still at risk as a result of having had the disease. Losses from the population as a result of case fatalities would then be removed from this compartment, (rather than from the infectious compartment) leaving the average duration of infection as $1/\gamma$.

The most important conclusion to be drawn from this work is that the proportion of each cohort that needs to be vaccinated in order to eradicate the disease is no greater in developing than in industrialized countries. This leaves two problems to be overcome if effective vaccination campaigns and eventual eradication are to be achieved. The first of these is inadequate infrastructure, leading to vaccine waste through breakdown of the cold-chain and other practical problems in the organisation of vaccination campaigns. This is not a problem upon which this work can shed any light. The second of the two difficulties is the so-called 'window' problem briefly mentioned in the last section. In a situation where a significant number of cases occur before the age at which all individuals have lost their maternally derived antibodies, there is no age at which a whole cohort can be successfully vaccinated. A choice must therefore be made as to whether to vaccinate after maternal antibodies have waned and risk high mortality from cases in the very young, or to vaccinate at an earlier age and waste vaccine on individuals who do not seroconvert because they are still protected by maternal antibodies. An evaluation of a measles vaccination campaign in Yaounde (McBean, 1976) revealed that only 17% of vaccine doses resulted in protection of a child, whilst the other 83% were wasted as a result of these two problems. Since vaccination will act to shift the age distribution of cases upwards, this second problem should be alleviated as vaccination begins to have its effect. The average age at infection will rise and the age span during which vaccination is best administered will broaden.

Finally, although eradication will only be achieved as a result of huge efforts to overcome practical difficulties, so as to immunise more than 95% of each cohort, reductions in mortality - a result of the shift in the age distribution of cases - should be achieved by much lower levels of immunisation coverage.

Acknowledgements

This work was supported in full by the Rockefeller Foundation to whom we should like to offer our grateful thanks.

References

Aaby, P., Bukh, J., Lisse, I., & Smits, A. (1983) Measles mortality, state of nutrition, and family structure: A community study from Guinea-Bissau. The Journal of Infectious Diseases 147, 693-701

Abdurrahman, M.B., Greenwood, B.M., Olafimihan, O.,& Whitle, H.C., (1982) Measles antibody levels from birth to 9 months of age in Nigerian infants. African Journal of Medical Sciences 11, 113-115

Anderson, R.M., Grenfell, B.T., & May, R.M. (1984) Oscillatory fluctuations in the incidence of infectious disease and the impact of vaccination : time series analysis. Journal of Hygiene 93, 587-608

Anderson, R.M., & May, R.M. (1982) Directly transmitted infectious disease: control by vaccination. Science 215, 1053-60

Anderson, R.M., & May, R.M. (1985) Vaccination against microparasitic infections: Age specific transmission rates. Journal of Hygiene 94, 365-436

Bailey, N.T.J. (1975). The Mathematical Theory of Infectious Diseases and its Applications. London : Griffin.

Bhau, L.N.R., Madhavan, H.N., & Agarwal, S.C. (1979) Serological survey of measles virus infection in children in Pondicherry area. Indian Journal of Medical Research 69, 634-638

Billewicz, W.Z. & McGregor, I.A. (1981) The demography of two African (Gambian) villages, 1951-75. Journal of Biosocial Sciences 13, 219-240

Black F.L. (1959) Measles antibody in the population of New Haven, Conneticut. Journal of Immunology 83, 74-83

Boue, A. (1964) Contribution a l'etude serologique de l'epidemiologie de la rougeole au Senegal. Bulletin de la Societe Medical d'Afrique Noire de Langue Francais 9, 253-254

Collins S.D. (1929) Age Incidence of the common communicable diseases of children. United States Public Health Reports 44, 763-828

Dietz, K. (1975) Transmission and control of arbovirus diseases. In Epidemiology (ed. D. Ludwig & K.L. Cooke), pp. 104-121. Philadelphia: Society for Industrial and Applied Mathematics.

Golubjatnikov, R., Elsea, W.R., & Leppla, L. (1971) Measles and rubella hemagglutination-inhibition antibody patterns in Mexican and Paraguayan children. The American Journal of Tropical Medicine and Hygeine 20, 958-963

Guyer,B., & McBean, A.M. (1981) The epidemiology and control of measles in Yaounde, Cameroun, 1968-1975. International Journal of Epidemiology 10, 263-269

Helmholz, R.C., & Seck, M. (1975) The epidemiology of measles in rural Senegal before and after mass vaccination. The West African Medical Journal 23, 137-140

Henderson, R.H. (1984) Vaccine preventable diseases of children : The problem. Bellagio Conference to Protect the Worlds Children, Working Papers

John, T.J., & Jesudoss, E.S. (1973) A survey of measles antibody in children. Indian Pediatrics 10, 65-66

McBean, A.M. (1976) Evaluation of a mass measles immunization campaign in Yaounde, Cammeroun. Transactions of the Royal Society of Tropical Medicine and Hygiene. 70, 206-212

May, R.M., & Anderson, R.M. (1985) Endemic infections in growing populations. Mathematical Biosciences (in press)

Morley, D.C. (1962) Measles in Nigeria American Journal of Diseases of Children 103, 230-233

Morley, D.C. (1969) Severe measles in the tropics. 1. British medical Journal i, 293-300

Morley, D.C. (1974) Measles in the developing world. Proceddings of the Royal Society of Medicine 67, 1112-1115

Pollard, J.H. (1973) Mathematical Models for the Growth of Human Populations. Cambridge University Press.

Ristori, C., Boccardo, H., Borgono, J.M., & Armijo, R. (1962) Medical importance of measles in Chile. American Journal of Diseases of Children. 103, 236-241

Schenzle, D. (1984) Control of virus transmission in age structured populations, in Mathematics in Biology & Medicine (V. Capasso, Ed),Springer, Berlin.

Ueda, S., Okuno,Y., Sangkawibha, N., Jayavasu, J., & Tuchinda, P. (1967) Studies on measles in Thailand. 1. Seroepidemiological examination. Biken Journal 10, 129-133

U.S. Agency for International Development (1977) Age Specific Fertility Rates and other Demographic Data for Countries and Regions of the World. Washington D.C.

W.H.O. (1979) E.P.I. Kenya. Weekly Epidemiological Record 54, 337-339

Measurement and Estimation in Heterogeneous Populations

A.I. Yashin
J.W. Vaupel

International Institute for Applied Systems Analysis
Laxenburg, Austria

1. INTRODUCTION

Individuals differ in their susceptibility to various causes of morbidity and mortality. Epidemiologists are accustomed to thinking about this heterogeneity in terms of "risk factors" and "relative risks". Some of the heterogeneity among individuals is genetic in origin and some is acquired as a result of individual behaviour (like cigarette smoking) or environmental exposure (to, say, water pollution). The levels of the risks faced by an individual change over time as the individual ages, changes his behaviour and is exposed to different conditions.

Many biological, medical, and epidemiological studies focus on measuring various risk factors and on linking these factors to observed rates of disease and death. Analyzing how mortality depends on blood pressure, on alcohol consumption or on education level is clearly important.

Heterogeneity analysis, broadly defined, is concerned with understanding the dynamics of the evolution of some hazard rate (like the incidence of mortality) in a population whose members differ in their susceptibility or frailty. Sometimes all the relevant risk factors are observed and the task is to sort out their importance; the method of regression analysis developed by Cox [1,2] is frequently used for this purpose. Very often, however, the variables and processes that are observed, i.e., for which data are available, represent only a portion of the relevant risk factors.

Such hidden heterogeneity is usually ignored in biomedical and epidemiological studies. Recent research, however, indicates that hidden factors can have a major and often surprising impact on the dynamics of mortality and morbidity (see [3,4,5,6] for examples). Furthermore, it has been shown by Ridder and Verbakel [7] that ignoring hidden heterogeneity leads to biased estimates of the importance of observed risk factors, if standard methods such as Cox's partial likelihood approach or maximum likelihood approaches are used. The principal focus of heterogeneity analysis, narrowly defined, is to develop methods that appropriately account for the effects of hidden heterogeneity on the dynamics of mortality and morbidity.

Even if a risk factor is unobserved in some study, information about it may be available from previous studies. A key question thus is, "How can this ancillary information be used in measurement and estimation?". In this paper we survey some recent research in heterogeneity analysis that addresses this question.

2. A SIMPLE MODEL OF HETEROGENEITY

Mathematically the simplest case of heterogeneity in mortality can be represented in terms of the properties of the probability distributions of two random variables (T,Z), where T is interpreted as a death time and Z as "frailty"or "relative risk". The variable Z can be interpreted as arising from a biological, environmental, or social economical factor that influences mortality. The joint distribution function for T and Z will be specified if, for instance, both the conditional distribution function for T given Z and the distribution of Z are known.

Assume that the conditional distribution function of T given Z can be represented in the form

$$P(T \le t \mid Z) = 1 - e^{-\int_0^t \mu(x,Z)dx}$$

where $\mu(x,Z)$ can be interpreted as an age-specific mortality rate for individuals with frailty Z. If $\bar{\mu}(x)$ characterizes the unconditional distribution function by the equality

$$P(T \le t) = 1 - e^{-\int_0^t \bar{\mu}(x)dx} ,$$

then the following relationship holds between $\mu(x,Z)$ and $\bar{\mu}(x)$

$$\bar{\mu}(x) = E(\mu(x,Z) \mid T > x) . \qquad (1)$$

Various applications of this formula were analyzed in [4,5].

3. CONSTANT HETEROGENEITY

Assume that $\mu(x,Z) = Z\mu(x)$ and that Z is a random variable with the Gamma distribution function $F(\lambda,k)$. Recall that the distribution density in this case $f(z)$, is given by the following formula

$$f(z) = \lambda^k z^{k-1} e^{-\lambda z} / \Gamma(k) .$$

By applying formula (1) to this case, it was shown in [3] and [4] that

$$\bar{\mu}(x) = \mu(x)\bar{z}(x)$$

where

$$\bar{z}(x) = \frac{k}{\lambda + \int_0^x \mu(u)du} .$$

This formula for $\bar{z}(x)$ (which can be interpreted as the average frailty among those who survive) indicates that average frailty decreases with age, as the result of selection. It turns out that this property is true in general, i.e. for an arbitrary-distributed non-negative risk factor. More exactly, for the derivative of $\bar{z}(x)$ we have

$$\frac{d\bar{z}(x)}{dx} = -\mu(x)\sigma_z^2(x) < 0 ,$$

where $\sigma^2(x)$ is the conditional variance of z among the individuals in the population who are alive at time x.

4. WHEN HETEROGENEITY EVOLVES OVER TIME

It turns out that even if the mortality rate is influenced by a stochastic process Z_t, the relationship between $\bar{\mu}(t)$ and $\mu(t,Z_t)$ is the same as in (1)

$$\bar{\mu}(t) = E(\mu(t,Z_t) \mid T > t) \quad . \tag{2}$$

For some particular forms of stochastic processes the conditional mathematical expectation on the right-hand side of (2) can be calculated.

Assume for instance that Z_t is the finite-state continuous-time jumping Markov process with the transition intensities $q_{ij}(t)$ and initial probabilities $\pi_j(0), j = \overline{1,N}$. Then,

$$\bar{\mu}(t) = \sum_{i=1}^{N} \mu(t,i)\pi_i(t) \quad , \tag{3}$$

where $\pi_i(t)$ are the solutions of the following equations [8]

$$\frac{d\pi_i(t)}{dt} = \sum_{j=1}^{N} q_{ji}(t)\pi_j(t) + \pi_i(t)\left[\sum_{j=1}^{N} \mu(t,j)\pi_j(t) - \mu(t,i)\right] \quad , \pi_i(0) \quad . \tag{4}$$

Assume now that $\mu(t,Z_t)$ can be represented in the form

$$\mu(t,Z_t) = Z_t \mu(t) \tag{5}$$

where $Z_t = Y_t^2$, and the stochastic process Y_t satisfies the following stochastic differential equation

$$dY_t = [a_0(t) + a_1(t)Y_t]dt + b(t)dW_t \ , \ Y_0 \quad , \tag{6}$$

where Y_0 is a normally distributed random variable with the mean m_0 and variance γ_0. It turns out that in this case the following formula for $\bar{\mu}(t)$ is true [9]

$$\bar{\mu}(t) = \mu(t)(m_t^2 + \gamma_t) \quad , \tag{7}$$

where m_t and γ_t are the solutions of the following nonlinear equations

$$\frac{dm_t}{dt} = a_0(t) + a_1(t)m_t - 2m_t\gamma_t\mu(t) \ , \quad m_0 \tag{8}$$

$$\frac{d\gamma_t}{dt} = 2a_1(t)\gamma_t + b^2(t) - 2\gamma_t^2\mu(t) \ , \ \gamma_0 \quad . \tag{9}$$

Equations (8) and (9) are nonlinear ordinary differential equations that can be solved numerically if the coefficients $a_0(t)$, $a_1(t)$, $b(t)$, $\mu(t)$ are specified.

5. MEASUREMENTS AND ESTIMATION

Suppose that the mortality rate depends on some observed vector of covariates $x = (x_1,\ldots,x_l)$ and can be represented in the form

$$\mu(\alpha,t,x) = \lambda_0(t)e^{\alpha' x} \quad .$$

Such a form of the hazard rate is commonly used to implement Cox's partial likelihood approach for the estimation of the parameters α.

If one has information about death times of n individuals in the cohort and the covariates related to these individuals, then Cox suggested maximizing the function to get the parameter estimates, where R_i is the set of the individuals at risk at time t_i.

In practice, however, not all factors that influence the mortality rate are observed. What kind of effects can one expect from these hidden influential variables and processes on the parameter estimation? The answer to this question depends on what is known about the unobservables.

Assume, for instance, that the mortality rate for an individual depends not only on an observed vector of covariates x but also from some unobserved stochastic process z_t. Suppose $\mu(\alpha,t,x,z_t)$ can be represented in the form

$$\mu(\alpha,t,x,z_t) = \lambda_0(t)e^{\alpha' x} z_t \quad ,$$

where z_t is a finite-state continuous-time Markov process with the transition intensities $q_{ij}(\alpha,t)$ depending on the unknown parameter vector $\alpha = (\alpha_1, \ldots, \alpha_k)$. Another model for $\mu(\alpha,t,x,z_t)$ can be specified when $z_t = y_t^2$ and y_t satisfy equation (6) with unknown parameters in the coefficients $a_0(\alpha,t)$, $a_1(\alpha,t)$, $b(\alpha,t)$.

The right-hand side of equations (4), (8) and (9) will also depend on the parameters α and produce the solutions $\pi_j(\alpha,t)$, $m_t(\alpha)$, and $\gamma_t(\alpha)$

$$\frac{d\pi_i(\alpha,t)}{dt} = \sum_{j=1}^{N} q_{ji}(\alpha,t)\pi_j(\alpha,t) + \pi_i(\alpha,t)\left[\sum_{j=1}^{N} \mu(\alpha,t,j)\pi_j(\alpha,t) - \mu(\alpha,t,i)\right] , \tag{4'}$$

$$\frac{dm_t(\alpha)}{dt} = a_0(\alpha,t) + a_1(\alpha,t)m_t(\alpha) - 2\mu(\alpha,t)\gamma(\alpha,t)m_t(\alpha) , \tag{8'}$$

$$\frac{d\gamma_t(\alpha)}{dt} = 2a_1(\alpha,t)\gamma_t(\alpha) - 2\gamma_t^2(\alpha)\mu(\alpha,t) . \tag{9'}$$

For both of these cases one can write the likelihood function in the form

$$L = \prod_{i=1}^{n} \bar{\mu}(t_i,\alpha)e^{-\int_0^{t_i} \bar{\mu}(x,\alpha)dx} , \tag{10}$$

where t_i, $i = 1,\ldots,n$ are the observed death times for individuals. Note that $\bar{\mu}(t,\alpha)$ can be specified in terms of $\pi_j(t,\alpha)$, given by the equations (4) or in terms of $m_t(\alpha)$ and $\gamma_t(\alpha)$ given by equations (8') and (9').

6. MORE INFORMATION ABOUT HIDDEN PROCESSES

Sometimes not only data about death but also some additional measurements of the influential processes are available. In this case again the maximum likelihood procedure can be used for parameter estimation. The form of the likelihood function should depend not only on the mortality data but also on the data about observable variables.

If Z_t is finite-state jumping Markov process with transition coefficient $q_{ij}(\alpha,t)$, and $T_1,T_2,\ldots$ are the times when the state of this process is observed, then for the likelihood function one still has formula (10) where

$$\bar{\mu}(\alpha,t) = \sum_{i=1}^{N} \pi_i(\alpha,t)\mu_i(\alpha,t)$$

and $\pi_i(\alpha,t)$ satisfies equation (4') on the intervals $[T_k,T_{k+1}[$, with the initial conditions

$$\pi_i(\alpha,T_k) = \delta_{i,X_k} \quad ,$$

where X_k is the state of the process Z_t observed at time T_k.

If the process Y_t from equation (6) can be observed in discrete times $T_1, T_2, \ldots$, then for the likelihood function one can write formula (10) where

$$\overline{\mu}(t,\alpha) = \mu(t,\alpha)(m_t^2(\alpha) + \gamma_t(\alpha))$$

and m_t and γ_t are the solutions of the following system of nonlinear equations (8') and (9'). These equations should be solved on the time interval $[T_i, T_{i+1}[$, with the initial conditions m_{T_i}, γ_{T_i}, defining from the equalities

$$m_{T_i} = Y_{T_i} \quad ,$$

$$\gamma_{T_i} = 0 \quad .$$

7. HIDDEN HETEROGENEITY IN LONGITUDINAL DATA

Suppose one needs to analyze survival data for a certain population such that the duration of life for any individual in the cohort is the functional of the two-component process $Z(t) = X(t), Y(t)$. Let the data which are available consist of the results of measurements of component $X(t)$ at some fixed times for the population cohort consisting of n individuals. Let $X_i(t_1), \ldots, X_i(t_k)$ be data related to the i-th individual. Assume that both measured and unmeasured processes influence the mortality rate and this impact is specified as a quadratic form of both $X(t)$ and $Y(t)$, that is

$$\mu(t, X(t), Y(t)) = (X'(t) Y'(t)) \begin{pmatrix} Q_{11}(t), & Q_{12}(t) \\ Q_{21}(t), & Q_{22}(t) \end{pmatrix} \begin{pmatrix} X(t) \\ Y(t) \end{pmatrix} + \mu_0(t)$$

where $Q_{11}(t)$, $Q_{22}(t)$ are positive-definite symmetric matrices and

$$Q_{12}'(t) = Q_{21}(t) \quad .$$

Note that one can always find the vector-function F and function G, such that the mortality rate $\mu(t,X,Y)$ can be represented in the form

$$\mu(t,X,Y) = (Y - F)' Q_{22}(t)(Y - F) + G$$

where F and G are the functions of t and X

$$F(t,X) = Q_{22}^{-1}(t) Q_{21}(t) X$$

$$G(t,X) = X' Q_{11}(t) X - X' Q_{12}(t) Q_{22}^{-1}(t) Q_{21}(t) X + \mu_0(t) \quad .$$

Assume that the problem is to estimate the elements of the matrix Q on the base of data $X_i(t_1 \wedge T_i), \ldots, X_i(t_k \wedge T_i)$, $i = \overline{1,n}$, where T_i are the observed death times and

$$Q = \begin{pmatrix} Q_{11} & Q_{12} \\ Q_{21} & Q_{22} \end{pmatrix} \quad .$$

Note that some parameters specifying the evolution of the process $Y(t)$ might also be known.

Assume that processes $X(t)$ and $Y(t)$ are the solutions of the following linear stochastic differential equations

$$d\begin{bmatrix} Y(t) \\ X(t) \end{bmatrix} = \left[\begin{bmatrix} a_{01}(t) \\ a_{02}(t) \end{bmatrix} + \begin{bmatrix} a_{11}(t) & a_{12}(t) \\ a_{22}(t) & a_{22}(t) \end{bmatrix}\begin{bmatrix} Y(t) \\ X(t) \end{bmatrix}\right] dt + \begin{bmatrix} b(t) \\ B(t) \end{bmatrix} d\begin{bmatrix} W_{1t} \\ W_{2t} \end{bmatrix}$$

where Q_{1t} and W_{2t} are vector-valued Wiener processes, independent of initial values $X(0), Y(0)$, and $b(t), B(t)$ are matrices having the appropriate sizes.

For notational simplicity, we will omit index i related to some particular individual in the notations related to $X_i(t)$.

Let $\hat{x}(t)$ denote the vector $X(t_1), X(t_2), \ldots, X(t_j(t))$, where

$$t_j(t) = sup\{t_m : t_m < t\} \ .$$

Define the conditional survival function $S(t, \hat{x})$ with the help of the equality

$$S(t, \hat{x}) = P(T > t \mid \hat{x}(t))$$

and let

$$\bar{\mu}(t, \hat{x}(t)) = -\frac{\partial}{\partial t} \ln S(t, \hat{x}) \ .$$

The problem is to find the form of $\bar{\mu}(t, \hat{x}(t))$.

The following theorem about the form of $\bar{\mu}(t, \hat{x}(t))$ is true.

Theorem. Let the processes $X(t)$ and $Y(t)$ be defined as above. Then $\bar{\mu}(t, \hat{x}(t))$ can be represented in the form

$$\bar{\mu}(t, \hat{x}(t)) = (m'(t) - F'(t, \hat{x}))Q(t)(m(t) - F(t, \hat{x})) + Sp(Q(t)\gamma(t)) + \mu_0(t)$$

where $m(t) = \begin{bmatrix} m_1(t) \\ m_2(t) \end{bmatrix}$ $\gamma(t) = \begin{bmatrix} \gamma_{11}(t) & \gamma_{12}(t) \\ \gamma_{21}(t) & \gamma_{22}(t) \end{bmatrix}$ on the intervals $t_j \le t < t_{j+1}$ satisfy the equations

$$\frac{dm(t)}{dt} = a_0(t) + a(t)m(t) - 2\gamma(t)Q(t)m(t)$$

$$\frac{d\gamma(t)}{dt} = a(t)\gamma(t) + \gamma(t)a^*(t) + b(t)b^*(t) - 2\gamma(t)Q(t)\gamma(t)$$

where

$$a_0(t) = \begin{bmatrix} a_{01}(t) \\ a_{02}(t) \end{bmatrix} \ .$$

$$a(t) = \begin{bmatrix} a_{11}(t), & a_{12}(t) \\ a_{21}(t), & a_{22}(t) \end{bmatrix}$$

$$m(t) = \begin{bmatrix} m_1(t) \\ m_2(t) \end{bmatrix}$$

$$\gamma(t) = \begin{bmatrix} \gamma_{11}(t), & \gamma_{12}(t) \\ \gamma_{21}(t), & \gamma_{22}(t) \end{bmatrix} .$$

At time t_j, $j = 1,\ldots,k$, the initial values for these equations are

$$m_1(t_j) = m_1(t_j^-) + \gamma_{12}(t_j^-)\gamma_{22}^{-1}(t_j^-)(X(t_j) - m_2(t_j^-))$$

$$m_2(t_j) = X(t_j)$$

$$\gamma_{11}(t_j) = \gamma_{11}(t_j^-) - \gamma_{12}(t_j^-)\gamma_{22}^{-1}(t_j^-)\gamma_{21}(t_j)$$

$$\gamma_{22}(t_j) = 0$$

$$\gamma_{12}(t_j) = \gamma_{21}(t_j) = 0 \quad .$$

The proof of this theorem can be done using for instance the approach developed in [10].

8. ESTIMATION OF UNKNOWN PARAMETERS IN THE CASE OF PARTLY OBSERVED STOCHASTIC PROCESSES

If the unknown parameters not only represent the mortality rate but also characterize the coefficients of the stochastic processes that influence mortality and are partly observed, then there is one more opportunity to extract information about parameters by including some additional terms in the likelihood ratio function.

In the case of heterogeneity in longitudinal data as described above, the uncertainty (unknown parameters) invalues only the coefficients of the mortality function $Q(\alpha,t)$, $\mu_0(\alpha,t)$. The likelihood function in the case of the data concerned with n individuals will look as before

$$L = \prod_{i=1}^{n} \bar{\mu}(\alpha,t_i,\hat{x}(t_i))e^{-\int_0^{t_i} \bar{\mu}(\alpha,u,\hat{x}(u))du} \quad .$$

Stallard [11] noticed that if the unknown parameters also indicate the probabilistic characteristics of the partly observed process, then the likelihood function should include the additional term related to these observed components. Taking into account this remark the formula for the likelihood function takes the form [11]

$$L = \prod_{i=1}^{n} \mu(\alpha, t_i, \hat{x}(t_i)) e^{-\int_0^{t_i} \mu(\alpha, u, x(u)) du} \, .$$

$$\times \prod_{j=0}^{K_i} |\gamma_{i22}(t_j^-, \alpha)|^{-\frac{1}{2}} \exp\left\{ -\frac{1}{2} [X_i(t_j) - m_{i2}(t_j^-, \alpha, \hat{x}(t_j^-))] \right.$$

$$\left. \times \gamma_{i22}^{-1}(t_j^-, \alpha) [X_i(t_j) - m_{i2}(t_j^-, \alpha, \hat{x}_i(t_j^-))] \right\} ,$$

where the equations for m and γ are given in the previous section.

9. CONCLUSION

Nearly all biomedical and epidemiological studies of the influence of risk factors on the dynamics of mortality and morbidity have ignored unobserved risk factors. Sometimes the effects of hidden heterogeneity are small and can be ignored, but in many cases hidden heterogeneity can substantially alter risk dynamics and can result in biased parameter estimates. This paper has presented some approaches for taking the effects of hidden heterogeneity into account, with emphasis on cases where ancillary information from previous studies is available. Some first efforts have been made to apply some of these approaches in epidemiological research [12,13] but the field is still fresh and largely unplowed.

References

1. D.R. Cox, "Regression Models and Life Tables," *Journal of Royal Statistical Society* **B 34**, pp.187-220 (1972).

2. D.R. Cox, "Partial Likelihood," *Biometrika* **A 62**, pp.269-276 (1975).

3. J.W. Vaupel, K. Manton, and E. Stallard, "The Impact of Heterogeneity in Individual Frailty on the Dynamics of Mortality," *Demography* **16**, pp.439-454 (1979).

4. J.W. Vaupel and A.I. Yashin, *The Deviant Dynamics of Death in Heterogeneous Populations, RR-83-1*, International Institute for Applied Systems Analysis, Laxenburg, Austria (1983). An abridged version is in Nancy Tuma (ed.) *Sociological Methodology 1985*, Jossey-Bass, San Francisco.

5. J.W. Vaupel and A.I. Yashin, *Heterogeneity's Ruses: Some Surprising Effects of Selection on Population Dynamics*, Forthcoming in *The American Statistician*, September 1985, 1984.

6. A. Yashin and J. Vaupel, *Heterogeneity and Competing Risk: Understanding Changes in Cause-Specific Mortality*, International Institute for Applied Systems Analysis, Laxenburg, Austria (1985). Forthcoming Working Paper

7. G. Ridder and W. Verbakel, *On the Estimation of the Proportional Hazard Model in the Presence of Unobserved Heterogeneity, Report AE 22/83*, Faculty of Actuarial Science and Econometrics, University of Amsterdam, the Netherlands (1985).

8. A.I. Yashin, *Evaluation of Danger or How Knowledge Transforms Hazard Rates. WP-83-101*, International Institute for Applied Systems Analysis, Laxenburg, Austria (1983).

9. A.I. Yashin, *Dynamics in Survival Analysis: Conditional Gaussian Property Versus Cameron-Martin Formula. WP-84-107*, International Institute for Applied Systems Analysis, Laxenburg, Austria (1984).

10. A.I. Yashin, K.G. Manton, and J.W. Vaupel, *Mortality and Aging in a Heterogeneous Population: A Stochastic Process Model with Observed and Unobserved Variables. WP-83-81*, International Institute for Applied Systems Analysis, Laxenburg, Austria (1983).

11. A. Yashin, K. Manton, and E. Stallard, *Evaluating the Effects of Observed and Unobserved Diffusion Processes in Survival Analysis of Longitudinal Data*, Forthcoming in *Journal of Applied Probability*, 1985.

12. K.G. Manton and E. Stallard, "A Population-Based Model of Respiratory Cancer Incidence, Progression, Diagnosis, Treatment and Mortality," *Computers and Biomedical Research*(15), pp.342-360 (1982).

13. K.G. Manton and E. Stallard, in *Recent Trends in Mortality Analysis* , Academic Press, Orlando, Florida (1984).

PART V

DIVERSE TOPICS

ON MIGRATORY LYMPHOCYTE MODELS[1]

R. R. Mohler[2], Z. Farooqi and T. Heilig
Department of Electrical and Computer Engineering
Oregon State University
Corvallis, OR 97331

Abstract

Linear time-delay models are developed and compared to other models for the circulation of lymphocytes throughout the immune system. A building-block synthesis of the lymphatic system is presented. The models mimick experimental tracer data for rats, but more extensive data is needed to do a good job of parameter estimation.

1. INTRODUCTION

This paper attempts to describe the dynamic behavior of circulating lymphocytes as a base for the understanding of the organ-distributed immune function. In particular new mathematical models are presented, simulated and compared to other models in their ability to mimick experimental tracer data for rats.

It is intended that the development of such a model will be used for predictive purposes in experimental planning. Eventually such modelling, analysis and experimentation may have an impact on tumor control, cancer and immunology in general. In the long run, such research could relate system control theory to effective immunotherapy and chemotherapy. Radiation and chemotherapy adversely affects the immune response in a manner which may be similar to pollutant effects. Systemic immune research could help explain such effects and provide a base for improved treatment.

[1] Research sponsored by NSF Grant No. ECS-8215724.

[2] NAVELEX Professor of Electrical and Computer Engineering, Naval Postgraduate School, Monterey, CA 93943 during 1984-85.

An excellent introduction to immunology is given by Roitt [1], and a treatment of more detailed aspects of its theory is edited by Bell, et al [2]. An overview of mathematical system theory in immunology and in disease control is given by Mohler, Bruni and Gandolfi [3] and by Marchuk [4] and [5], respectively.

Lymphocyte migration to a site of infection and preferential lymphocyte "homing" have been a factor for growth of interest in circulation of lymphocytes. See Roitt [1] and deSousa [6]. These being relatively long-lived cells a portion of them recirculates. Experiments have been done to look at the quantitative aspects of this recirculating pool. The data for the present paper was obtained from one such experiment, Smith and Ford [7].

Apparently, there is a need to better understand migratory patterns of immune mechanisms. A preliminary, three-compartment, humoral model is studied by Mohler, et al [3], [8], [9]. The present analysis studies only lymphocyte migration which is basic to the humoral process but includes mostly thymus-derived T cells. Also included here are twelve compartments and extensive experimental data.

2. EXPERIMENTAL SUMMARY

Details of the experiment from which the data is derived are given by Smith and Ford [7]. Briefly, the data were taken from a uniform strain of rats as near to the natural physiological state as possible. Lymphocytes were taken from the thoracic duct of a donor, radioactively labelled in vitro, passaged from blood to lymph in an intermediate rat and finally injected into a series of recipients for examination at thirteen time points from one minute to one day. Thirteen tissues were examined from sacrificed rats at each time.

To better understand the system dimensions, it is interesting to note that 180 rats (AO female) were used in the experiment with blood sampled and cells injected on the venous side of the right heart. The total pool of recirculating lymphocytes number about $1.2(10)^9$ with about $40(10)^6$/hour circulating through the thoracic duct and other efferent lymphatics each (see Fig. 1). The coeliac LN weigh only about 8 mg out of a total LN weight of 700 to 800 mg.

At 1, 2 and 5 minutes after injection most of the labelled cells are in blood, lungs and liver, [7]. Concentrations in these compartments subsided during the ensuing 25 minutes as more cells entered the spleen, lymph nodes and Peyer's patches where they peaked between 1 and 18 hours. The migratory pattern of lymphocytes is summarized in Fig. 1 with experimental data compared to model-simulated data in Figs. 2 to 4 for spleen, bone marrow and lungs which exemplify the other organs.

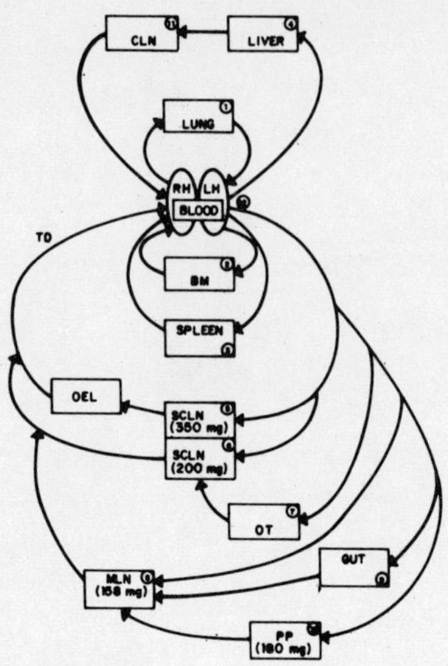

Figure 1. Lymphocyte Circulation

3. CIRCULATORY LYMPHOCYTE

The models studied here consist of separate compartments and states for blood, bone marrow, lungs, liver, spleen, lymph nodes, Peyer's patches, gut and miscellaneous tissues. The lymph nodes were further broken down into mesenteric, coeliac, subcutaneous, right and left popliteal, and deep and superficial cervical lymph nodes for certain data collection.

Each of these organs can be treated as separate compartments with a percent of lymphocytes in that organ as its state. Many of the lymph nodes serve very similar functions and bear the same relation to blood and other organs so that they can be lumped together into a single compartment labeled subcutaneous lymph nodes. This was done with popliteal LN, deep and superficial cervical LN. They form the SCLN in Fig. 1. This compartment has been divided into two subcompartments, one of which drains the miscellaneous tissues and the other does not.

The most common approach to compartmental models assumes lumped time-invariant linearity with diffusions proportional to the concentration differences between the compartments. A slight generalization of this leads to the nonlinear, time-variant linear and time-invariant models derived by Mohler, Farooqi and Heilig [8].

Here a new linear model is presented which considers time delays in the transport of lymphocytes between certain compartments. The state equations which evolve are given as follows:

$$\dot{x}_1(t) = \alpha_1 x_{12}(t) - \beta_1 x_1(t)$$

$$\dot{x}_2(t) = \alpha_2 x_{12}(t) - \beta_2 x_2(t) - \gamma_2 x_2(t-\tau_2)$$

$$\dot{x}_3(t) = \alpha_3 x_{12}(t) - \beta_3 x_3(t) - \gamma_3 x_3(t-\tau_3)$$

$$\dot{x}_4(t) = \alpha_4 x_{12}(t) - \beta_4 x_4(t) - \gamma_4 x_4(t-\tau_4)$$

$$\dot{x}_5(t) = \alpha_5 x_{12}(t) - \beta_5 x_5(t) - \gamma_5 x_5(t-\tau_5)$$

$$\dot{x}_6(t) = \alpha_6 x_{12}(t) + \beta_7 x_7(t) + \gamma_7 x_7(t-\tau_7) - \beta_6 x_6(t) - \gamma_6 x_6(t-\tau_6)$$

$$\dot{x}_7(t) = \alpha_7 x_{12}(t) - \beta_7 x_7(t) - \gamma_7 x_7(t-\tau_7)$$

$$\dot{x}_8(t) = \alpha_8 x_{12}(t) + \beta_9 x_9(t) + \gamma_9 x_9(t-\tau_9) + \beta_{10} x_{10}(t) + \gamma_{10} x_{10}(t-\tau_{10}) - \beta_8 x_8(t) - \gamma_8 x_8(t-\tau_8)$$

$$\dot{x}_9(t) = \alpha_9 x_{12}(t) - \beta_9 x_9(t) - \gamma_9 x_9(t-\tau_9)$$

$$\dot{x}_{10}(t) = \alpha_{10} x_{12}(t) - \beta_{10} x_{10}(t) - \gamma_{10} x_{10}(t-\tau_{10})$$

$$\dot{x}_{11}(t) = \beta_4 x_4(t) + \gamma_4 x_4(t-\tau_4) - \beta_{11} x_{11}(t) - \gamma_{11} x_{11}(t-\tau_{11})$$

$$\dot{x}_{12}(t) = -\left[\dot{x}_1(t) + \dot{x}_2(t) + \dot{x}_3(t) + \dot{x}_5(t)\right] - (\alpha_4 + \alpha_6 + \alpha_7 + \alpha_8 + \alpha_9 + \alpha_{10}) x_{12}(t) + \beta_6 x_6(t) + \beta_8 x_8(t) + \beta_{11} x_{11}(t) + \gamma_6 x_6(t-\tau_6) + \gamma_8 x_8(t-\tau_8) + \gamma_{11} x_{11}(t-\tau_{11})$$

$$x_{13}(t) = x_5(t) + x_6(t)$$

The subscripts refer to the following:

1 = lungs	7 = miscellaneous tissues
2 = bone marrow	8 = mesenteric LN
3 = spleen	9 = gut
4 = liver	10 = Peyer's Patches
5 = SCLN with efferent lymphatics	11 = coeliac LN
6 = SCLN with other tissues	12 = blood

13 = SCLN, Total

The parameters α_i, β_i, γ_i (i=1, 12) represent directional permeabilities that are proportional to flow rates in the various circulatory vessels and organs in different regions of the body. τ_i (i=2, ... 11) represent discrete time delays in different organs. In all compartments other than the lungs and the blood there are two components to the output, one consisting of those lymphocytes that enter the compartment and are just 'flushed out' and the other consisting of those that stay in the compartment for some time before leaving it. The average period of this sojourn is the basis of time delays in this model.

The values of the parameters used are seen in Table I.

i	1	2	3	4	5	6	7	8	9	10	11
α_i	1.0	.01	.1	.3	.016	.005	.05	.006	.02	.012	
β_i	.8	.015	.0007	.3	.0001	.008	.002	.0006	.03	.001	0.7
γ_i	-	.004	.0075	.0005	.0027	.0065	.0004	.0035	.0005	.0023	.001
τ_i	-	250	60	60	180	150	300	150	150	180	180

Table I. Model Parametric Values

The simulation results for spleen, bone marrow and lungs are compared with the experimental data in Figs. 2-4. Lymph node pathways are shown in Fig. 5.

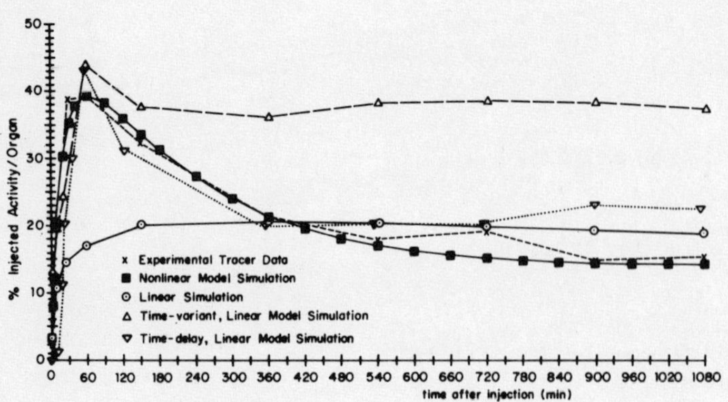

Fig. 2. Rat Spleen Lymphocyte Response

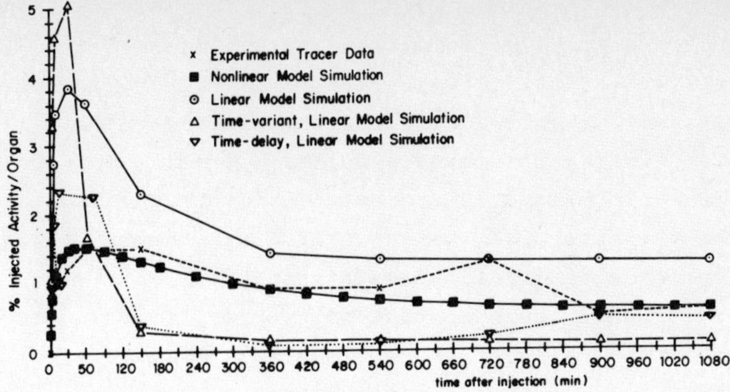

Fig. 3. Rat Bone-Marrow, Lymphocyte Response

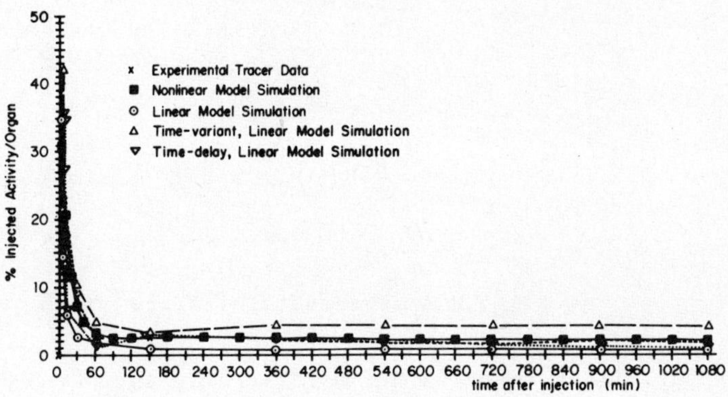

Fig. 4. Rat Lungs, Lymphocyte Response

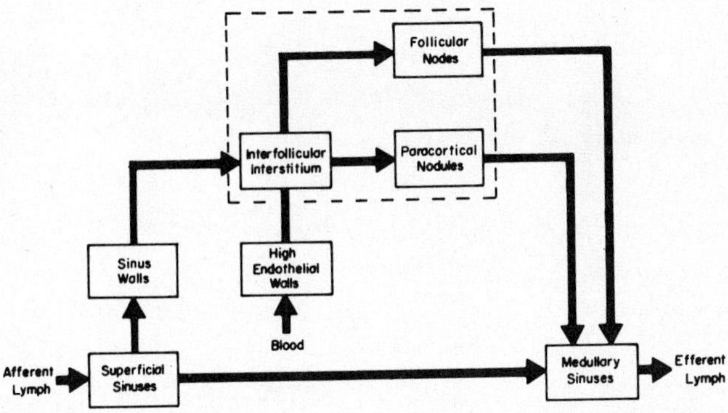

Fig. 5. Lymphocyte Pathways Through a Lymph Node

In general the fit of the model is quite close to the data. The state equations used here are time-invariant, linear, delay differential equations. It is interesting to compare the results obtained here with those in [8], which are reproduced here for the sake of convenience. The present model gives a better approximation to the real system than the two previous linear models.

Because of the nature of the radiolabeling process mostly T-cells were studied in the experiment by Smith and Ford [7]. B-cells and T-cells do not experience the same time delays in different compartments. For example, the time delays for B-cells are much larger for B-cells than T-cells in the lymph nodes. In this paper lymphocytes have been treated as one broad category of cells and have not been separated into T- and B-cells. Time-delays in the model are thus approximations for the broad category and not for one of the sub-categories. This will have to wait until data is available on T-cells and B-cells separately. That will also result in a better fit to the real system. For instance, then two delay terms could be used in the equations for SCLN, one term for T-cells and one for B-cells. Thus more statistical data needs to be collected for a more complete model of lymphocyte recirculation.

While the nonlinear model seems to mimick lymphocyte circulation most accurately, the time-delay linear model does approximate the following experimental results. After a rapid lymphocyte exchange with the <u>lungs</u> during the first couple minutes after injection, the level of blood lymphocytes decreases for the next hour with a half life of approximately 16 minutes. As lymphocytes return to <u>blood</u> (particularly from spleen), the exponential decay ceases between 1 and 2.5 hours after injection followed by a slow rise to near equilibrium at 6 hours onward. Localization of lymphocytes in the <u>liver</u> is somewhat similar to blood in its time response, but has a slower terminal decay of approximately a 24-minute half life. Approximately 40 percent of the injected lymphocytes are found in the <u>spleen</u> at the 30 minute mark. This is followed by a decay mode of approximately 300-minute half life. <u>LN lymphocytes</u> gradually build up to almost 60 percent in about 18 hours. <u>MLN and SCLN</u> responses have similar shape. <u>Peyer's patch level</u> builds up to about 7 percent in about 1.5 hours. Modeling of the liver is particularly complicated due apparently to three independent phenomena involving the lymphocyte migration.

First, there is intravascular pooling similar to lungs which results in rapid initial response. Then there is genuine recirculation blood to liver to coeliac LN, to thoracic duct and back to blood again. Finally, there is an accumulation of dying cells in liver which involves only about 1% to 2% of the total population per day. Still, the latter can be a substantial part of the liver response itself. This may very well account for the long term error which was found between the model simulation and certain other compartments such as liver.

4. LYMPH NODE MODEL

Lymph nodes are the only lymphoid organs placed in the course of lymphatic vessels. While tonsils, spleen and thymus have only efferent lymphatics, lymph nodes have both afferent and efferent lymph vessels [10]. Generally, lymph nodes are the entrance port for lymphocytes crossing from blood to lymph. As shown in Fig. 1, lymphatic vessels collect cells which leave the blood in tissue. Consequently, these cells are passed through a chain of lymph nodes prior to their return to blood via the thoracic duct. In some cases, lymphocytes seem to find their way into lymph by direct entry to lymph nodes.

Based on information available in the literature [11], [12] lymph node lymphocyte pathways may be represented by Fig. 5. While lymph nodes are conventionally divided into superficial cortex, deep cortex and medulla, these regions merge into one another with no clear boundaries. Thus, they are inappropriate compartments for studies which rely on tracer measurements. Both T and B cells enter the lymph node by crossing walls of the high endothelial venules, HEV. T cells either remain in the paracortex surrounding the HEV or move to nearby paracortical nodules. Meanwhile, B cells (of the lymphocyte population) migrate to primary follicles and to lymphocyte corona in the superficial cortex [12].

A detailed derivation of the lymph node model will be given in another publication. Briefly, however, the model is of form identical to that above comprising a linear time-delay set of ordinary differential equations. For each node (whether subcutaneous, mesenteric, coeliac or whatever), the basic model takes the following form:

$$\dot{x}_h(t) = \alpha_h x_{12}(t) - \beta_h x_h(t)$$

$$\dot{x}_s(t) = \alpha_s x_{12}(t) - \beta_s x_s(t)$$

$$\dot{x}_{i1}(t) = \alpha_i[x_h(t) - x_h(t-\tau_i)]$$

$$\dot{x}_{i2}(t) = \alpha_i x_h(t-\tau_i) - \beta_{i2} x_{i2}(t)$$

$$\dot{x}_{p1}(t) = (1-f_p)\alpha_p x_{i2}(t) + f_q\alpha_p x_{i2}(t-\tau_p) - \beta_p x_{p1}(t)$$

$$\dot{x}_{p2}(t) = f_p\alpha_p[x_{i2}(t) - x_{i2}(t-\tau_p)]$$

$$\dot{x}_{f1}(t) = (1-f_p)\alpha_f x_i(t) + f_p\alpha_f(x_i-\tau_f) - \beta_f x_{f1}(t)$$

$$\dot{x}_{f2}(t) = f_p\alpha_f[x_i(t) - x_i(t-\tau_f)]$$

$$\dot{x}_m(t) = \alpha_m x_{p1}(t) - \beta_m x_m(t)$$

Here, subscripts refer to the following:

h = high endothelial walls,
s = superficial sinuses,
i = interfollicular interstitum,
p = paracortical nodules,
f = follicular nodes,
m = medullary sinuses.

f_p is the fraction of delayed cells in paracortical nodules and follicular nodes. As before, the parameters depend on appropriate lymph or blood flow rates, compartmental volumes and resistances.

While a few of the parameters such as for high endothelial walls (HEW) and medullary sinuses are reasonably well determined, the same is not true for cortex parameters. Unfortunately, experimental results are extremely limited.

Fig. 6 shows a comparison of the model simulation, with the various compartmental populations summed up, relative to the previous experimental results of Smith and Ford [7]. It was found that this total lymph node response is very insensitive with respect to changes in the time delays τ_i, τ_p, τ_f. The corresponding simulated responses for the various lymph node compartments are given in Figs. 7 and 8. Labelled lymphocyte population was broken down in T and B cells for the medullary sinuses, since separate relative values of α_m and β_m are available for T and B cells.

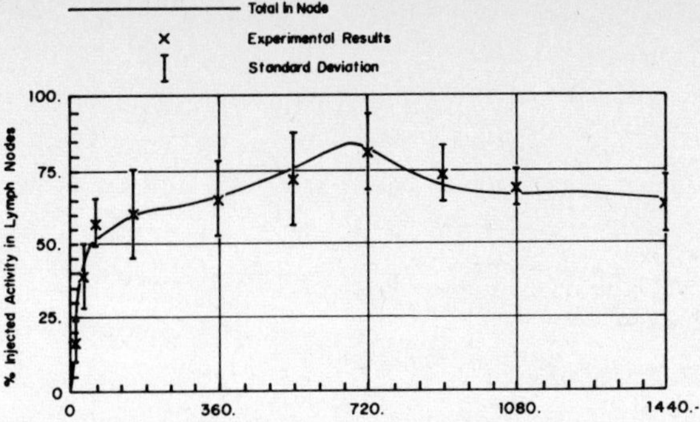

Fig. 6. Comparison of Lymph Node Experimental Data and Simulation

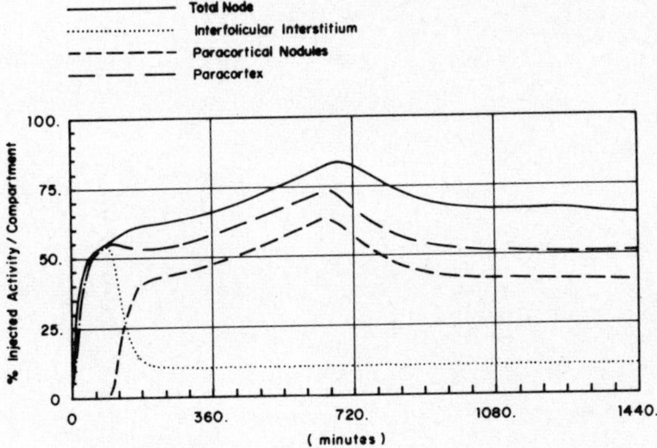

Fig. 7. Simulation of Lymphocyte Response in Node Compartments

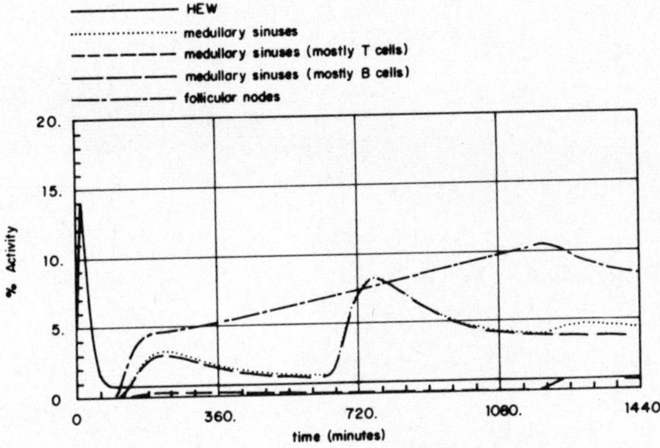

Fig. 8. Simulation for Particular Nodes

After injection of labelled thoracic-duct cells, there is a steep rise in population during the first sixty minutes, corresponding to the exponential fall in blood. When the concentration in blood reaches equilibrium, the rise slows significantly, but is maintained until 12 hours after injection. Then a slow descent continues toward equilibrium about 24 hours after injection. The simulation matches the data quite accurately.

The population of HEW cells rises sharply after injection to reach a peak only 20 minutes later. Then a steep decline results in an approximate equilibrium value of 1% after only two hours. This is consistent with qualitative descriptions [12]. The peak in the paracortex is reached only slightly before that of the total lymph node population - about 10 hours after injection. It would be expected to be similar since a majority reside in the paracortex. Inspecting the interfollicular-intestitium region of the cortex, an initial sharp rise to a peak at 90 minutes is observed which is followed by an exponential decay toward equilibrium after about three hours. The uptake in paracortical nodules - reaching maxima at 11 and 20 hours, respectively.

Medullar sinuses show a small population increase at about two hours after injection reaching a first peak at four hours, followed by a second peak about eight hours later. The latter is due to the release of cells from the paracortical nodes.

5. COMPARTMENTAL IMMUNE MODEL

The review here follows that of Mohler, Bruni and Gandolfi [3]. While the above discussion deals with lymphocyte circulation, the long-range interest is in total immune circulation and at the same time its time response to antigen stimulation. Here, a preliminary humoral model is reviewed as an indication of complicated experiments which will be required.

The qualitative aspects of lymphocyte traffic and their relevance to certain mechanisms of immunoregulation has attracted much attention, particularly emphasized recently by De Lisi [13], Bell [14], and Sprent [15]; though none of these references presents a mathematical model. However, Hammond [16] developed a mathematical model for the circulatory lymphocytes in the spleen using marginal zone, white pulp, and red pulp as compartments.

A compartmentation of the immune system according to the most relevant organs includes bone marrow, blood, spleen, thymus, lymph, and lymph nodes, and gut-associated lymphoid tissue (GALT). GALT includes the tonsils, small intestinal Peyer's patches, appendix, and peritoneal cavity. Bone marrow is the source of multipotential stem cells or precursor cells for the immune process. Spleen and lymph nodes are important locations of antibody-antigen reactions. Blood and lymph are important transport media but also represent significant storage of cells and molecules. Stem cells migrate from bone marrow to thymus and spleen, back via blood to GALT and lymph and back to blood again.

For keeping the model as tractable as possible and for lack of consistent experimental data, not all details of the migration patterns are taken into account, but more refined models are being developed. In what follows, the basic assumptions are:

1) The GALT compartment is neglected since one of the most significant roles of GALT is for generation of a particular class of antibodies, IgA, which is not considered in this paper.

2) Plasma cells (fully differentiated lymphocytes) and antigens do not recirculate in the blood compartment.

3) T cells and macrophages are assumed to be present in sufficient quantity to induce the normal immune response, but their dynamics are neglected, and consequently the thymus is neglected.

4) The product of antibody-antigen reaction, that is, the immune complex, is assumed to be removed shortly after it is formed. Consequently, the immune complex density is not considered.

5) No distinction according to different classes of antibodies is made here.

The state equations for the multicompartmental model are presented in this section assuming that during the migration of lymphocytes and molecules, the process dynamics to varying degrees may be approximated throughout the compartments similar to the single-compartment B model derived in [3]. Here an explanation of notations is in order. The first subscript on the variables 1, 2, 3, 4 refers to immunocompetent cells, plasma cells, antibody and antigens, respectively. The second subscripts b, s, 1, 0, stands for blood, spleen, lymph and lymph nodes, and external compartments, respectively.

Then the immune system is approximated by appropriate initial states and

$$\frac{dx_{1b}}{dt} = a_{1bs}x_{1s} + a_{1bl}x_{1l} - (a_{1sb} + a_{1lb} + a_{10b})x_{1b} + v_1$$

$$\frac{dx_{1s}}{dt} = a_{1sb}x_{1b} - (a_{1bs} + a_{10s})x_{1s} + \alpha p_{ss}(1-2p_{ds})x_{1s}$$

$$\frac{dx_{1l}}{dt} = a_{1lb}x_{1b} - (a_{1bl} + a_{10l})x_{1l} + \alpha p_{sl}(1-2p_{dl})x_{1l}$$

$$\frac{dx_{2s}}{dt} = 2\alpha p_{ss}p_{ds}x_{1s} - a_{20s}x_{2s}$$

$$\frac{dx_{2l}}{dt} = 2\alpha p_{sl}p_{dl}x_{1l} - a_{20l}x_{2l}$$

$$\frac{dx_{3b}}{dt} = a_{3bl}x_{3l} - (a_{3lb} + a_{30b})x_{3b}$$

$$\frac{dx_{3s}}{dt} = a'x_{2s} - kcx_{4s}x_{3s} - (a_{3ls} + a_{30s})x_{3s}$$

$$\frac{dx_{3l}}{dt} = a'x_{2l} - kcx_{4l}x_{3l} + a_{3lb}x_{3b} + a_{3ls}x_{3s} - (a_{3bl} + a_{30l})x_{3l}$$

$$\frac{dx_{4s}}{dt} = a_{40s}x_{4s} - kc_k x_{3s}x_{4s}$$

$$\frac{dx_{4l}}{dt} = a_{40l}x_{4l} - kc_k x_{3l}x_{4l}$$

where a_{kji} denotes the transfer rate coefficient of material k to jth compartment from ith compartment. Other parameters in the model are defined above and by

p_{ss}, p_{sl} probability that antigen stimulates cell, in the spleen and lymph node, respectively;

p_{ds}, p_{dl} probability that an ICC differentiates into a plasma cell in spleen and lymph node, respectively.

These probability terms are approximated in [3] as appropriate for spleen and lymph. Antigen stimulation is introduced by initial conditions.

A simulation of the compartmental model for mouse injected with a common experimental antigen, sheep red blood cells (SRBC), is presented in [3]. A comparison of the model simulation with the experimental data for a mouse with an inoperative spleen and a healthy mouse is given in [3]. The major differences between the simulation and the experimental antibody level, seem to be from a switchover in antibody class which the model neglects.

A sensitivity analysis of the models and simulation shows the following:

1) removal of the spleen results in an attenuation of antibody production by about a factor of three;

2) k is a most critical parameter, while c cannot be dropped in most cases, it need not be estimated accurately;

3) p_s, α, α', τ_1, and τ_4 are somewhat critical with the other parameters of less significance in defining model dynamics.

It should be noted that the humoral immune system involves relatively fast and relatively slow modes of response creating a very stiff process with interesting numerical integration problems for the computer simulation if association and dissociation are considered. Conventional Runge-Kutta integration algorithms were not found effective unless instant equilibrium in association and dissociation are assumed. An adaptive Gear [17] algorithm, however, was found to be very effective.

Following [18], [19], conditions of compartmental accessibility may be derived which are necessary for a minimum model realization from input-output tracer data. It is readily seen from standard linear system controllability and observability conditions for the tracer dynamics that the blood compartment is excellent for tracer insertion and observation. The spleen or the lymph, however, are not recommended as single compartments of accessibility as a consequence of the relatively small particle migration from spleen to lymph directly.

It is obvious that future models should consider switchover. Also, memory cells have been shown to recirculate throughout the lymphoid system, playing key role in immunity and enhanced secondary response. Time delays in certain organs (such as for B cells in spleen) are significant. Conceptually, it is not difficult to include these complications with the compartmental model shown above. However, there is a lack of consistent data to determine key parameters for such a model at this time. Special problem analyses may very well require subcompartmentation of spleen and lymph nodes. For example, certain tumors develop at specific nodes and T-B-Mϕ interactions occurring for only a short period of time take place in the white pulp compartment of the spleen. Also, the lungs receive a high concentration of lymphocytes early in the response, and are important in the early removal of antigen. An intensified program of collaboration between analysts and experimenters is necessary to better understand these processes.

6. CONCLUSION

It is seen that linear time-delay differential equations mimick the experimental data for lymphocyte distribution of rats within the accuracy of the data available. Unfortunately more extensive data is required to do an adequate job of parameter estimation, and such data is not readily obtained. This is particularly true for the lymph node compartments presented here as a building-block synthesis of the lymphatic system. Eventually, it is hoped that data will be available to check models for dynamic behavior of antibodies and antigen as well as T and B lymphocytes. Such a model is reviewed in Section 5.

ACKNOWLEDGEMENT

The authors wish to express their gratitude for the experimental cooperation of Professor Bill Ford (University of Manchester Medical School) and his associates. And, at the same time, to express our bereavement at the recent sudden death of Professor Ford. The profession has lost a great man.

REFERENCES

[1] I. Roitt, Essential Immunology, Blackwell Scientific, Oxford and London, 1974.

[2] G. I. Bell, A. S. Perelson and G. H. Pimbley, Jr., (eds.), Theoretical Immunology, Marcel Dekker, New York, 1978.

[3] R. R. Mohler, C. Bruni and A. Gandolfi, "A Systems Approach to Immunology," IEEE Proc. 68, 964-990, 1980.

[4] G. I. Marchuk, Mathematical Models in Immunology, Science Press, Moscow, 1980 (In Russian; English version, Optimization Software, Publication Division, distributed by Springer-Verlap, New York, 1984).

[5] G. I. Marchuk, Mathematical Modeling in Immunology and Medicine, North Holland, Amsterdam, 1983.

[6] M. DeSousa, Lymphocyte Circulation, John Wiley, Chicester, U.K., 1981.

[7] M. E. Smith and W. L. Ford, "The Recirculating Lymphocyte Pool of the Rat: A systematic description of the migratory behaviour of recirculating lymphocytes," Immunology 49, pp. 83-94, 1983.

[8] R. R. Mohler, Z. Farooqi and T. Heilig, "An Immune Lymphocyte Circulation Model," in System Modeling and Optimization (Proc. 11th IFIP Conf.), Springer-Verlag, New York, 1984.

[9] R. R. Mohler and C. F. Barton, "Compartmental Control Model of the Immune Process," Proc. 8th IFIP Optimiz. Conf., Springer-Verlag, New York, 1978.

[10] J. M. Yoffey and F. C. Courtice, Lymphatics, Lymph and the Lymphomyeloid Complex, Academic Press, London, 1970.

[11] S. Fossum, M. E. Smith and W. L. Ford, "The Recirculation of T and B Lymphocytes in the Athymic Nude Rat," Scand. J. Immun. 17, pp. 551-557, 1983.

[12] P. Nieuwenhuis and W. L. Ford, "Comparative Migration of B and T Lymphocytes in the Rat Spleen and Lymph Nodes," Cell. Immun. 23, pp. 254-267, 1976.

[13] C. De Lisi, "Some mathematical problems in the initiation and regulation of the Immune Response," Math Biosci., Vol. 35, pp. 1-26, 1977.

[14] G. I. Bell, "Lymphocyte traffic patterns and cell-cell interactions," in Theoretical Immunology, pp. 341-375, 1978.

[15] J. Sprent, "Circulating T and B lymphocytes of the mouse, I, migratory properties," Cell Immunol., Vol. 7, pp. 10-39, 1973.

[16] B. J. Hammond, "A compartmental analysis of circulatory lymphocytes in the spleen," Cell Tissue Kinet., Vol. 5, pp. 153-169, 1975.

[17] C. W. Gear, "DIFSUB for solution of ordinary differential equations," Comm. ACM, Vol. 14, pp. 185-190, 1971.

[18] R. R. Mohler, "Biological modeling with variable compartmental structures," IEEE Trans. Automat. Contr., Vol. AC-19, pp. 922-926, 1974.

[19] W. D. Smith and R. R. Mohler, "Necessary and sufficient conditions in the tracer determination of compartmental system order," J. Theor. Biol., Vol. 57, pp. 1-21, 1976.

PROCEDURE FOR EVALUATION OF A LIQUID PHASE RADIOIMMUNOASSAY DETERMINING IMMUNE COMPLEXES IN SERA

C. Łaba[1], H. Haas[2], J.T. Jodkowski[3], A. Lange[1]

[1]Dept. of Clinical Immunology, Institute of Immunology and Experimental Therapy, Polish Academy of Sciences, Wrocław, Poland

[2]Borstel Research Institute, 2061 Borstel, FRG

[3]Dept. of Physical Chemistry, Medical School of Wrocław, Wrocław, Poland

INTRODUCTION

Employment of the optimal mathematical procedure for determining a standard curve is essential for a proper evaluation of laboratory tests. These test results are then frequently calculated with the use of a standard curve, which expresses the relationship between the dose and response. This approach is also used in a liquid phase radioimmunoassay which employes binding of iodinated (^{125}I) Clq as a measure of the presence of immunological complexes in serum samples. The present work describes our approach for calculation of the predicted variance - which is a rational for giving weights to empirical points composing the standard curve.

THE RADIOIMMUNOASSAY DOSE - RESPONSE CURVE

Fourteen of twenty-two curves reflecting the relationship between the dose (standardized human IgG aggregates) and response (fraction of ^{125}I·C1q bound) showed sigmoidal shape. Furthermore, in eight tests the standard curves were partly sigmoidal but did not reach the upper or lower asmptote. Our test result curves are described by the following formula:

$$Y_1 = \frac{a - d}{1 + \left(\frac{X_1}{c}\right)^b} + d \qquad (1)$$

where Y_1 - response, X_1 - dose, a - upper asymptote, d - lower asymptote, b - slope, c - midpoint.

The amount of ^{125}I·C1q precipitated by trichloroacid is used as a measure of the total precipitable amount of C1q (B_{max}). Mathematically this represents the upper asymptote. The lower asymptote is approximated by the value of 0 . The response seen at different concentrations of standard aggregates can be expressed as the fraction of B_{max} .

$$\hat{Y} = \frac{Y_1}{a} \qquad (2)$$

where Y_1 - response, a - upper asymptote.

The logistic transformation of Y at different ranges of response ($Y_1 \ldots Y_M$) makes the dose-response curve linear. Therefore the curve can be plotted with the use of the linear least squares method. This enables the calculation of the two other parameters of the sigmoidal curve - slope and midpoint (Gaines Das and Tydeman, 1982; Laughton and Miles, 1977).

Gaines Das and Tydeman (1982) recently offered several possibilities of the logistic transformation. In our test the transformation described by the following formula was the most suitable:

$$Y = \log \frac{\log (\hat{Y} \cdot 100)}{2 - \log (\hat{Y} \cdot 100)} \tag{3}$$

$$X = \log (X_1) \tag{4}$$

With this transformation the dose - response regression varied from 0.94 - 0.99 .

THE PREDICTED VARIANCE CALCULATION

In C1q radioimmunoassay the empirical variance did not simply follow the magnitude of response. This called for applying a weighted - procedure to the variance calculation according to the formula:

$$\mathrm{VAR}(\hat{Y}) = \frac{\sum\limits_{I=1}^{N} Y_1^2 (I) - N \cdot \bar{Y}_1^2}{(N - 1) \cdot \bar{Y}_1^2} \tag{5}$$

where:

$$\bar{Y} = \frac{1}{N} \sum_{I=1}^{N} Y_1 (I) \tag{6}$$

The relation between predicted variance $\mathrm{VAR}(\acute{Y})$ versus Y predicted ($\acute{Y}$) is expressed by the equation given by Rodbard and Hutt (1974):

$$\mathrm{VAR}(\acute{Y}) = a_0 + a_1 \acute{Y} + a_2 \acute{Y}^2 \tag{7}$$

where:

$$\acute{Y} = 10^{-\frac{2}{1 + 10^{(\alpha \cdot X + \beta)}}} \tag{8}$$

α - slope, β - intercept, $a_1 = a_2$.

The significance of the various terms of the equation depends upon the characteristic of the test which is under study.

As in other test systems (Chen et al., 1980) a_0 - is represented by the variance of negative control [CONTR(-)]:

$$a_0 = \mathrm{VAR}\ [\mathrm{CONTR}(-)] \tag{9}$$

a_1 - can be calculated as a difference between the variance of B_{max} and variance of negative control.

$$a_1 = VAR(B_{max}) - VAR[CONTR(-)] \tag{10}$$

The predicted weighted variances at different points along the standard curve either when calculated with one as an exponent equaling $[VAR(\dot{Y}) = a_0 + a_1\dot{Y}]$ or two as an exponent equaling $[VAR(\dot{Y}) = a_0 + a_2\dot{Y}^2]$ are from 1.1 to 3.0 and from 1.2 to 5.0 times higher as compared to the empirical variances respectively. Therefore, we looked for the exponent which when used for predicted variance estimation could secure the optimal fittness between predicted and empirical variance. This was achived when the following formulas were employed.

$$VAR(\dot{Y}) = a_0 + a_1\dot{Y}^{IP2} \tag{11}$$

where:

$$IP2 = \begin{cases} \dfrac{VAR(B_{max})}{\frac{1}{M}\sum\limits_{J=1}^{M} VAR[\hat{Y}(J)]} & \text{if } a_1 \geqslant 0 \\[2ex] \dfrac{\frac{1}{M}\sum\limits_{J=1}^{M} VAR[\hat{Y}(J)]}{VAR[CONTR(-)]} & \text{if } a_1 < 0 \end{cases}$$

The predicted variances calculated with the IP2 exponent fits better to the emprical values than do the calculations based on the assumption of either constant linear or quadratic proportionality between variance and the response as it is seen from Table 1.

WEIGHTING AND DETERMINATION OF THE FINAL RESULT

Knowing the predicted variance of previously suggested formulas (11), allowed a determination of weights calculation. Similarly, we employed the known procedure (Rodbard and Hutt, 1974) for determination of the regression of curve parameters, with allowance for the weights of particular measurements at the specific standard curve points, based upon the iterative method described by the formulae:

$$Y(J) = 10^{-\frac{2}{1+10^{[\alpha\cdot X(J)+\beta]}}} \tag{12}$$

$$W(J) = \frac{\dot{Y}^2(J)\cdot[1 - \dot{Y}(J)]^2}{VAR[\dot{Y}(J)]} \tag{13}$$

$$L(J,I) = \alpha\cdot X(J) + \beta + \frac{\hat{Y}(J,I) - \dot{Y}(J)}{\dot{Y}(J)\circ[1 - \dot{Y}(J)]} \circ \frac{1}{\ln 10} \tag{14}$$

The slope of the weighted regression line - α, intercept point with the axis of ordinates - β, and correlation coefficient - r, are determined by means of the method of least squares for weighted linear regression with repetitions. At the end of the procedure the content of immunological complexes in sera is calculated. This content in the serum investigated is expressed by the formula:

$$C = 10^{\frac{Y-\beta}{\alpha}} \tag{15}$$

where Y - response for the serum under investigation expressed by the transformation described in formula (3), α - slope, β - intercept.

To make all the calculations possible a computer program was written in FORTRAN which is described in details elsewhere (Łaba et al., 1986).

CONCLUSION

Twelve tests were evaluated with the use of the above procedure and by that described by Gaines Das and Tydeman (1982). The standard curves were plotted with the use of two methods. From these curves the results were read, which corresponded to the B/B_{max} fractions ranging from 0.05 to 0.9. The differences in reading, when two curves were used, were negligible at the lower range of fractions from 0.05 to 0.7. There was some difference at higher B/B_{max} range (>0.7), however, small and statistically non-significant [$t_{0.05(22)} = 2.074$, $0.031 \leq t_s \leq 0.360$].

This comparison gives credit to our presently described approach to the predictive variance calculation. Calculated predictive variance can be further used in the iterative method of weighted regression curve determination.

SUMMARY

Statistical evaluation of the liquid phase radioimmunoassay, which employes binding of labelled C1q (^{125}I·C1q) as a measure of the presence of immunological complexes in serum samples, was made.

The curve representing the relationship between the dose (standardized human IgG aggregates) and response (fraction of ^{125}I·C1q) was sigmoidal or partly sigmoidal and after logistic transformation was linear and could be plotted with the use of the least squares method. This allowed calculation of the two other parameters of the sigmoidal curve (slope and midpoint).

A procedure for calculating predictive variance was worked out. This procedure uses the relation between the higher value of two evaluated variances - the variance of B_{max} and the variance of negative control - and the mean empirical variance of the response to different doses of standard aggregates, for a calculation of the exponent for Y predicted. The predictive variance was further used for weighting of points of a standard curve.

TABLE 1

Options of predicted variance	Statistical significance of difference	
	N.S.	0.05
$a_0 + a_1 Y^{IP2}$	14	1
$a_0 + a_1 Y$	8	7
$a_0 + a_2 Y^2$	7	8

The statistical evaluation (Student - t test for pairs) of differences between empirical and predicted variances (calculated according to the listed formulas) in 15 independent experiments.

REFERENCES

1 Chen, L-W., Heminger, L., Maxon, H.R., Tsay, J.Y. (1980) Non-specific binding as a source of error in thyrotropin radioimmunoassay with polyethylene glycol as separating agent. Clin. Chem. 26:487-490.

2 Gaines Das, R.E., Tydeman, M.S. (1982) Iterative weighted regression analysis of logit responses. A computer program for analysis of bioassays and immunoassays. Computer Programs in Biomedicine 15:13-22.

3 Laughton, E., Miles, M. (1977) Immunoradiometric assay (IRMA) and two-side IRMA systems. In: Abraham, G.A., Handbook of radioimmunoassay. Marcel Dekker, New York 131-177

4 Łaba, C., Haas, H., Jodkowski, J.T., Lange, A. (1986) Statistical analysis of a liquid phase radioimmunoassay for immune complex determination. Arch. Arch. Immunol. Ther. Exp., in press

5 Rodbard, D., Hutt, D.M. (1974) Statistical analysis of radioimmunoassays and immunoradiometric (labelled antibody) assays: A generalized weighted, iterative, least squares method for logistic curve fitting. In: Radioimmunoassay and Related procedures in Medicine. Proceedings of a Symposium, Istanbul 1973, Vol.I., IAEA, Vienna 165-192

APPLICATION OF MATHEMATICAL MODELS IN THE MEMBRANE ELECTROPHYSIOLOGY OF MACROPHAGES

Can Ince

Department of Infectious Diseases, University Hospital, 2333 AA Leiden, The Netherlands.

Introduction

In most cells there is a transmembrane potential difference, called a resting membrane potential (about -70 mV) arising from the unequal distributions of ions across the cell membrane and the selective permeability of the cell membrane for the various ion species. In nerve and muscle cells a sudden change in the ionic permeability of the membrane causes a rapid all-or-nothing change in membrane potential called an action potential. In nerve cells the action potential forms the basic information-carrying signal and in muscles cells it evokes cell contraction (27).

In 1952, on the basis of electrophysiolgical experiments on the giant axon of the squid, Hodgkin and Huxley formulated a series of equations to describe the membrane conductance changes underlying the occurrence of the action potential (15). These equations, called the Hodgkin-Huxley equations, are still applied in the field of membrane electrophysiology and are consistent with the notion that changes in the membrane conductance giving rise to the action potential are the result of the collective behavior of individual transmembrane proteins called ion channels, which can be in either a conducting or in a non-conducting state. The existence of such ion channels was recently established by the use of the patch clamp technique introduced by Neher and Sackmann (14,36). This technique makes it possible to measure transmembrane currents passing through individual ion channels as they open and close (i.e. as they change from a conducting to a non-conducting state). Analysis of the kinetics of channel activity has led to the development of mathematical models representing the behavior of ion channels (1,3,4,17). This means that for membrane electrophysiological studies, mathematical models can be applied to macroscopic membrane conductance changes as well as to the underlying activity of single ion channels. The results from such mathematical considerations provide a theoretical basis for the analysis of membrane electrophysiological phenonmena leading to predictions that can be verified experimentally.

Phagocytic cells form an important part of the host-defence system due to their ability to recognize, phagocytose, kill and digest invading pathogens. There are two lines of phagocytes, one polymorphonuclear and the other mononuclear. Both cell lines originate in the bone marrow and later enter the blood circulation. The mononuclear phagocytes in the circulation, called monocytes, migrate to the tissues, where they mature into macrophages (41). Besides their capacity to endocytose (i.e. phagocytose and pinocytose) micro-organisms, fluid, cell debris, foreign bodies and tumor cells, macrophages can produce a wide array of humoral factors. Recent investigations concerning the characteristics and physiology of mononuclear phagocytes have been reported in the proceedings of the IVth International Conference on Mononuclear Phagocytes (40).

Macrophages have numerous surface receptors supplying them with information about their environment and enabling them to interact with other cells, micro-organisms and humoral factors. Most of the above-mentioned functions are receptor-mediated, and the binding of ligands to macrophages is the first step in the activation of these cells. Since transmembrane electrical currents carried by ions are known to form an important link between ligand-receptor interaction and the activation of cell functions in many other cell types, it is conceivable that the same is the case for mononuclear phagocytes. Before this point can be investigated, however, the resting electrophysiological properties of mononuclear phagocytes need to be defined. For this purpose mononuclear phagocytes of human origin, i.e. peripheral blood monocytes, were used. In vitro culture of human monocytes for periods longer than one week results in increased cell size and differentiation of these monocytes into macrophage-like cells. Such cultured human monocytes were used for the experiments reported here.

This paper gives a brief review of work done on the characterization of some basic electrophysiological properties of cultured human monocytes, mathematical models being used to support experimental results. Since the two main techniques for electrical measurements on single cells are based on microelectrode and patch clamp measurements, the use of these methods in the study of mononuclear phagocytes are discussed separetely.

Transmembrane potential measurements with intracellular microelectrodes

In characterizing membrane electrophysiological properties of mononuclear phagocytes it is important to first establish the value of the resting membrane potential of these cells. Conventionally, membrane potential measurements are made with saline-filled open-tipped glass pipettes (called microelectrodes) with a tip diameter smaller than 0.2 µm. Impalement of a cell with this kind of electrode provides an intracellular measuring point, allowing measurement of the transmembrane potential (Fig. 1A). Such measurements in macrophages have shown that endocytosis of latex beads (26) and exposure to substances that induce chemotaxis (11) (i.e., directed cell movement along a concentration gradient of a chemoattractant) causes changes in the membrane potential. In alveolar macrophages changes in the membrane potential precede the production of super oxide by these cells (2). Macrophages can show free-running oscillatory membrane potential changes, which have been found to arise from modulation of the membrane conductance for potassium caused by cyclic changes in intracellular concentration of calcium ions (7,12,19,37,38). Action potentials have also been described in cultured human monocytes (33).

Penetration of small cells with microelectrodes can inflict damage on the cell, leading to unreliable measurements. Until recently, measurement of a sustained potential over a given period after microelectrode penetration was seen as an indication that transmembrane microelectrode induced leakages had not occurred and its value was taken as the value of the pre-impalement membrane potential. Nevertheless, values obtained in small cells can suffer from inaccuracy due to a transmembrane shunt arising from the hydration mantle (estimated to be about 100 Å thick) surrounding the intracellular microelectrode (Fig. 1A). If the resistance R_s of this shunt (about 100 Mohm) is less than or of the same order of magnitude as the membrane resistance R_m (as is the case for small cells), the pre-impalement resting membrane potential will be underestimated and a source of error introduced into measurements (14,25,28).

A method to estimate the pre-impalement membrane potential of small cells that takes into account the presence of the microelectrode induced transmembrane shunt, was introduced by Lassen et al., who worked with ascites tumor cells (28). Using a microelectrode with a fast response time (i.e., $T_e = R_e C_e < 0.1$ msec), these authors measured the fast potential transient occuring in the initial milliseconds after microelectrode entry into the cell. A schematic representation of an intracellular microelectrode measurement with an equivalent circuit superimposed on it is shown in Fig. 1A. Prior to cell impalement (and the introduction of R_s) the membrane capacitance C_m is charged up to the resting membrane potential (E_m). When the microelectrode is driven into the cell and R_s introduced, the charged C_m will discharge from E_m to a new steady state potential level (E_s) with a time course determined by the time constants of the impaled membrane (including the shunt components) and of the microelectrode. The ability of the voltage amplifier to detect this discharge is limited by the response time of the microelectrode (T_e). If, however, the time constant of the microelectrode is sufficiently smaller than that of the cell membrane, the discharge of E_m upon the introduction of R_s by the microelectrode can be measured. Small microelectrode time constants can be achieved by the use of an electronic technique called capacitance compensation. Under these conditions the potential transient recorded by the voltage amplifier in the initial milliseconds after microelectrode penetration is characterized by a rapid negative-going potential transient reaching a peak value (E_p) and followed by a slower depolarizing (positive-going) transient caused by the discharge of C_m, to a steady state potential E_s (Fig. 1B). The best approximation of E_m directly measurable by a microelectrode is therefore E_p.

To assess the usefulness of fast potential transient measurements in the estimation of pre-impalement resting membrane potentials, an analytical expression for the fast potential transient is needed. Application of Kirchoff's laws to the circuit illustrated in Fig. 1A gives the following differential equation for the potential transient (V_e) measured by the amplifier upon cell penetration by a microelectrode and the instantaneous introduction of the shunt resistance R_s at time t=0:

$$T_m T_e \frac{d^2V_e}{dt^2} + (T_m + T_c + BT_e)\frac{dV_e}{dt} + BV_e = \frac{R_m}{R_s} E_d + E_m \qquad (1)$$

in which $T_m = R_m C_m$, $T_e = R_e C_e$, $T_c = R_m C_e$, $B = (R_s + R_m)/R_s$, Ed is a diffusion potential, and R_s is the resistance of the microelectrode induced shunt. A peak potential E_p is reached when $dV_e/dt=0$. In the steady state situation (i.e., $t \rightarrow \infty$) eq. 1 reduces to:

$$V_e = E_s = \frac{E_m R_s + E_d R_m}{R_m + R_s} \tag{2}$$

and shows the influence of microelectrode-induced components (R_s and E_d) on steady state potential measurements. On this basis it can be concluded that steady state potential measurements can only give a reliable measure of the pre-impalement resting membrane potential when $R_s \gg R_m$.

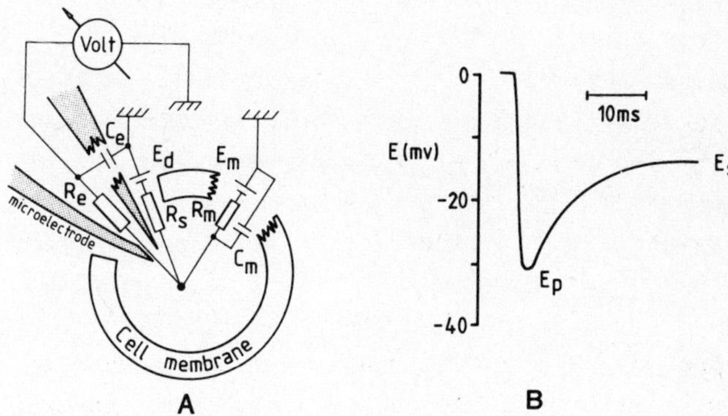

Fig.1. Microelectrode measurements on single cells. (A) The introduction of a microelectrode into a cell induces a transmembrane shunt. The microelectrode has a tip resistance R_e and an electrode capacitance C_e. The hydration mantle surrounding the electrode provides a transmembrane shunt with a resistance R_s. The unequal ionic concentrations across the shunt also produce a diffusion potential E_d. The electric parameters of the cell include the resting membrane potential E_m, a membrane resistance R_m, and capacitance C_m. (B) When R_m is of the same order of magnitude or larger than R_s a peaked potential transient is seen during the initial milliseconds after microelectrode entry into the cell. The potential transient rapidly reaches a peak potential E_p and is followed by a slower positive-going transient to a steady state potential E_s. Provided the time constant of the electrode is sufficiently small, E_p will provide a good measure of the pre-impalement resting membrane potential of the cell.

However close the approximation of E_m, the value of E_p will always be an underestimation of the pre-impalement resting potential because of the change in potential across C_m while C_e charges up. Analysis of equation (1) shows that when microelectrodes are used with timeconstants of less than 0.1 ms, E_p, although an underestimation, provides a good estimate of the pre-implament membrane potential of cells as small as macrophages. Experimental evidence that E_p is an accurate measure of E_m within 10 mV was provided by experiments in which membrane potential measurement with the patch clamp technique was combined with intracellular microelectrode impalement (24). Patch clamp measurements do not suffer from the ill effects of an R_s and allow the measurement of E_m prior to cell penetration by the microelectrode.

Impalement transients measured in mononuclear phagocytes of various origin revealed that E_p was more negative than the sustained potential E_s. This observation led to the conclusion that the pre-impalement membrane potential of mononuclear phagocytes is more negative than had previously been assumed on the basis of sustained potential measurements (25).

The values of the resting membrane potentials of cultured human monocytes as determined by peak potential measurements lie between -30 and -50 mV (24,25,37). These values are less negative than those usually reported for nerve and muscle cells (around -70 mV), which suggests that the ionic basis of the resting membrane potential of cultured human monocytes differs from that usually asssociated with nerve or muscle cells.

The knowledge that the peak potential is a good measure of the resting membrane potential led us to use the constant field equation (13,16) to investigate the ionic basis of the resting membrane potential of cultured human monocytes. This equation rests on the assumption that there is a linear potential decline across the cell membrane, and relates the resting membrane potential to the intra- and extracellular concentrations of monovalent ions and the permeability of the cell membrane for them. The constant field equation is given by:

$$E_m = \frac{RT}{F} \ln \frac{P_K K_e + P_{Na} Na_e + P_{Cl} Cl_i}{P_K K_i + P_{Na} Na_i + P_{Cl} Cl_e} \quad (3)$$

in which E_m is the resting membrane potential, R the gas constant, T the temperature in K, F is Faraday's constant, and K_e, Na_e, and Cl_e the extracellular and K_i, Na_i, and Cl_i the intracellular concentrations of K^+, Na^+ and Cl^-, respectively. P_K, P_{Na}, and P_{Cl} give the permeability of the cell membrane to K^+, Na^+, and Cl^- ions, respectively.

To find out whether this equation adequately describes the ionic basis of the resting membrane potential of cultured human monocytes, values of its parameters were determined. First, the intracellular concentrations of K^+, Na^+, and Cl^- were determined biochemically in terms of the mean cell size, water content, and the K^+, Na^+, and Cl^- contents of monocytes in suspension. The experimentally obtained values for K_i, Na_i, and Cl_i in human monocytes were 130, 30, and 120 mM, respectively. Next, determination of membrane potentials by measurement of E_p under various extracellular ionic conditions gave values for P_{Na}/P_K and P_{Cl}/P_K, of 0.05 and 0.33, respectively.

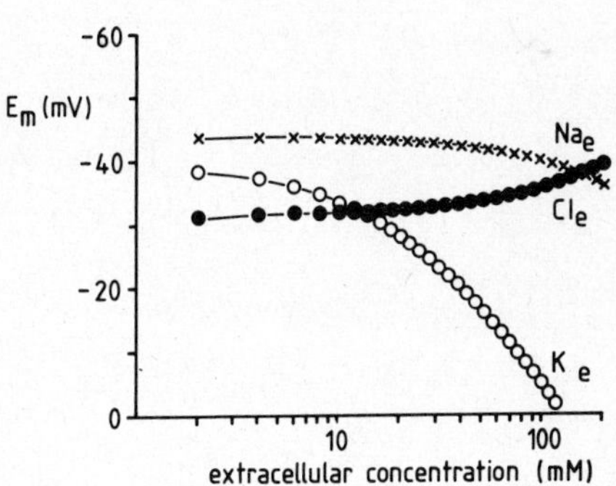

Fig 2. Calculations of the resting membrane potential of cultured human monocytes as a function of the extracellular concentration of monovalent ions (K_e, Na_e, and Cl_e). Three curves are shown for each of which the concentration of a different ion type (indicated next to each curve) is varied (indicated on the x axis), and, using the constant field equation, the resting membrane potential (E_m) was calculated (y axis). Values for the parameters used in the the constant field equation were obtained experimentally and were 121, 21, 106 mM for K_i, Na_i, and Cl_i, respectively, and 0.05 and 0.23 for P_{Na}/P_K and P_{Cl}/P_K, respectively.

With these values for P_{Na} / P_K, P_{Cl} /PK, Ki, Na_i, and Cl_i, E_m was calculated with the constant field equation (eq. 3) for three experiments, in each of which one of the ionic concentrations was varied and the remaining ionic concentrations were kept constant. The results of these calculations are shown in Fig.2. Experiments in which K_e, Na_e, and Cl_e were varied by using membrane-impermeable substitutes for these ions showed good agreement (within 10 mV) with the theoretically derived curves shown in Fig. 2 (21). The results of these studies revealed that the main difference between the ionic basis of the resting membrane potential of cultured human monocytes and that of nerve and muscle cells is the relatively high intracellular chloride concentration in the former combined with a membrane permeability to chloride close to that of potassium. The use of fast potential transient recordings to determine the resting membrane potential and the description of this potential by the constant field equation show the usefulness of mathematical descriptions in the characterization of the resting membrane electrophysiological properties of cultured human monocytes.

Patch clamp measurements of single ion channel activity

The limitations imposed on electrophysiological investigation of single cells by the presence of a microelectrode-induced shunt were abolished by the introduction of the patch clamp technique by Neher and Sakmann (14,36,39). Because a discussion of the many aspects of this powerful technique would take us beyond the scope of this paper, the reader is referred to the literature (14,18,39).

The patch clamp technique has recently been applied to mononuclear phagocytes (9,10,22-24,44,45). In brief, patch clamp measurements are performed with saline-filled fire-polished suction glass micro-pipettes (patch electrode) with slightly larger tip diameters (1 to 5 μm) than those of microelectrodes. The patch electrode is placed on the surface of the cell and suction is applied to it, which seals off a patch of the cell membrane from the extracellular environment (Fig. 3A). Under suitable conditions the seal can have a resistance in the the giga ohm range and is therefore referred to as a giga seal. This seal provides favorable electrical conditions for the measurement of currents, and sensitive current amplifiers can detect currents flowing through single ion channels.

Quantal changes in current are observed when the ion channels open and close. If a number of such transmembrane proteins are present under the patch, step-like current fluctuations are measured (Fig. 3B). Control of the kinetics of the alternating behavior of the opening and closing channel is provided by, e.g., the membrane potential or specific ligands (such as acetycholine). Ligand-receptor binding can therefore be investigated in great detail with the patch clamp technique (4).

The cumulative effects of channel activity over the entire cell membrane can also be measured with the patch clamp technique by breaking the membrane patch; this is done by applying an extra suction pulse. In a whole-cell configuration of this kind the macroscopic transmembrane currents can be measured (14). Thus, patch clamp measurements can be used to investigate the dependence of macroscopic membrane currents on the activity of single ion channels (31,34). Combination of patch clamp and microelectrode measurements in cultured human monocytes revealed correlation between changes in the microelectrode-measured membrane potential and enhanced channel activity measured with a patch electrode in the same cell (24).

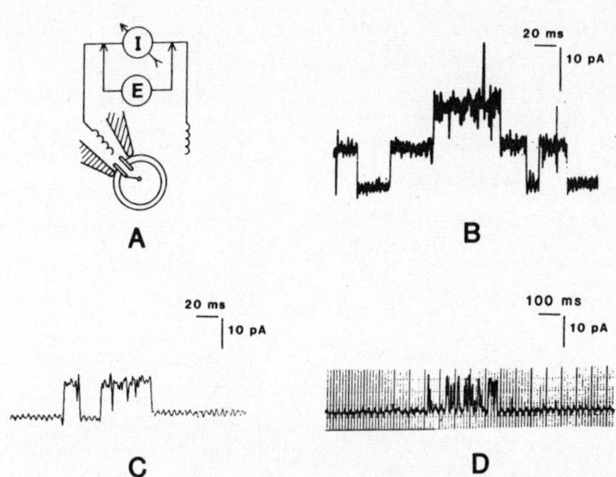

Fig 3. Single ionic channel measurements measurements performed in cultured human monocytes by use of the patch clamp technique. (A) A schematic representation of a patch clamp measurement shows how ionic channel activity can be measured without disrupting the cell. (B) When more than one channel is present under the patch step-like curent changes are measured. (C) Under certain conditions the noise produced by ions passing through the open channel is registered. (D) Due to the presence of more than one closed or open state in channels, burst-like opening of the channel can sometimes be observed.

Mean channel open and close times and the probability that a channel will be in a particular state under a number of conditions, can be used to construct models of the kinetics of channel activity. The observation that the binding of IgG (a sub-class of immunoglobulins) to its membrane receptor forms an ion channel (43) and that extracellular IgG stimulates the ability of human monocytes to kill micro-organisms intracellularly (30) are examples of the possiblities offered by patch clamp measurements for the study of the function of receptor-ligand binding in cells of the host-defence system.

Single channel measurements can also provide information concerning the movement of ions through an ion channel. As can be seen in Fig. 3C, enhanced noise levels are sometimes observed when an ion channel is open. These fluctuations occur as a result of the passage of ions through the channel and could reflect fluctuations in channel structure (29). Fluctuation analysis of such noise signals could provide additional information on the kinetics of ion channel activity (29). Analysis of the membrane noise of whole cells, for example, can be used to obtain information about the kinectic parameters of membrane conductance changes (42).

Analysis of the conditions that determine the kinectics of channel activity can provide information about the mechanisms by which the state of the channel is changed. For example, the use of Markov processes to describe the kinetics of channel behavior (3,17) has confirmed the general opinion that an ion channel forms a transmembrane tunnel in which there are a number of gates that can close or open. Such models predict a phenomenon called bursting sometimes seen in single channel activity (Fig. 3D) (4).

A related application of single channel measurement that is also relevant to the study of host-defence mechanisms is the finding that pathogens such as Neisseria gonorrhoeae and Neisseria meningitidis (32) and toxins such as diphtheria toxin (6) incorporate ion channels called porins into the membrane of host cells. It is speculated that such pathogens incorporate porins into host cells to affect their permeability thereby enabling the pathogen to enter the host cell (32). Thus various types of transmembrane proteins involved in host defence mechanisms seem to have ion channel-like structures. Electrophysiological techniques provide a tool for the study of the kinetics of such proteins.

Discussion

This brief review has shown some applications of mathematical models for the description of membrane electrophysiological processes in macrophages. Patch clamp measurements can provide detailed information concerning membrane events and provide an ideal basis for mathematical models of molecular mechanisms. Recent application of the patch clamp technique to cells involved in the host defence system has identified ion channel activity in human T lymphocytes (5,35) and monocytes (10,23,24) as well as in mouse peritoneal macrophages (44,45) and spleen macrophages (9) and mouse B lymphocytes (8). The precise role of such ion channels in the functional activity of these cells is poorly understood, but further research should provide information about relationships between the functioning of cells involved in host defence and membrane electrophysiological processes. Such studies can be expected to generate a basis for theoretical models of the molecular biology of host-defence mechanisms.

Acknowledgements

The work described in this paper was mainly carried out at the Department of Physiology, University of Leiden, the Netherlands.

C.Ince is supported by the Foundation for Medical Research (FUNGO), which is subsidized in part by the Netherlands Orginization for the Advancement of Pure Research (ZWO).

Thanks are extended to B. van Duijn, B. Thio, J.T. van Dissel, A. Coremans and E. van Bavel for their help in experiments, J. van de Gevel for preparation of cells, K. Versluis for electronic support, and Drs. P.C.J. Leijh and D.L. Ypey for their critical reading of the manuscript.

REFERENCES

1. Aldritch RW, Yellen, G. Nonstationary channel kinectics.1983. In: Single-Channel Recording, eds. B. Sakmann and E. Neher, publ. Plenum Press, New York, pp pp287-299.

2. Cameron, AR, Nelson, J, Forman, HJ. 1983. Depolarization and increased conductance precede superoxide release by concanavalin A-stimulated rat alveolar macrophages. Proc. Natl. Acad. Sci. USA. 80:3726-3728.

3. Colquhoun, D, Hawkes, AG. 1983. The principles of the stochastic interpretation of ion-channel mechanisms. In: Single-Channel Recording, eds. B.Sakmann and E. Neher, publ. Plenum Press, New York, pp 135-177.

4. Colquhoun, D, Sackmann, B. 1983. Bursts of openings in transmittor-activated ion channels. In: Single-Channel Recording, eds. B.Sakmann and E. Neher, publ. Plenum Press, New York, pp 345-364.

5. DeCoursey, TE, Chandy, KG, Gupta, S, Cahalan, MD. 1984. Voltage-gated K^+ channels in human T lymphocytes: a role in mitogenesis. Nature 307:465-468.

6. Donovon, JJ, Simon, MI, Draper, RK, Montal, M. 1981. Diptheria toxin forms transmembrane channels in planer lipid bilayer. Proc. Natl. Acad. Sci., USA. 78:172-176.

7. Dos Reis, GA, Oliveira-Castro, GM. 1977. Electrophysiology of phagocytic membranes I. Potassium-dependent slow membrane hyperpolarizations in mice macrophages. Biochim. Biophy. Acta. 469:257-263.

8. Fukushima, Y, Hagiwara, S.1985. Currents carried by monovalent cations through calcium channels in mouse neoplastic B lymphocytes. J. Physiol. 358:255-284.

9. Gallin, EK. 1984. Electrophysiological properties of macrophages. Fed. Proc. 43:2385.

10. Gallin, EK. 1984. Calcium and voltage-activated potassium channels in human macrophages. Biophy.J. 46:821-827.

11. Gallin, EK, Gallin JI. 1977. Interaction of chemotactic factors with human macrophages: Induction of transmembrane potentials. J.Cell Biol. 75:277-289.

12. Gallin, EK, Wiederhold, ML, Lipsky, PE, Rosenthal, AS. 1975. Spontaneous and induced membrane potential hyperpolarizations in macrophages. J. Cell. Physiol. 86:653-661.

13. Goldman, DE. 1943. Potential impedance and rectification in membranes. J. Gen. Physiol. 27,37-60.

14. Hamill, OP, Marty, A, Neher, E, Sakmann, B, Sigworth FJ. 1981. Improved patch-clamp techniques for high resolution current recording from cells and cell-free membrane patches. Pflugers Arch. 391:85-100.

15. Hodgkin, AL, Huxley AF. 1952. A quantative description of the membrane current and its application to conduction and excitation in nerve. J. Physiol. (Lond). 117:500-544.

16. Hodgkin, AL, Katz, B. 1949. The effect of sodium ions on the electrical activity of the giant axon of the squid. J. Physiol. 108:37-77.

17. Horn, R , Lange, K. 1983. Estimating kinectic constants from single channel data. Biophy. J. 43:207-223.

18. Ince, C. 1985. Introduction to the electrophysiology of mononuclear phagocytes. In: Mononuclear phagocytes. Characteristics, Physiology and Function, ed. R. Van Furth), Martinus Nijhoff Publishers, Boston, Dordrecht, Lancaster.Chap.38, pp 361-368.

19. Ince, C, Leijh, PCJ, Meijer, J, Van Bavel, E, Ypey, DL. 1984. Oscillatory hyperpolarizations and resting membrane potentials of mouse fibroblast and macrophage cell lines. J. Physiol. 352:625-635.

20. Ince, C, Leijh, PCJ, Thio, B, Van Duijn, B, Ypey, DL. 1985. Identification of a Na/K pump in cultured human monocytes. J. Physiol. (in press).

21. Ince, C, Thio, B, Van Duijn, B, Van Dissel J.T., Ypey, DL, Leijh, PCJ. 1985. Intracellular concentrations of K^+, Na^+ and Cl^- and the ionic basis of the resting membrane potential in human monocytes. (submitted).

22. Ince, C, Van Dissel, J, Diesselhoff, MMC. 1985. A teflon culture dish for high magnification observations and measurements from single cells. Pflugers Arch. 403:240-244.

23. Ince, C, Van Duijn, B, Ypey, DL, Leijh, PCJ (1984). A small conductance K^+ -channel in cultured human monocytes. In: Book of Abstracts 8th International Biophysics Congress, Abstr. .

24. Ince, C, Ypey, DL. 1985. Membrane hyperpolarizations and ionic channels in cultured human monocytes. In: Mononuclear phagocytes. Characteristics, Physiology and Function,ed. R.Van Furth, Martinus Nijhoff Publishers, Boston, Dordrecht, Lancaster.Chap. 39, pp 369-337.

25. Ince, C, Ypey, DL, Van Furth, R, Verveen, AA. 1983. Estimation of the membrane potential of cultured macrophages from the fast potential transient upon microelectrode entry. J. Cell Biol. 96:796-801.

26. Kouri, J, Noa, M, Diaz, B, Niubo, E. 1980. Hyperpolarisation of rat peritoneal macrophages phagocytosing latex particles. Nature 283:868-69.

27. Kuffler, SW, Nicholls, JG. 1977. From Neuron to Brain, Pub. Sinaur Associates, Inc., Sunderland, Mass.

28. Lassen, UV, Nielsen, AMT, Pape, L, Simonsen, LO. 1971. The membrane potential of Ehrlich ascites tumor cells. Microelectrode measurements and their critical evaluation. J. Membrane Biol. 6:269-288.

29. Lauger, P. 1983. Conformational changes of ionic channels. In: Single-Channel Recording, eds. B.Sakmann and E. Neher, publ. Plenum Press, New York, pp 177-189.

30. Leijh, PCJ, van den Barselaar, M, van Zwet, TL, Daha, MR,van Furth, R. 1979. Requirement of extracellular complement and immunoglobulin for intracellular killing of micro-organisms by human monocytes. J. Clin. Invest. 63:772-784.

31. Lux, Neher, E, Marty, A. 1981. Single channel activity associated with the calcium dependent outward current inHelix Pomatia. Pflugers Archiv, 389:293-295.

32. Lynch, EC, Blake, MS, Gotschlich, Mauro, A. 1984. Spontaneously transferred from whole cells and reconstituted from puroified proteins of Neisseria gonorrhoeae and Neisseria meningitidis. Biophys. J. 45:104-107.

33. MacCann, FV, Cole, JJ, Guyre, PM, Russel, JAG. 1983. Action potentials in macrophages derived from human monocytes. Science 199:991-993.

34. Maruyama, Y, Peterson, OH, Flanagan,P ,Pearson, GT. 1983. Quantification of Ca2+-activated K+ channels under hormonal control in pancreas acinar cells. Nature 305:228-232.

35. Matteson, DR, Deutsch, C. 1984. K channels in T lymphocytes: a patch clamp study using monoclonal antibody adhesion. Nature 307:468-471.

36. Neher, E, Sackmann, B. 1976. Single channel currents recorded from membrane of denervated frog muscle fibres. Nature (Lond.) 260:799-802.

37. Oliveira-Castro, GM. 1983. Ca^{2+}-sensative K^{+} channels in phagocytic cell membranes.Cell Calcium 4:475-492.

38. Persechini, PM, Araujo, EG, Oliveira-Castro, GM. 1981. Electrophysiology of phagocytic membranes: induction of slow hyperpolarizations in macrophages and macrophage polykaryons by intracellular calcium injection. J.Membrane Biol. 81-90.

39. Sakmann, B, Neher, E. (eds). 1983. Single-Channel Recording, Publishers. Plenum Press, New York.

40. Van Furth, R (ed). 1985. Mononuclear Phagocytes: Characteristics, Physiology and Function. Publishers: Martinus Nijhoff Publ., Boston, Dordrecht, Lancester.

41. Van Furth, R, Cohn, ZA, Hirsch, JG, Humphrey, JH, Spector, WG, Langevoort. 1972. The mononuclear phagocyte system. a new classification of macrophages, monocytes and their precursor cells. Bull WHO 46:845.

42. Verveen, AA, DeFelice, LJ. 1974. Membrane noise. In: Progress in Biophysics and Molecular Biology. 28:189-265.

43. Young, JDE, Unkeless, JC, Young, TM, Mauro, A, Cohn, ZA 1983. Role for a mouse IgGFc receptor as a ligand-dependent ion channel. Nature 306:186-189.

44. Ypey, DL, Clapham, DE. 1983. Development of a delayed outward-rectifying K+ conductance in cultured mouse peritoneal macrophages. Proc.Natl.Acad.Sci. 81:3083-3087.

45. Ypey, DL, Clapham, DE, Ince, C. 1985. Potassium channels and conductance in cultured mouse peritoneal macrophages. In: Mononuclear phagocytes. Characteristics, Physiology and Function, ed. R. Van Furth, Martinus Nijhoff Publishers, Boston, Dordrecht, Lancaster.Chap.41, pp 389-396.

Linking mathematics and biology

Journal of

Mathematical Biology

Subscription Information:
ISSN 0303-6812 Title No. 285
1986, Vol. 24 (6 issues)
For Subscribers outside North America: DM 596,– plus carriage charges.
For Subscribers in USA, Canada and Mexico:
US $ 237.00 (includes postage and handling).

For sample copies or instructions for authors, please contact one of the addresses listed below

Springer-Verlag
Berlin Heidelberg
New York Tokyo

Editorial Board:

K. P. Hadeler, Tübingen;. S. A. Levin, Ithaca (Managing Editors); H. T. Banks, Providence; J. D. Cowan, Chicago; J. Gani, Santa Barbara; F. C. Hoppensteadt, Salt Lake City; D. Ludwig, Vancouver; J. D. Murray, Oxford; T. Nagylaki, Chicago; L. A. Segel, Rehovot

The **Journal of Mathematical Biology** serves as a meeting ground for mathematics and biology. It publishes papers ranging from those which provide new theoretical formulations of current biological issue, to those which use substantive mathematical techniques in solving biological problems. It is must reading for the biologist interested in theoretical questions, and for the mathematician seeking new problems and new inspiration from biological applications.
Among the fields addressed regularly in the journal are population genetics, ecology, epidemiology, demography, physiology, cell biology, morphogenesis, chemistry, and physics.

Selected articles from recent issues:

W. L. Keith, R. H. Rand: 1:1 and 2:1 phase entrainment in a system of two coupled limit cycle oscillators.
S. Karlin, S. Lessard: On the optimal sex-ratio: A stability analysis based on a characterization for one-locus multiallele viability models.
S. Ellner: Asymptotic behavior of some stochastic difference equation population models.
O. Dlakmann, H. J. A. M. Heijmans, H. R. Thieme: On the stability of the cell size distribution.
A. Hunding: Bifurcations of nonlinear reaction-diffusion systems in oblate spheroids.
J. K. Hale, A. S. Somolinos: Competition for fluctuating nutrient.
M. Bertsch, M. E. Gurtin, D. Hilhorst, L. A. Peletier: On interacting populations that disperse to avoid crowding: The effect of a sedentary colony.
Y. Iwasa, E. Taramoto: Branching-diffusion model for the formation of distributional patterns in populations.

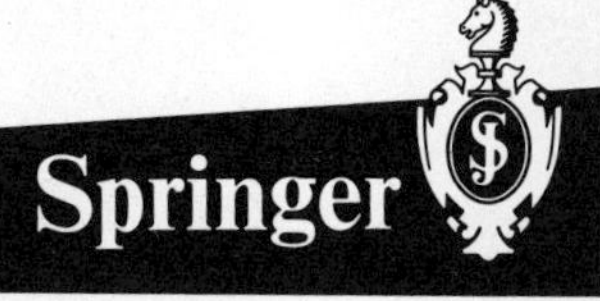

Biomathematics

Managing Editor: **S.A. Levin**

Editorial Board: **M. Arbib, H.J. Bremermann, J. Cowan, W.M. Hirsch, J. Karlin, J. Keller, K. Krickeberg, R.C. Lewontin, R.M. May, J.D. Murray, A. Perelson, T. Poggio, L.A. Segel**

Volume 17

Mathematical Ecology

An Introduction

Editors: **Th. G. Hallam, S. A. Levin**

1986. Approx. 87 figures. Approx. 495 pages
ISBN 3-540-13631-2

Contents: Introduction. - Physiological and Behavioral Ecology. - Population Ecology. - Communities and Ecosystems. - Applied Mathematical Ecology. - Subject Index.

Volume 16

Complexity, Language, and Life: Mathematical Approaches

Editors: **J.L. Casti, A. Karlqvist**

1986. XIII, 281 pages. ISBN 3-540-16180-5

Contents: Allowing, forbidding, but nor requiring: a mathematic for human world. - A theory of stars in complex systems. - Pictures as complex systems. - A survey of replicator equations. - Darwinian evolution in ecosystems: a survey of some ideas and difficulties together with some possible solutions. - On system complexity: identification, measurement, and management. - On information and complexity. - Organs and tools; a common theory of morphogenesis. - The language of life. - Universal principles of measurement and language functions in evolving systems.

Volume 15
D.L. DeAngelis, W. Post, C.C. Travis

Positive Feedback in Natural Systems

1986. 90 figures. Approx. 305 pages. ISBN 3-540-15942-8

Contents: Introduction. - The Mathematics of Positive Feedback. - Physical Systems. - Evolutionary Processes. - Organisms Physiology and Behavior. - Resource Utilization by Organisms. - Social Behavior. - Mutualistic and Competitive Systems. - Age-Structured Populations. - Spatially Heterogeneous Systems: Islands and Patchy Regions. - Spatially Heterogeneous Ecosystems; Pattern Formation. - Disease and Pest Outbreaks. - The Ecosystem and Succession. - References. - Appendices A to H.

Springer-Verlag
Berlin Heidelberg
New York Tokyo

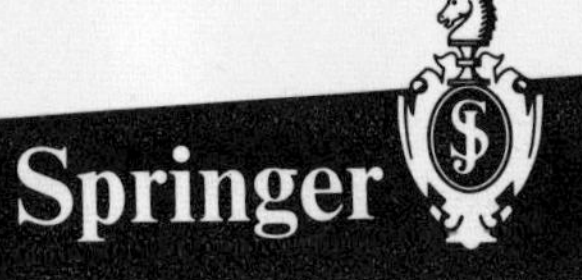